Exam Preparation in

ENT and Head-Neck Surgery

with Many Easy to Remember One-liners

Exam Preparation in
ENT and
Head-Neck
Surgery

with Many Easy to Remember One-liners

JP Purohit MBBS, MS

Professor and Head
Department of ENT and Head–Neck Surgery
Maharani Laxmi Bai Medical College
Jhansi
Uttar Pradesh

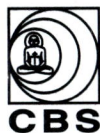

CBS

CBS Publishers & Distributors Pvt Ltd

New Delhi • Bengaluru • Chennai • Kochi • Kolkata • Mumbai
Bhopal • Bhubaneswar • Hyderabad • Jharkhand • Nagpur • Patna • Pune • Uttarakhand • Dhaka (Bangladesh)

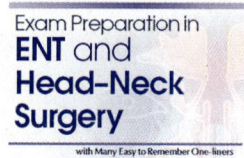

Exam Preparation in
ENT and
Head–Neck Surgery

with Many Easy to Remember One-liners

ISBN: 978-93-88108-42-3

Copyright © Author and Publisher

First Edition: 2019

Published by Satish Kumar Jain and produced by Varun Jain for

CBS Publishers & Distributors Pvt Ltd
4819/XI Prahlad Street, 24 Ansari Road, Daryaganj, New Delhi 110 002, India.
Ph: 23289259, 23266861, 23266867   Fax: 011-23243014   Website: www.cbspd.com
e-mail: delhi@cbspd.com; cbspubs@airtelmail.in.

Corporate Office: 204 FIE, Industrial Area, Patparganj, Delhi 110 092
Ph: 4934 4934   Fax: 4934 4935   e-mail: publishing@cbspd.com; publicity@cbspd.com

Branches

- **Bengaluru:** Seema House 2975, 17th Cross, K.R. Road,
  Banasankari 2nd Stage, Bengaluru 560 070, Karnataka
  Ph: +91-80-26771678/79   Fax: +91-80-26771680   e-mail: bangalore@cbspd.com
- **Chennai:** 7, Subbaraya Street, Shenoy Nagar, Chennai 600 030, Tamil Nadu
  Ph: +91-44-26680620, 26681266   Fax: +91-44-42032115   e-mail: chennai@cbspd.com
- **Kochi:** 42/1325, 1326, Power House Road, Opposite KSEB Power House,
  Ernakulam 682 018, Kochi, Kerala
  Ph: +91-484-4059061-65   Fax: +91-484-4059065   e-mail: kochi@cbspd.com
- **Kolkata:** 6/B, Ground Floor, Rameswar Shaw Road, Kolkata-700 014, West Bengal
  Ph: +91-33-22891126, 22891127, 22891128   e-mail: kolkata@cbspd.com
- **Mumbai:** 83-C, Dr E Moses Road, Worli, Mumbai-400018, Maharashtra
  Ph: +91-22-24902340/41   Fax: +91-22-24902342   e-mail: mumbai@cbspd.com

Representatives

• **Bhopal**	0-8319310552	• **Bhubaneswar**	0-9911037372	• **Hyderabad**	0-9885175004
• **Jharkhand**	0-9811541605	• **Nagpur**	0-9021734563	• **Patna**	0-9334159340
• **Pune**	0-9623451994	• **Uttarakhand**	0-9716462459	• **Dhaka (Bangladesh)**	01912-003485

Printed at Goyal Offset Printers, GT Karnal Road, Industrial Area, Delhi, India

Contributors

JP Purohit MS (ENT)
Professor and Head
Department of ENT and Head–Neck Surgery
MLB Medical College
Jhansi, UP

Kartikeya Purohit MS (ENT)
Senior Resident
MLB Medical College
Jhansi, UP

Shiva S MS (ENT)
Senior Resident
MLB Medical College
Jhansi, UP

Preface

ENT is a subject to undergraduate medical students in their third professional or final professional part first and at the end of it they have to appear for their examination. If they want to have a career in ENT, they can do MS, DLO or DNB, all of which need the students to appear in passing out examination to obtain the degree. This book is written to help the students to prepare easily for their examinations. In this book, the students can find many important facts and answers of questions commonly asked during practical *viva voce* examination, compiled together at the same place which reduces the revision time significantly. Certain special topics like vertigo, vestibulo-ocular reflex arc, facial nerve, tympanoplasty technique in detail, bleeding disorders, post-tonsillectomy bleedings, lymphoma and its management, spaces, triangles, and syndromes have been added. High-yielding topics, thyroid lesions and management, in short, pharmacology in ENT, post-cancer surgery reconstructions and Virchow-Robin space, and the commonest route of spread of otogenic brain infection have been discussed in short and easy to revise form just before the examination.

This book will be continuously improved from time to time in the future editions. Any suggestions and healthy criticism to improve the quality of the book are most welcome from the readers.

JP Purohit

Acknowledgements

In preparing this book, I wish to thank everyone, especially senior consultant Dr SK Kashyap, Professor, who has an excellent aptitude for good research and during our postgraduate classes he gave stimulus to write a book which should be helpful in revising ENT during the eleventh hour of examination. I wish to thank Dr Jitendra Singh Yadav, Associate Professor, my ex-student and a lion hearted surgeon, and junior residents of Department of ENT and Head–Neck Surgery, MLB Medical College, Jhansi, Uttar Pradesh.

I got the inspiration to write this book from my teachers Prof SK Kackar (*Ex-Director, AIIMS*), Dr (Prof) D Dayal and Dr (Prof) SC Mishra, Department of ENT, King George Medical College, Lucknow. I shall always be grateful for the blessings and motivation they have provided me during my residency and chief residency. Dr Siva S has taken special interests and spent a lot of time in editing, rewriting and improving the quality of illustrations and drawings for this book. I am thankful to Dr SP Singh, ex-Professor and Head, Department of Biochemistry, for his timely guidance. I am thankful to Dr VK Sharma in giving valuable information about general pathology and histopathology related to ENT.

I also express our gratefulness to Dr JC Passi, Director, MAMC, New Delhi; Dr NN Mathur, Professor (ENT), Principal and Director, VMMC, New Delhi; Dr Dharmendra Gupta, Professor and Head, Department of ENT, SNMC, Agra; Dr Anupam Mishra, Professor, KGMC Lucknow; Dr AK Jain, Professor and Head, GRMC, Gwalior; Dr VP Narvey, Associate Professor, GRMC, Gwalior; Dr S Vaidya, Professor, RD Gardi MC, Ujjain; Dr Brajendra Baser, Professor, Sri Aurobindo Medical College, Indore; Dr S Varshney, Professor and Head, AIIMS, Rishikesh; Dr SS Bisht, Professor and Head, HIMS, Jolly Grant, Dehradun; Dr Sandeep Kaushik, Professor, GSVM Medical College; Dr Vineet Sharma, Associate Professor, SRMS IMS, Bareilly; and Dr SK Kannaujiya, Associate Professor, GSVM Medical College, Kanpur; for encouraging me from time to time to write this book.

Last, I would like to give my special thanks to my wife, Mrs Fabuli Purohit, and my sons Dr Karthikeya Purohit who also contributed in part in writing this book and Mr Krishna P Purohit and my daughter-in-law Dr Kena Joshi Purohit, for sparing valuable time for me and bearing all the hardships given to them during the preparation of this book.

J P Purohit

Contents

Section 3 Oral Cavity and Throat

Section 4 Laryngology, Head and Neck and Miscellaneous Topics

Otology

CHAPTER 1

Clinical Anatomy of Ear and Physiology of Hearing and Balance

EMBRYOLOGY OF EAR

Timeline for the development of ear (in weeks)

Development	Cochlea	Vestibular labyrinth	Middle ear	External auditory meatus	Pinna
Begins	3rd	3rd	3rd	8th	6th
Completes	20th	20th	20th	28th	20th

EXTERNAL EAR

Pinna

1st and 2nd branchial arch mesoderm thickens to form the six "Hillocks of His" which finally unite to form pinna. Tragus and anterior crus of helix develop from the first arch and the rest of the pinna develops from the 2nd arch.

External Auditory Canal (EAC)

It develops from dorsal aspect of 1st branchial cleft. It becomes a solid core by second month of IUL and by 7th month, canal forms completely with tympanic membrane.

Tympanic Membrane

The endoderm of tubotympanic recess fuses with the lateral ectoderm of 1st cleft with an intact layer of mesoderm in between to form the tympanic membrane. This is how TM has all three germ layers.

Ear Ossicles

Ossicles develop from

Mesoderm of 1st branchial arch

- Known as Meckel's cartilage
- Malleus except handle
- Incus except lenticular process.

Mesoderm of 2nd branchial arch
- Known as Reichert's cartilage
- Handle of malleus
- Lenticular process of incus
- Superstructure of stapes.

Stapes footplate develops from
- Otic capsule which develops from ectoderm.

Middle Ear Muscles

Stapedius—from 2nd arch mesoderm, thus innervated by facial nerve.

Tensor tympani—from 1st arch mesoderm, thus innervated by mandibular nerve.

Middle ear, eustachian tube and tympanic cavity linings are formed by endoderm of the first pharyngeal pouch.

Inner Ear

Membranous labyrinth develops from the ectoderm of otic placode. Bony labyrinth forms from the mesoderm. Inner ear development is not dependent on the development of rest of the ear. This may be the reason for presence of normal inner ear anatomy even in cases of complete aural atresia. But many a time, congenital deafness can be related to 1st and 2nd arch anomalies.

Mastoid develops from: 1st branchial pouch and dorsal end of 2nd branchial pouch.

Korner's septum: It is a remnant of petrosquamous suture line which may cause difficulty in locating the antrum. Many a times it is mistaken as lateral semi-circular canal by young surgeons.

Conditions Associated with Development of Ear

Preauricular sinus: It occurs due to failure of fusion of 1st and 2nd hillocks. It is found at the ascending limb of helix. The patient commonly presents with repeated infections and abscess formation in the sinus tract.

Sinus tract excision is to be done after the active phase of infection subsides. During surgery for pre-auricular sinus, one should be careful not to injure the facial nerve branches and superficial temporal artery branches as there can be many ramifications of the sinus tract. The sinus tract never goes deep to the temporalis fascia.

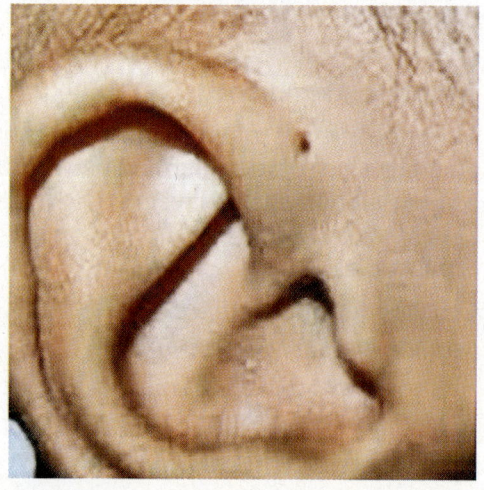

Collaural fistula: It occurs due to failure of obliteration of ventral aspect of 1st branchial cleft. Upper end of the fistula opens in external auditory canal, lobule or concha and lower end is seen between angle of mandible and sternomastoid muscle. Complete excision of the tract is warranted.

Microtia and Anotia: They are developmentally small external ears. There are four types 1–4; of which type 4 is anotia. Detailed radiological study of middle ear and inner ear development is necessary before planning for correction. Associated other systemic congenital anomalies should be kept in the mind. Surgical correction is usually done after the age of 4 years.

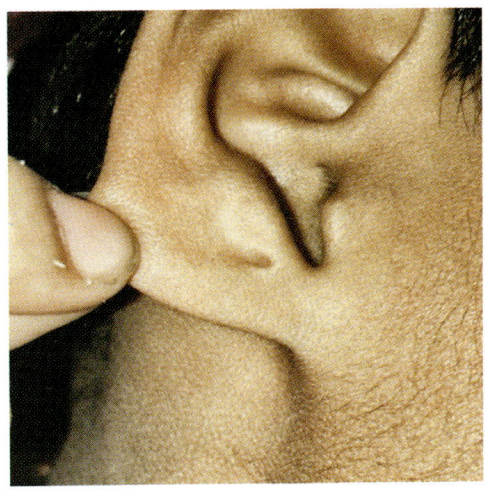

Aural atresia: It can be congenital or acquired following a trauma or infection. Congenital atresia is due to failed closure of 1st branchial cleft and pouch. It might be associated with a spectrum of other congenital abnormalities. Surgery is preferably done at 5–6 years of age. Till surgery, patient is given hearing aid to help language development.

Inner ear congenital malformations: Inner ear development anomalies are classified into membranous and bony. They result in congenital sensorineural hearing loss. Most cases are membranous labyrinth malformation (80%). There will be inner hair cell defect which cannot be detected by CT scans. Patients are managed with hearing aids or cochlear implant based on the severity of hearing loss.

Anatomically Significant Areas

Tragus: It is a cartilaginous projection in front of EAC. This cartilage can be used to harvest graft for ossiculoplasty.

Fissure of Santorini: It is a defect in cartilaginous part of EAC through which infections or tumors can travel from EAC to parotid space and vice versa.

Foramen of Huschke (also called "foramen tympanicum"): It is a defect in bony EAC. It might be communicating with temporomandibular joint space. In most cases this condition is asymptomatic.

Incisura terminalis: This area is between tragus and crux of helix and is devoid of cartilage. This is the site for endaural incision and meatoplasty.

Cymba concha: It is related medially to suprameatal triangle (Macewan's triangle) where mastoid tenderness is palpated. Other sites to palpate mastoid tenderness are mastoid tip (tip cell suppuration) and posterior part of mastoid (mastoid emissary vein thrombophlebitis).

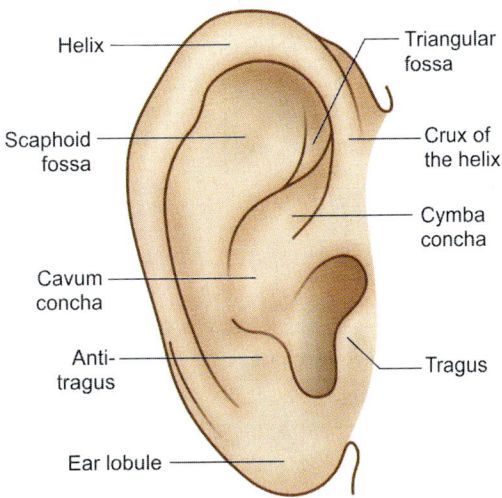

External Auditory Canal

Length of EAC
- Total—24 mm in adults.
- Lateral 1/3rd (8 mm) is cartilaginous part.
- Medial 2/3rd (16 mm) is bony part.

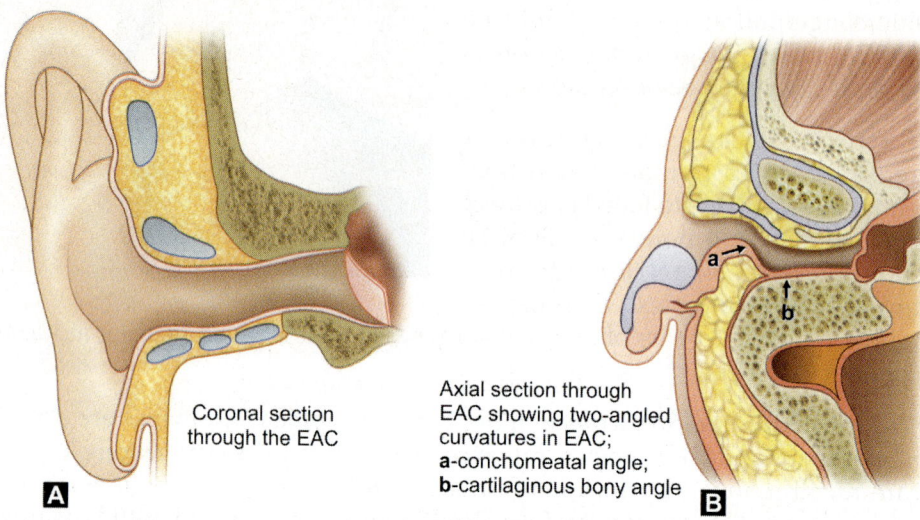

Coronal section
through the EAC

Axial section through
EAC showing two-angled
curvatures in EAC;
a-conchomeatal angle;
b-cartilaginous bony angle

A **B**

Adults: Cartilaginous EAC is directed medial, upwards and anterior.

Bony EAC is directed medial, downwards and anterior.

To examine the EAC and pinna, pinna should be pulled backwards and upwards, so that EAC becomes straight to visualize the tympanic membrane. Bony overhangs in the EAC will not be corrected by this action.

Children: Auricle is pulled downwards and backwards.

Isthmus of EAC: Narrowest portion of EAC; found 6 mm lateral to annulus. Bony cartilaginous junction is the 2nd narrowest point.

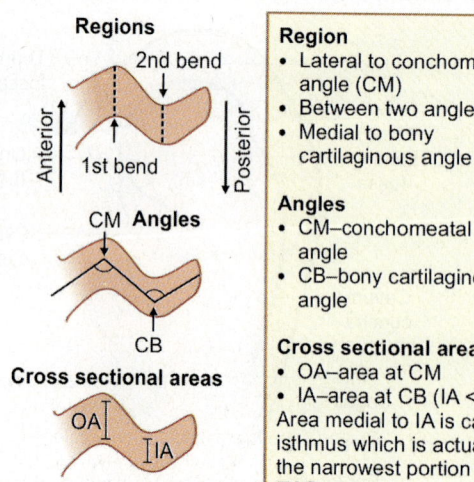

Regions
2nd bend

Anterior

1st bend

Posterior

CM **Angles**

CB

Cross sectional areas

OA

IA

Region
- Lateral to conchomeatal angle (CM)
- Between two angles
- Medial to bony cartilaginous angle (CB)

Angles
- CM–conchomeatal angle
- CB–bony cartilaginous angle

Cross sectional areas
- OA–area at CM
- IA–area at CB (IA < OA)
Area medial to IA is called isthmus which is actually the narrowest portion in EAC.

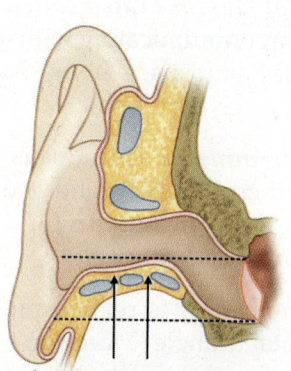

Anterior displacement

Axial section of EAC showing the posterior wall anterior displacement due to more conchomeatal angle; seen more in elderly; sometimes can cause hearing loss

Anterior recess: Prominence of anterior EAC wall narrows the canal and thus a recess is formed at the medial most part, called anterior recess. Here collection of pus, wax or foreign body lodgement can occur, which is difficult to clean without microscope.

Vascular supply to Pinna and EAC: Post-auricular artery and superficial temporal artery.

Nerve supply to pinna:

1. Most of the medial surface (2/3rd) + Posterior part of lateral surface is supplied by greater auricular nerve.
2. Upper part of medial surface is supplied by lesser occipital nerve.
3. Tragus, helix is supplied by auriculotemporal nerve.
4. Concha by vagus (Arnold's nerve) along with communicating branches from facial nerve (note in Hitselberger's sign mentioned in the text).

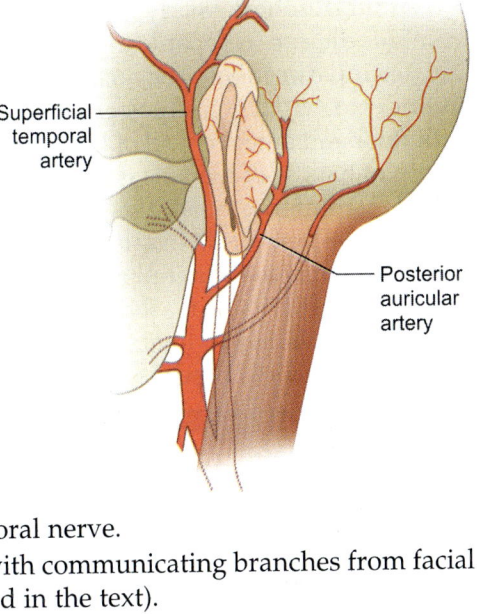

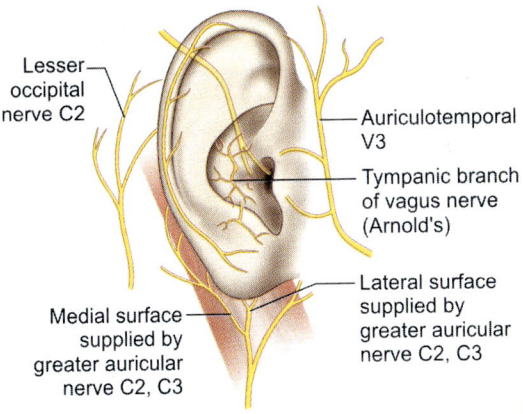

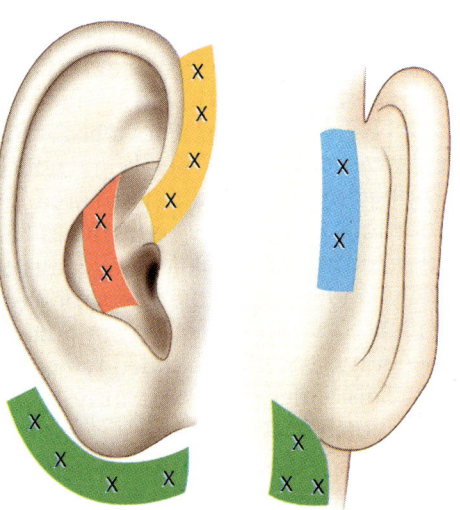

The "X" marked points are the sites of injection of local anesthetic drug to anesthetize the pinna.
Yellow-auriculo-temporal nerve; Red-Arnold's nerve;
Blue-lesser occipital nerve; Green-greater auricular nerve.

Tympanic Membrane

It is a thin, elliptical, pearly grey and semi-transparent membrane that separates EAC from middle ear. Tympanic membrane is placed obliquely in EAC in both horizontal and vertical directions. The angulations to the EAC vary from 29 degrees (inferior and anterior) to 140 degrees (posterior and superior). It makes an angle of 40–55 degrees with floor and anterior wall of EAC. Its maximum convexity is found at umbo—where the tip of handle of malleus is attached. Cone of light reflected from the umbo is seen in its anteroinferior quadrant. Tympanic membrane is 9–10 mm in height, 8–9 mm in width. Thickness of TM varies at different sites—it is thickest at the anterosuperior quadrant and near the annulus (0.09 mm) and thinnest at the posterosuperior quadrant (0.055 mm). This is the reason for traumatic rupture of TM being more common at the posterior quadrants. Its total surface area is 85 mm^2 out of which only 2/3rd is vibrating. Total weight of TM tissue is 14 mg.

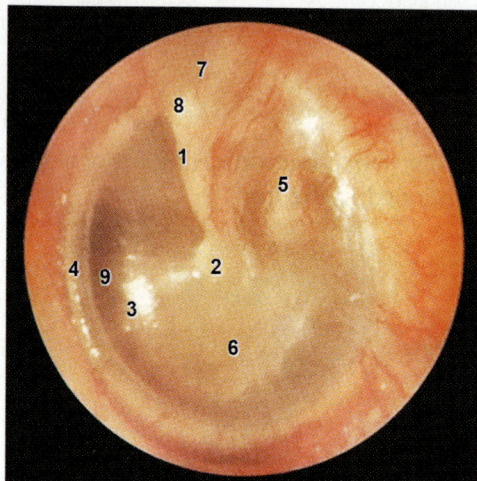

1. Handle of malleus
2. Umbo
3. Cone of light
4. Annulus tympanicus
5. Shadow of long process of incus
6. Pars tensa
7. Pars flaccida
8. Lateral process of malleus
9. Shadow of eustachian tube

Left tympanic membrane

Tympanic membrane is divided into: (1) Pars tensa; and (2) Pars flaccida (Shrapnell's membrane). Pars tensa is the larger lower part of the membrane which is peripherally thickened to form annulus tympanicus. Annulus continues as anterior and posterior malleolar ligaments which go and attach to the lateral process of malleus. Annulus is placed in a bony groove in tympanic bone called tympanic sulcus. This is deficient superiorly to the form of Notch of Rivinus.

Tympanic membrane consists of 3 layers: (1) Outer epidermal layer (posterosuperior quadrant has more squamous cells); (2) Middle fibrous layer with outer radial and inner circular

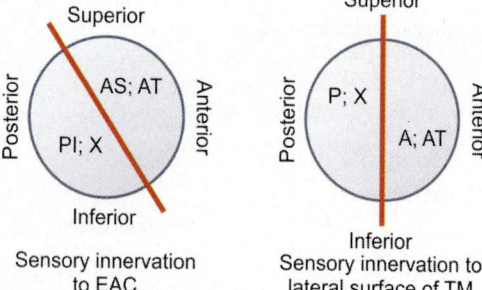

Sensory innervation to EAC

Sensory innervation to lateral surface of TM

Left pic: Posterior and inferior walls (PI) supplied by vagus (X); Anterior and superior walls (AS) by auriculotemporal nerve (AT). Right pic: Posterior half (P) of lateral surface of TM by vagus (X); Anterior half (A) of lateral surface of TM by auriculotemporal nerve (AT) inner surface of TM is supplied by tympanic branch of glosso-pharyngeal nerve (Jacobson's nerve).

tangential fibers; and (3) Inner mucosal layer. Handle of malleus is incorporated in middle layer of tympanic membrane. Pars flaccida is devoid of middle fibrous layer.

Migration of squamous epithelium in the lateral surface of TM starts at the umbo and goes on laterally to EAC. The rate of migration in the TM surface is 0.05 mm/day. Whereas the rate of migration in the EAC is 1 mm/day.

Ossicles

Malleus: The most lateral ossicle

- 7.5–9 mm in size.
- It has head, neck, handle, lateral process and anterior process.
- Facet for articulation with incus is present posteromedially.

Incus: Has body, short process, long process and lentiform process which articulate with stapes.

- Long process of incus has delicate structure and tenuous blood supply thus causing this, the commonly eroded ossicle in CSOM.

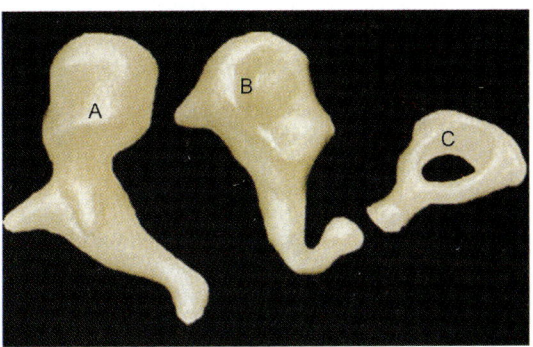

(A)—Malleus; (B)—Incus; (C)—Stapes

Stapes: Has head, neck, two crura and footplate.
- Posterior crus is long, thick and curved than anterior crus.
- Measurement of footplate—3 mm, 1.4 mm
- Measurement of oval window—3.25 mm, 1.75 mm
- Footplate is surrounded by annular ligament.

What is columella? Fishes have only single ossicle called columella. This is because sound travels faster in water than air.

MIDDLE EAR

Middle ear cleft includes:
- Middle ear,
- Eustachian tube,
- Aditus,
- Antrum—the biggest air cell of mastoid and
- Other mastoid air cells.

Volume of middle ear cleft varies between 1 and 30 ml with an average of 6.5 ml. Total surface area of middle ear cleft mucosa is around 50–250 cm^2 with an average of 105 cm^2.

Walls of the Middle Ear (Structures/Landmarks)

Anterior wall
- Canal for tensor tympani
- Eustachian tube opening

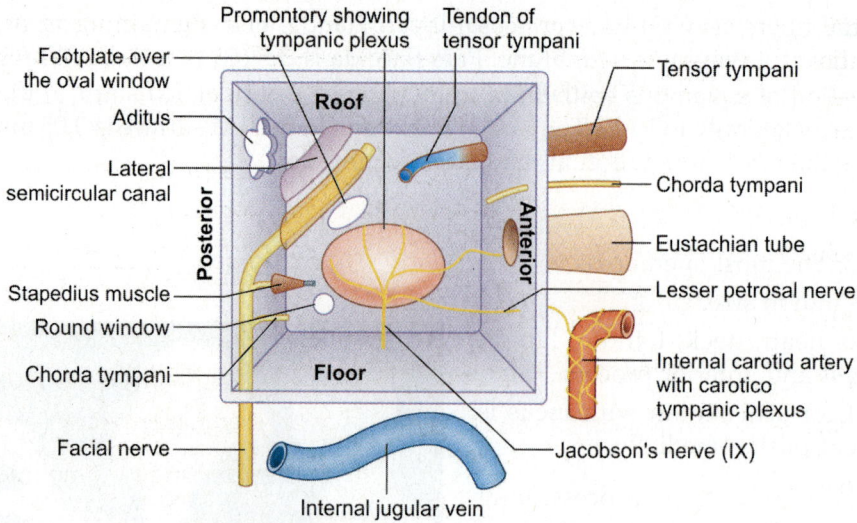

Structures related to the walls of the middle ear

- Canal of Huguier/iter chorda anterius (for chorda tympani)
- Glaserian fissure/petrotympanic fissure (for anterior malleolar ligament and anterior tympanic artery)
- Anteroinferiorly internal carotid artery

Posterior wall: Aditus ad antrum, fossa includes pyramid, supra and infrapyramidal recess and facial recess.

Lateral wall: Scutum, tympanic membrane and tympanic bone.

Medial wall
- Promontory, oval window, round window, sinus tympani
- Ponticulus and subiculum
- Processus cochleariformis
- Horizontal part of facial nerve
- Cog and medial wall of attic

Roof: Tegmen tympanum.

Floor: Bone over the jugular bulb. Sometimes the bony covering may be absent and jugular bulb can be dehiscent.

Mastoid antrum: Biggest and most consistent air cell in the mastoid. Lies 1–1.5 cm medial to the suprameatal triangle. When seen through the postaural approach, it is located immediately posterosuperior and medial to the spine of Henle. It opens into middle ear through aditus ad antrum.

Histology of Middle Ear Cleft
- Mastoid antrum and posterior tympanum—flat cuboidal/endothelial cells in 87.5% cases. Tall cuboidal cells with some cilia are seen around the facial nerve prominence.

- Posterior tympanum—60% cases are flat cuboidal cell. Remaining is stratified cuboidal epithelium with cilia.
- Epitympanic recess—stratified cuboidal epithelium with cilia. In 15% cases goblet cells are present.
- Promontory—stratified columnar epithelium with cilia. Cilia are not as dense as above.
- Medial surface of tympanic membrane—non-ciliated cuboidal epithelium.
- Eustachian tube—histology varies at both ends. Near tympanic end, there is ciliated simple cuboidal or columnar. Near nasopharynx, there is ciliated pseudostratified columnar epithelium.

Protympanum: Part of tympanic cavity near eustachian tube opening.

Epitympanum: Part of middle ear above the level of tympanic membrane.

Mesotympanum: Part of tympanic cavity medially corresponding to tympanic membrane.

Hypotympanum: Part of tympanic cavity below the level of tympanic membrane.

Retrotympanum: Includes hidden areas like sinus tympani, suprapyramidal recess and facial recess.

Dimensions of Middle Ear

- Anteroposterior and vertical— 15 mm
- Epitympanum—6 mm
- Hypotympanum—4 mm
- At the level of umbo—2 mm (variable depending on the position of TM—Pindborg classification mentioned later-on in the text).

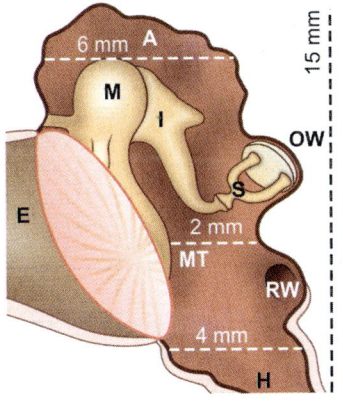

A: Attic
MT: Mesotympanum
H: Hypotympanum
E: EAC
M: Malleus
I: Incus
S: Stapes
OW: Oval window
RW: Round window

Scutum: Bony outer attic wall.

Subiculum: It is a posterior extension of promontory which separates the oval window from round window.

Ponticulus: It is a bony spicule which runs from promontory to pyramid, superior to subiculum.

Cog: Bony projection from tegmen found anterior to head of malleus lying posteromedial to processus cochleariformis.

Facial recess: A triangular space bounded by facial nerve medially, fossa incudis superiorly and chorda tympani laterally. It is the site for posterior tympanotomy. Angle between the facial nerve and chorda tympani is called *"mastoid threshold angle"*. Extended facial recess is reached by sacrificing the chorda tympani and this approach is used in glomus surgeries.

Sinus tympani: Also called infrapyramidal facial recess.

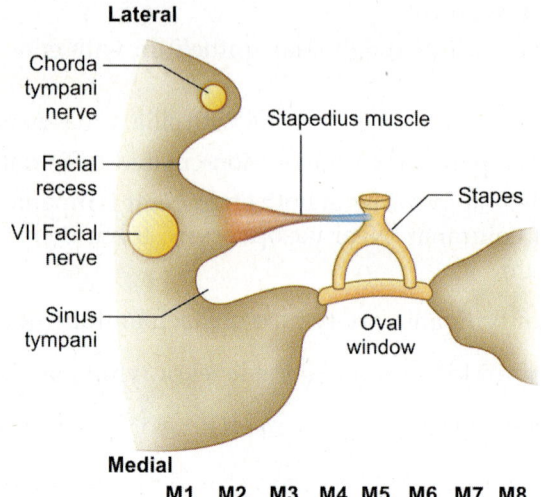

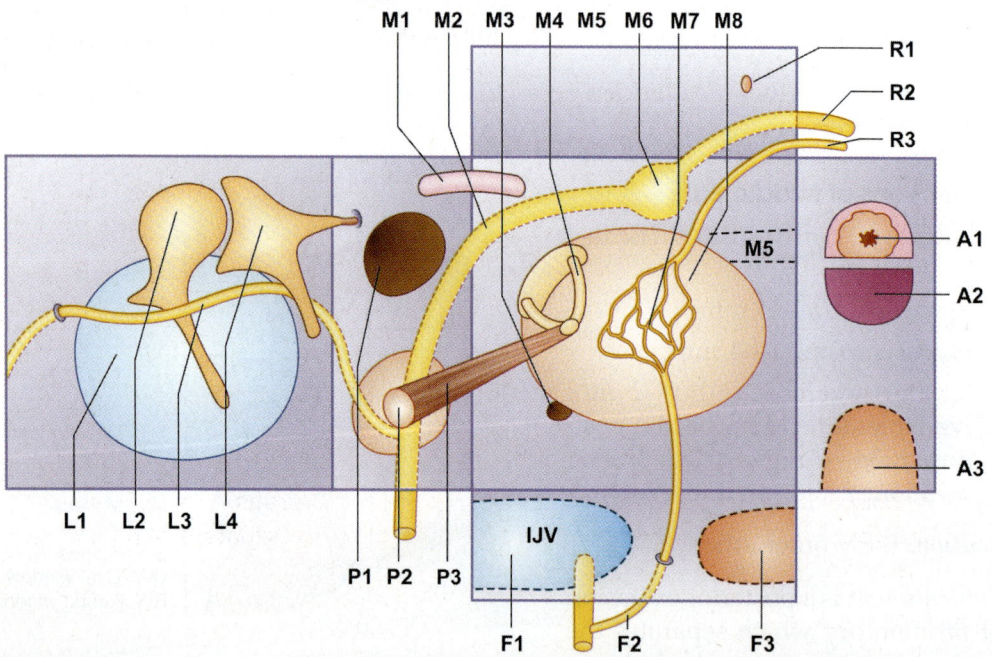

Anterior wall	Medial wall (cont.)	Roof
A1: Tensor tympani	M4: Stapes covering oval window	R1: Tegmen tympani
A2: Auditory tube	M5: Semicanal for tensor tympani	R2: Greater petrosal nerve
A3: Internal carotid artery (ICA)	M6: Geniculate ganglion	R3: Lesser petrosal nerve
Posterior wall	M7: Tympanic plexus	**Floor**
P1: Aditus	M8: Promontory	F1: Internal jugular vein (IJV)
P2: Pyramid	**Lateral wall**	F2: Tympanic branch of IX
P3: Stapedius	L1: Tympanic membrane	F3: Internal carotid artery (ICA)
Medial wall	L2: Malleus	
M1: Lateral semicircular canal	L3: Chorda tympani	
M2: Facial canal	L4: Incus	
M3: Round window (FC)	**Roof**	
	R1: Tegmen tympani	

Structures in relation to the walls of middle ear

Mucosal folds of middle ear

Pouches of von Troeltsch and other middle ear spaces

Connects Prussak's space to posterior mesotympanum

Eustachian tube

- Length—36 mm in adults
- Lateral—12 mm bony
- Medial—24 mm cartilaginous

Pharyngeal opening is located 1–1.5 cm behind and little below the posterior end of inferior turbinate.

- It is directed downwards, forwards and medial.
- Angle between bony and cartilaginous is 135°.

Muscles attached to eustachian tube are:

1. Tensor tympani
2. Levator palatini
3. Tensor palatini
4. Salpingopharyngeus

Parts of temporal bone: Squamous; mastoid; tympanic; petrous.

Styloid (but some recent literatures say that styloid is a separate bone and not a part of temporal bone).

Groups of Mastoid Air Cells

Groups of mastoid air cells	Location
1. Peri sinus cells	Cells around sigmoid sinus
2. Perilabyrinthine cells	Cells around the labyrinth—supralabyrinthine, infra-labyrinthine or retrolabyrinthine
3. Tegmen cells	Cells along tegmen tympani and antri
4. Zygomatic cells	Cells in the root of the zygoma
5. Petrous cells	Cells in the petrous apex
6. Peritubal cells	Cells around the eustachian tube
7. Retrofacial cells	Cells along the vertical segment of facial nerve
8. Tip cells	Cells in the mastoid tip—lateral and medial groups divided by digastric ridge
9. Periantral cells	Cells around the mastoid antrum
10. Squamous cells	Cells in the squamous temporal bone
11. Sinodural angle cells	Cells along sinodural angle
12. Hypotympanic cells	Cells above jugular bulb

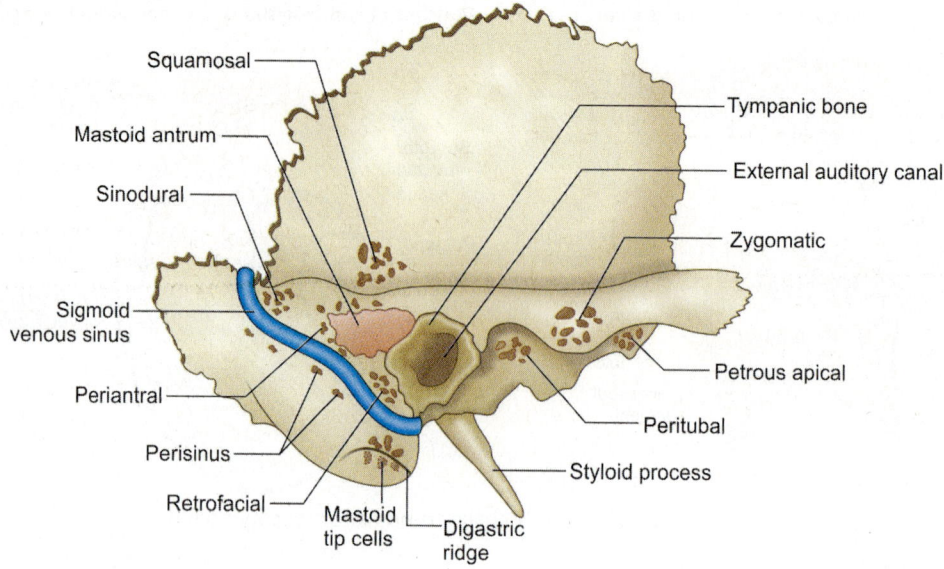

Squamosal

Mastoid antrum

Sinodural

Sigmoid venous sinus

Periantral

Perisinus

Retrofacial

Mastoid tip cells

Digastric ridge

Tympanic bone

External auditory canal

Zygomatic

Petrous apical

Peritubal

Styloid process

Mastoid tip cells (medial and lateral tip cells divided by digastric ridge)

These various groups of mastoid air cells communicate by the following tracts, viz. (1) Posterosuperior tract, (2) Posteromedial tract, (3) Sub-arcuate tract, (4) Perilabyrinthine tract and (5) Peritubal tract.

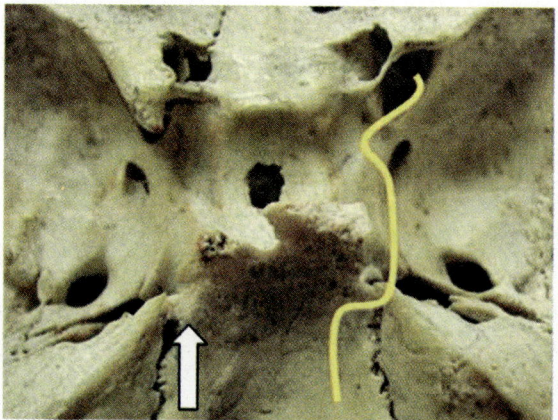

Dorello's canal—superior view of bilateral petrous apex and sellar region. Yellow line is the passage of abducens nerve and white arrows show Dorello's canal

INNER EAR

Cochlea—2½ turn; basal turn—high frequencies. Apex of cochlea—low frequencies. The cavity is divided into 3 compartments—scala vestibuli, scala media and scala tympani by Reissner's membrane and basal membrane where the hair cells rest.

Modiolus is the apical point of bone around which cochlea turns.

Helicotrema is the point where scala vestibuli communicates with scala tympani.

Inner and outer hair cells of cochlea: Inner hair cells are arranged in a single row; outer hair cells in 3 rows.

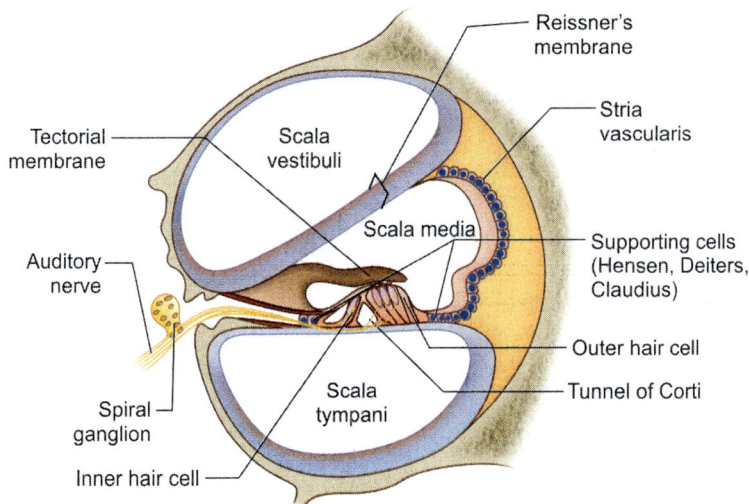

Organ of Corti has several supporting cells like Hensen's, Claudius, etc.

Ductus reuniens is the duct connecting cochlear duct and saccule.

Ampulla is the dilated end of semicircular canal (SCC) where sensory epithelium is located. There are 3 ampullae in respect to 3 SCC. The non-dilated ends of SCC are just 2 in number due to crus commune.

Crus commune is formed by union of non-ampulated ends of superior and posterior semicircular canals.

Macula—sensory epithelium present in utricle and saccule of vestibule. Calcium carbonate crystals (otoliths) are found attached to mucopolysaccharide gel of macula called otoconia. This is responsible for linear acceleration. Detachment of otolith from otoconic organ leads to BPPV.

Crista ampullaris is the end organ found in the ampulated ends of three SCC. They are responsible for sensing angular acceleration.

Kinocilium: Sensory epithelium in vestibular organs have hair cells. The single longest hair cell is called kinocilium.

Sterocilia: The smaller hair cells are called stereocilia.

Donaldson's line: An imaginary line passes along lateral SCC and one line along posterior SCC. Inferior to the intersection of these 2 lines is endolymphatic sac.

Dorello's canal: Formed by petroclinoid ligament, through this VI cranial nerve passes.

Gasserian ganglion: Ganglion of 5th cranial nerve present in close proximity to petrous apex.

In petrositis, VI CN at either Dorello's canal, gasserian ganglion or both is involved and this causes Gradenigo syndrome which is characterized by retro-orbital pain, VI nerve palsy and ear discharge.

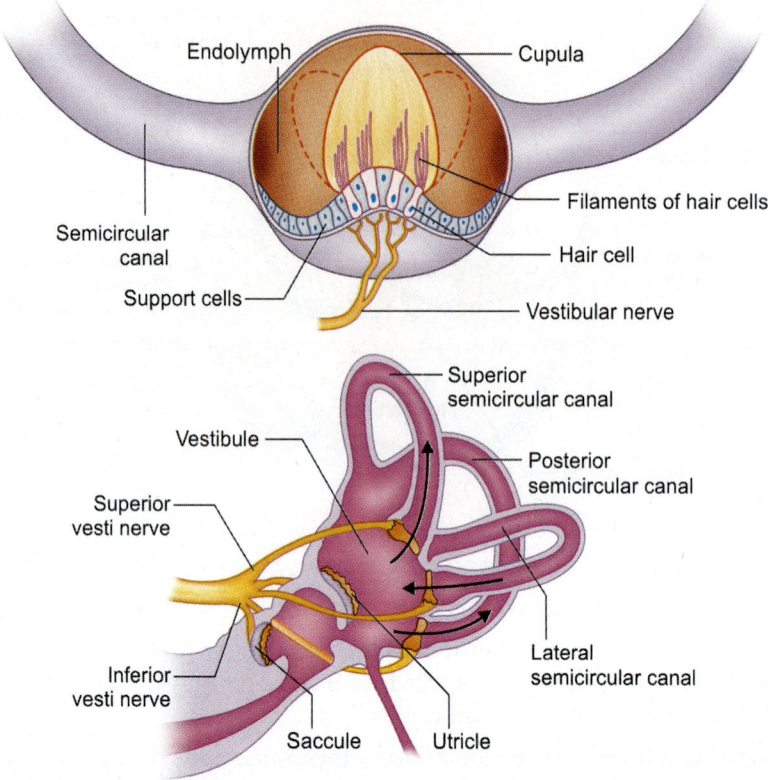

The direction of endolymph movement in vestibule causing depolarization

AUDIOLOGY

Theories of Hearing

1. **Place theory (Helmholtz):** Each pitch has its own loci in basilar membrane.
2. **Telephone theory (Rutherford):** Pitch is differentiated by the difference in individual nerve fiber firing rate.
3. **Volley theory (Wever):** Combination of the above 2 theories.
4. **Travelling wave theory (von Békésy):** (*Nobel Prize*). Amplitude of wave produced by a particular frequency sound at oval window reaches its maximum intensity at a particular point. Higher frequency at base and lower frequencies at apex.

Sound is a form of energy produced by an object possessing both inertia and elasticity. When it vibrates, it causes alternating compression and rarefaction of the surrounding media and sound is transmitted.

Speed of sound: 344 m/s in air. In water, sound travels four times faster. In bone sound travels even faster than in water. Speed of sound varies with media, temperature and pressure.

Frequency: Cycles (1 rarefaction and 1 compression) per second is the frequency of sound. Its SI unit is Hertz (Hz).

Intensity: Loudness of sound.

Decibel (dB)
- It is a unit by which intensity of sound is measured.
- 1/10 of Bel.
- 1 dB = 0.00002 dyne/cm^2.
- Named after Sir Alexander Graham Bell.
- It is a logarithmic value.

0 dB (audiometric zero): It is the mean auditory threshold in healthy individuals in the age group of 18–25 years. It is not quantitatively zero as dB is a log value.

–5 dB and –10 dB: Threshold even below 0 dB may be possible because in a group of randomly selected population, a few may hear much lower intensity than the mean levels.

Noise levels (intensity levels)
- Painful noise: 130 dB
- Discomfort to ear: >85 dB
- Truck horn: 110 dB
- Jet airline: 105 dB
- Heavy city traffic: 90 dB
- Office: 80 dB
- Car air horn: 70 dB
- Normal conversation: 60 dB
- Whispering: 30 dB
- Average living room in a home: 50 dB
- Hospital indoor where usual hearing tests are done: 35 dB
- Bedroom: 25 dB

Whisper and voice test
Conversation test (CV): Normal is 18–24 ft
- 30 dB hearing loss CV = 16–20 ft
- 40 dB hearing loss CV = 8–12 ft
- 50 dB hearing loss CV = 1–3 ft
- 60 dB hearing loss CV = 1 inch

Whisper test: Normal is 12 ft
- Conversational and whisper tests are done by voice of 40 dB loudness.
- Vocal index (VI) = (Conversation/Whisper) = 2:1
- In cases of conductive hearing loss, VI becomes 1:1
- Faint whisper: 20 dB
- Soft whisper: 30 dB
- Loud whisper: 50 dB
- Conversational voice: 60 dB
- Shout: 80 dB

Speech frequencies: 500, 1000, 2000 and 4000 Hz as most of human conversations falls under this range.

Pure tone sound: Sound produced when an object vibrates in fixed single frequency of C-band octave frequency.

Overtone: Frequencies that are above and multiples of fundamental frequency of an object are called overtones. They determine the quality of sound.

White noise (broad band or wide band): It contains all frequencies in equal proportion.

Narrow band: Narrow band of sound is 100–200 Hz below and above the test frequency.

Masking: Presence of one sound impairs the perception of the other. This is used to avoid the response from the non-test ear.

Indications of masking
* Bone conduction audiological studies.
* If the difference of air conduction and bone conduction is >40 dB.

Methods for masking
* Finger friction
* Barany box
* Maskers in audiometer
* Rustle of paper
* Rubbing of patient's hairs together in front of the ear.
  Inter-aural attenuation for air conduction: 45 dB.
  Inter-aural attenuation for bone conduction: 5 dB.

Fletcher index: It is the average hearing threshold at 500, 1000 and 2000 Hz.

Conductive deafness: Bone conduction (BC) is within normal range, i.e. 15–20 dB with an air bone (AB) gap >15 dB.

Sensorineural deafness: BC > 20 dB and air bone is ≤15 dB

Mixed deafness: BC ≥20 dB and air bone gap ≥15 dB

Role of outer hair cells in hearing: Modulation of the sound received by inner hair cells and convert them into perfect acoustic sound with classical sine wave.

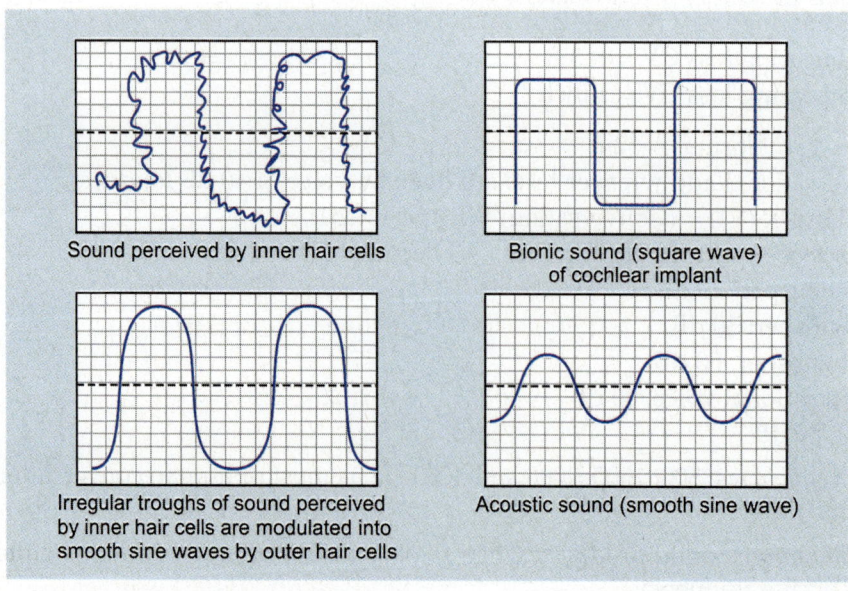

Sound perceived by inner hair cells

Bionic sound (square wave) of cochlear implant

Irregular troughs of sound perceived by inner hair cells are modulated into smooth sine waves by outer hair cells

Acoustic sound (smooth sine wave)

CHAPTER 2

Audiological Evaluation of the Patients

TUNING FORKS

Invented by John Shore in 1711.

Parts: Stem, base, shoulder and prongs.

Made up of nickel, stainless steel, copper or aluminium.

Frequencies of tuning fork commonly used in audiological tests are: 256, 512, 1024 and 2048 Hz; out of these 512 is the commonest because it is the one coming under speech frequencies and also does not produce overtones and has minimum tone decay.

Ideal time for the tuning fork to vibrate to have optimum results is 1 minute.

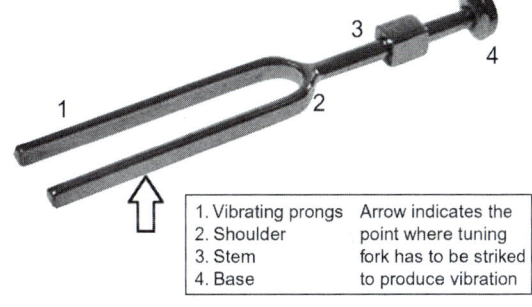

1. Vibrating prongs	Arrow indicates the
2. Shoulder	point where tuning
3. Stem	fork has to be striked
4. Base	to produce vibration

Commonly performed tests are: Rinne, Weber, absolute bone conduction, Schwabach, Bing's and Gelle.

Rinne Test (Sir Adolf Rinne, 1855)

It is to compare the air conduction (AC) versus bone conduction (BC) of the patient.
- Rinne +ve—normal hearing;
- Rinne –ve—conductive loss (BC > AC)
- Decreased Rinne +ve—SNHL (AC > BC, but both decreased)
- Infinite Rinne +ve—BC is 0, AC present—severe SNHL
- False Rinne –ve—BC > AC but Weber is lateralized to opposite ear—unilateral SNHL.

Weber's Test (EH Weber, 1834)

Sound from the tuning fork is lateralized to the diseased ear in conductive hearing loss or the normal ear in SNHL. Lateralization can occur with even 5 dB difference in hearing between the ears.

Theories of Weber's test are: Absence of ambient noise in conductive hearing loss.

Reverse conduction of sound from inner ear to environment does not happen in CHL.

Change of phase in CHL: All these factors let the bone conduction to be heard better in the CHL or normal ear.

Absolute Bone Conduction Test and Schwabach's Test

They are comparative tests where bone conduction of the patient is compared to that of the examiner. Schwabach's test involves not occluding the EAC. In case of SNHL the bone conduction of the patient will be less than the examiner's bone conduction.

Gelle Test

Increasing the pressure in EAC with Siegel's speculum reduces bone conduction in normal and SNHL (positive). But if stapes are fixed as in otosclerosis, no change will occur (negative).

Bing Test

In normal and SNHL, when EAC is occluded, BC increases (positive). No change occurs in conductive loss (negative).

Pure Tone Audiometry

Uses of pure tone audiogram:
- Baseline
- Medicolegal purpose
- Type and degree of deafness
- For advice of hearing aid

Average of thresholds of air and bone conduction is measured at frequencies 500, 1000, 2000 and 4000. Air-bone (A-B) gap is calculated. 10 dB A-B gap is considered as normal and surgery to correct the disease is done when A-B gap is 20 or >20 dB.

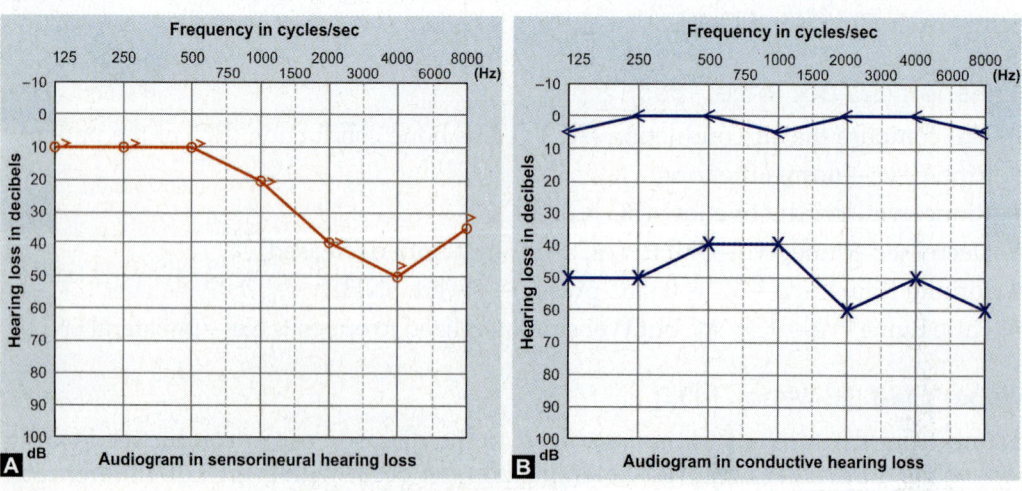

A   **Audiogram in sensorineural hearing loss**   B   **Audiogram in conductive hearing loss**

Type of Audiograms in Conductive Deafness

Left sloping—loss in lower frequencies seen in otosclerosis.

Right sloping—loss in higher frequencies seen in secretory otitis media.

Large A-B gap> 60 dB—ossicular dislocation.

Type of Audiograms in Sensorineural Deafness

Ascending—endolymphatic hydrops (Meniere)

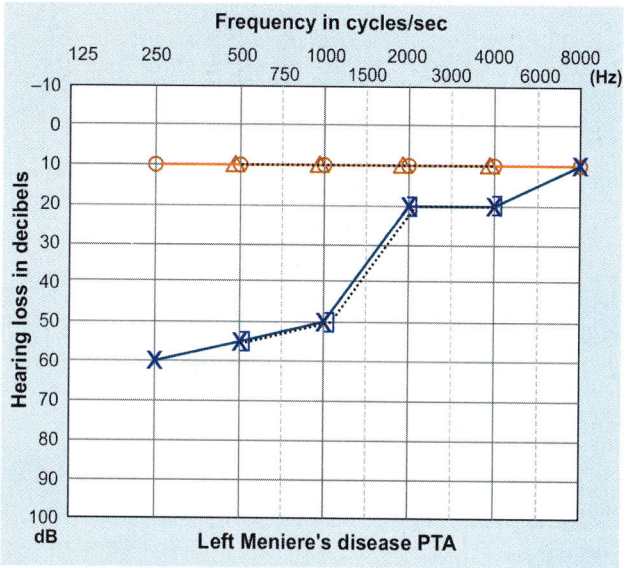

Left Meniere's disease PTA

Descending—ototoxicity

Both of the above can be found in presbycusis

Trough shape (U-shaped)—congenital SNHL

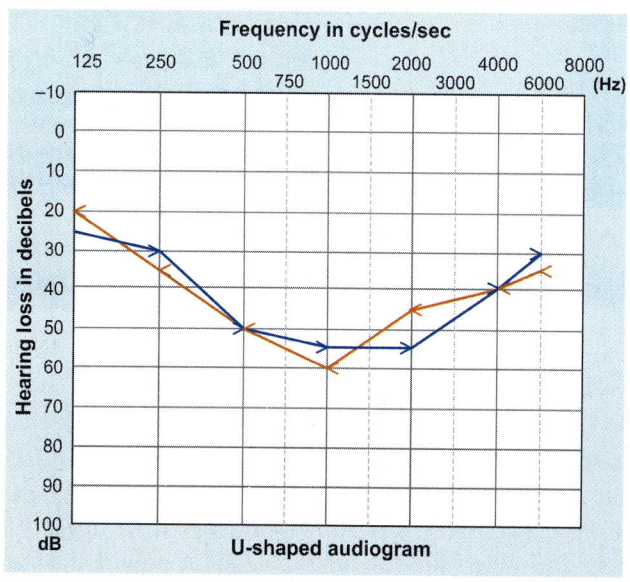

U-shaped audiogram

Dip in audiogram

At 4000 Hz in AC—acoustic trauma

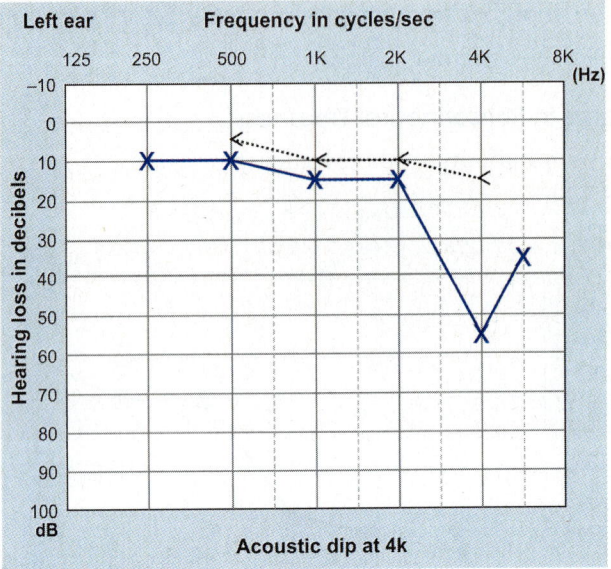

Acoustic dip at 4k

2000 Hz in BC—Carhart's notch otosclerosis

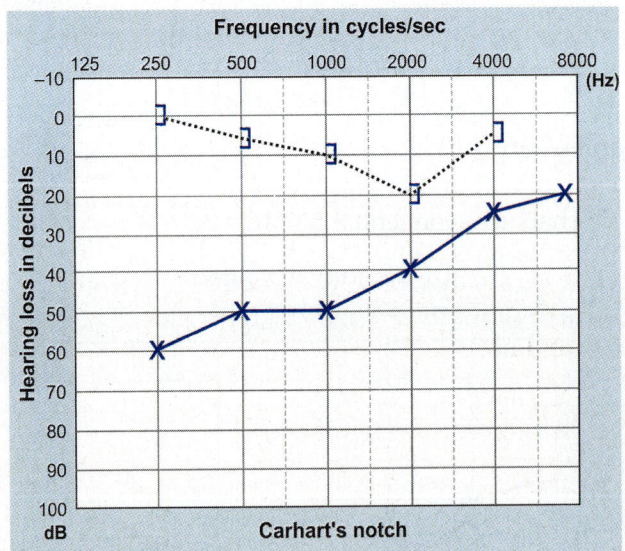

Carhart's notch

Bone conduction sound reaches the inner ear by the following three routes:
- Direct cochlear vibration due to skull bone vibration,
- By the vibration of ossicles which are suspended in the middle ear and
- By the sound entering the EAC and further conducted into the inner ear.

Out of these, last 2 routes are affected in ossicular fixation thus causing a dip in the bone conduction threshold, mainly at 2k frequency, called the *Carhart's notch*. This notch will disappear following stapes surgery. This is called *Carhart's effect*.

When there is any disparity between the tuning fork test results and PTA results, it is advised to go with tuning fork tests result rather than PTA result.

Recruitment: It is defined as an abnormally steep perception of loudness of sound which is disproportionate with intensity of sound.

Seen in cochlear pathology, e.g. presbycusis, Meniere's disease.

Tests for recruitment: ABLB (Fowler test), SISI, Metz's recruitment test.

Loudness discomfort level: It is level of sound at which discomfort in the ear is felt. 90–105 dB SL (sensation level).

Dynamic range: The difference (gap) between hearing level and loudness discomfort level. This gap is reduced in cochlear pathologies because of recruitment phenomenon. Patients with recruitment, i.e. poor dynamic ranges, are poor candidates for hearing aid as amplified sound produces discomfort in ear.

Tone decay test: It is slow decline in discharging frequency with time. It measures the nerve fatigue and associated with retro-cochlear lesion, e.g. acoustic neuroma.

Normally person can hear tone up to 60 seconds. However, in retro-cochlear lesions patients cease to hear early.

Speech audiometry: To test a patient's ability to understand the speech. In this spondee words are delivered and patient is asked to repeat these words.

Spondee words: They are phonetically balanced words. Two syllable words that have equal stress on both words, e.g. head-light, foot-ball, sun-light, sun-set, white-wash, arm-chair, ink-pot, air-plane.

Phonetically balanced words: Single syllable word, e.g. as, can, age, dish, din, bin, day.

Speech reception threshold (SRT): It is the intensity at which 50% of the words are repeated.

Speech discrimination score (SDS): In this test phonetically balanced words that are 30–40 dB above the SRT are delivered and percentage of repeated words are calculated. DS markedly reduces (<80%) is SN deafness especially neural type, whereas in conductive deafness and normal hearing DS would be 90–100%.

Impedance: It is the resistance encountered by the acoustic energy (sound) when it passes through the medium (auditory system).

It is due to the mixture of:

1. Stiffness of medium
2. Mass of medium
3. Friction

Compliance: It is the ease by which sound (in test it is 226 Hz) travels through the tympanic membrane and middle ear and is maximum when air pressure (in mm of water commonly –300 to +200) in middle ear and EAC is equal to normal atmospheric pressure. Compliance is measured in cubic cm.

Uses of impedance audiometry: For differential diagnosis of conductive deafness.

To detect the secretory otitis media.

Stepedial reflex can be used for:

- Topodiagnostic test for facial nerve
- Prognosis of facial nerve paralysis
- For recruitment
- Malingering
- Fracture of footplate of stapes
- To assess the eustachian tube.

Advantages of impedance audiometry:

- It is objective test.
- Can be done in children.
- Easy to perform and requires a little training.
- Can be used as screening tools in children.

Type of curves in impedance audiometry:

Type A: Normal

Type A_s: Compliance lower at ambient pressure, e.g. otosclerosis and fixed malleus, tympanosclerosis.

Type A_d: High compliance, e.g. ossicular discontinuity

Type B: Flat and no pressure changes, e.g. secretory otitis media and thick TM

Type C: Maximum compliance when pressure is negative, e.g. retracted TM.

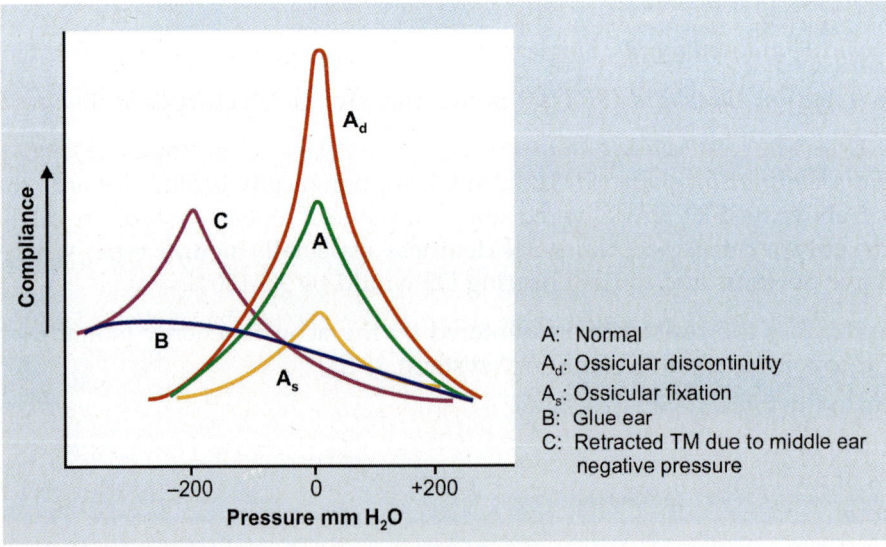

A: Normal
A_d: Ossicular discontinuity
A_s: Ossicular fixation
B: Glue ear
C: Retracted TM due to middle ear negative pressure

Brain Stem Evoked Response Audiometry (BERA)

Advantages

- Objective test
- Noninvasive
- Integrity of central pathways can be detected

Disadvantages
- Costly
- Time consuming

Uses
- Hearing threshold estimation
- Type of deafness
- Diagnosis of 8th cranial nerve pathologies
- Detection of malingering
- Mental retardation

Newborn screening in high-risk groups including:
- Birth asphyxia
- Intrauterine infection
- Neonatal hyperbilirubinemia
- Meningitis in early childhood
- Low birth weight babies

Evoke response audiometry can be divided into:
1. Electrocochleography 0–2 ms.
2. BERA 2–10 ms
3. Cortical evoke resp. audiometry 10–500 ms
    It has 3 divisions:
    a. AMEP (auditory middle evoked potentials) from 10 to 50 ms
    b. ALEP (auditory late latency or cortical evoked potentials) from 50 to 500 ms
    c. Postauricular myogenic response (PAM) from 10 to 30 ms and is part of AMEP.

Waves of BERA

There are seven waves in normal person, however, only first, third and fifth are stable and are clinically significant.

1. Cochlear nerve 2 ms
2. Cochlear nucleus
3. Superior olivary complex 4 ms
4. Lateral lemniscus
5. Inferior colliculus 6 ms most reliable
6. Medial geniculate body
7. Auditory radiations

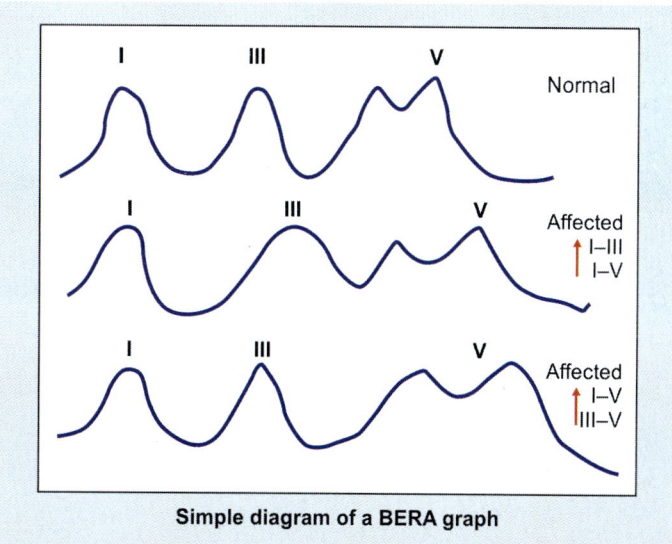

Simple diagram of a BERA graph

The morphology, latency and amplitude of these waves are important in different clinical situations.

Features of retro-cochlear lesions
- Wave I normal
- Wave IIIrd and wave IVth delayed
- Increased interaural latency of wave V >0.3 ms
- Increased interwave latency between I and V

Cortical evoked response audiometry (CERA): Similar to BERA; but the cortical responses are measured.

Otoacoustic emissions (OAE)/cochlear echoes/kemp echoes: Recording of sound generated from outer hair cells of organ of Corti. Screening test for congenital or neonatal sensorineural hearing loss.

Types
- Spontaneous (SOAE)
- Evoked (TEOAE or CEOAE, i.e. transient or single click evoked and DPOAE, i.e. distortion product to two click or stimuli evoked).
- Impaired cochlea does not make these sounds.

Electrocochleography (ECochG)
Diagnostic test for Meniere's disease.
- SP: AP = 0.45 N
- SP: AP = prolong in Meniere's disease.
- CCG—craniocorpography.

CHAPTER 3

Hearing Loss and Deafness

DEAF

The term should be applied only if there is no improvement in hearing with any kind of amplification (WHO).

WHO Classification of Deafness

Mild	26–40 dB
Moderate	41–55 dB
Moderately severe	56–70 dB
Severe	71–91 dB
Profound	>91 dB

Causes of Sensorineural Deafness

Congenital

Endogenous: Inherited, familial consanguinous marriages

Exogenous: Rubella, Rh incompatibility, birth asphyxia.

Toxic

Febrile illnesses: Measles, typhoid, mumps, influenza, pneumonia.

Drugs

Quinine, aminoglycosides, neomycin, kanamycin, salicylic acid, streptomycin, etc.
- Syphilis
- Skull trauma
- Concussion
- Labyrinthitis
- Acoustic neuroma
- Noise induced—onset is either sudden or gradual
- Central causes—multiple sclerosis
- Presbycusis
- Meniere's disease
- Psychogenic

Causes of conductive deafness (can lie at any point along the conductive tract)—external auditory canal (EAC).

Wax, polyp, foreign body, tumor, inflammation, etc.

Middle ear: Perforated/retracted TM, fluid or pus, otospongiosis, ossicular disruption, middle ear tympanosclerosis, etc.

Inner ear (rare): Superior semicircular canal dehiscence syndrome, large cochlear aqueduct mimicking otosclerosis, etc.

Causes of Sudden Hearing Loss

Vascular causes: Vasospasm, thromboembolism of end arteries
- Acoustic neuroma
- Noise trauma
- Otitic barotrauma
- Skull fracture, oval and round window rupture or perilymph fistula
- Viral infections
- Ototoxic drugs
- Concussion
- Labyrinthitis—purulent or serous
- Meniere's disease
- Psychogenic

Causes of Mixed Deafness

CSOM, secretory otitis media, otosclerosis.

Causes of reversible SN hearing loss: Meniere's disease, noise pollution, salicylate toxicity.

Treatable SN hearing loss: Cochlear otospongiosis, endolymphatic hydrops, syphilis.

Fluctuant hearing loss: Upper respiratory infection, secretory otitis media, eustachian tube functions, Meniere's disease, perilymph fistula.

Causes of Hearing Loss after Mastoid Surgery

Serous labyrinthitis, suppurative labyrinthitis, formalin treated gel foam, formalin treated sialastic sheet or PORP, perilymph fistula, excess movements at stapes, cutting burr touching the incus, noise-induced hearing loss due to sound generated by drilling.

Eustachian Tube Functions Testing

Valsalva maneuver, Toynbee test, Frenzel maneuver, politzerization, impedance, eustachian tube gush during swallowing.

OTOTOXICITY

Hearing loss secondary to drugs like salicylates, anti-malarial drugs like chloroquine, quinine, aminoglycosides [AG] (cochlear as well as vestibular), loop diuretics, macrolides, platinum drugs, etc. Drugs like streptomycin can become symptomatic even with single dose administration. It [AG] causes damage to outer hair cells by giant cell formation. But drugs like furosemide have transient damage. Once the drug is stopped, hearing loss improves. Patients develop hearing loss, vertigo and oscillopsia. Treatment is by auditory and vestibular rehabilitation. Regarding ototoxicity it is understood that preventing administration of ototoxic drugs is easier rather than futile efforts at reversing their effects after giving them.

PRESBYCUSIS

Old age hearing loss is known as presbycusis.

It is further divided into:

1. Conductive as the age advances beyond 50 the external auditory canal and pinna starts sagging down and obstruct the entry of sound leading to conductive hearing loss. There are senile changes in and around tympanic membrane like tympanosclerosis and hardening of tympanic annulus, can present as conductive hearing loss.
2. Cochlear or sensory hearing loss: Reason behind is either loss of outer or inner hair cells in basal turn of cochlea.
3. Strial presbycusis: It is because of declining metabolic functions of stria vascularis with ischaemia and diminished endolymph production.
4. Ganglionic presbycusis: Because of senile degeneration and ischemia, the spiral ganglion numbers drops from normal 34000 to below 13000 and patient experiences great problem in discriminating the speech.
5. Retrocochlear or neural: This is because of ischemia and deficiency of vitamin B_{12}, B_6 leading to neural sheath degeneration. This affects the nerve conduction causing problems in speech discrimination.
6. Cochlear conductive: This is due to decreased subcellular organelle functions without structural defects in the inner ear.

Most of the patients cannot be classified under any of the group as most of the time there is overlap of all changes and the condition is called intermediate presbycusis.

Treatment

1. Rule out renal, cardiac, hepatic diseases along with iron and B complex deficiencies.
2. B_1, B_6 and B_{12} supplements often (in India) along with iron supplements.
3. Most of the time these old people are addicted to tobacco/gutka/beedi. So, abstinence from addiction is advised.
4. Vasodilators to improve the micro-circulations like pyretinol, ixosuprine, cyclospasmol and complamina (nicotinic acid derivatives) are prescribed.
5. Hearing aid—multichannel aids are preferred and if it is BAHA, then feedback problem and further hearing loss due to it can be avoided. Hearing result with BAHA is very good.

CHAPTER 4

Diseases of External Ear

EAR WAX

Cartilaginous part of EAC has two types of glands:
1. Sebaceous gland
2. Ceruminous gland

When the number of sebaceous glands increases more than that of ceruminous gland, it results in hard wax formation.

When the number of ceruminous gland increases more than that of sebaceous gland, it results in no wax formation.

It is autosomal recessive trait.

WW → autosomal dominant → more ceruminous gland and ww (small letter w) → autosomal recessive → more sebaceous glands in EAC.

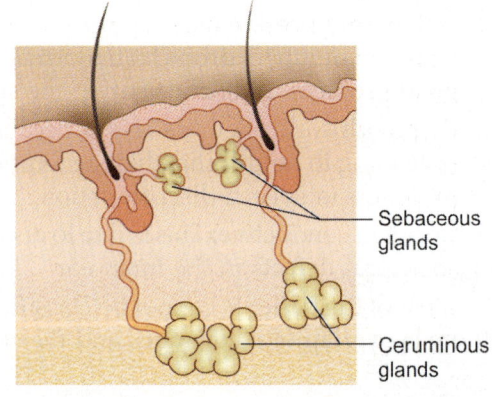

So WW → excessive ceruminous gland + less sebaceous glands and no wax formation.

Ww → 50% sebaceous gland + 50% ceruminous glands and wet wax formation.

ww → >50% sebaceous glands + <50% ceruminous glands and hard wax formation.

Sebaceous gland secretions are solute and ceruminous gland secretions act as solvent. When the EAC is totally occluded by wax, it can cause hearing loss up to 50 dB.

Keratosis Obturans

Painful condition where there is collection of desquamated cell debris along with wax in deeper part of EAC leading to bone erosion. This condition is more aggressive than cholesteatoma. It is associated with bronchiectasis and sinusitis.

Otitis Externa (Furunculosis)

Seen in cartilaginous EAC because of infection in hair follicles.

Staphylococcus aureus is the most common organism.

Treatment: 10% Ichthammol glycerin packing daily, drug should be freshly prepared

- Ichthammol local antiseptic
- Glycerin hygroscopic
- Packing immobilizes the EAC and thus less pain
- Oral antibiotics
- Analgesics

Recurrent Otitis Externa

Rule out diabetes or other immunocompromised states.

Look for finger nails and vestibule as source of infection.

Culture sensitivity of the causative organism to rule out drug resistance.

Singapore Ear/Tropical Ear

Diffuse otitis externa Pseudomonas, Staphylococcus, proteus.

Otomycosis

It is the fungal infection of the ear. It is seen more in moist and hot environmental conditions. Common in persons with narrow EAC, bony canal osteoma, etc.

Commonly involved organisms are *Aspergillus niger, Aspergillus fumigatus, Candida albicans.*

Drugs for otomycosis: Topical cotrimazole with or without keratolytic agents like 2% salicylic acid and topical anaesthetic agent.

Clotrimazole, itraconazole and voriconazole.

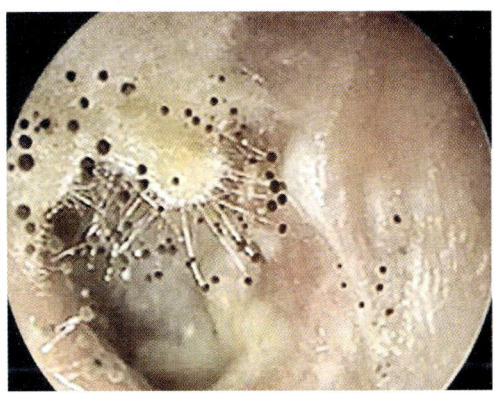

Otomicroscopic picture of otomycotic body where black colored spores are seen (most probably *Aspergillus niger* species)

Myringitis Bullosa

Viral infection of TM, Bleb seen on TM

Treatment: Antibiotics, analgesics

Bleb should not be punctured.

Malignant Otitis Externa

It is a locally destructive infection of EAC which can lead onto base of skull osteomyelitis.

Caused by *Pseudomonas aeruginosa.*

Predisposing factors: Diabetes uncontrolled, ageing and immunosuppression

Local destruction can involve mastoid, petrous apex, parotid, etc.

Multiple cranial nerve palsy, Vth to XII—the commonest one is facial nerve palsy.

Treatment: Antibiotics, debridement and management of underlying immunocompromised state.

Herpes Zoster Oticus

Involvement of 7th cranial nerve and external ear (Ramsay Hunt syndrome). On examination
- Severe pain in ear
- Vesicles in EAC and pinna
- Vesicle may be seen on palate, pharynx
- LMN facial nerve paralysis.

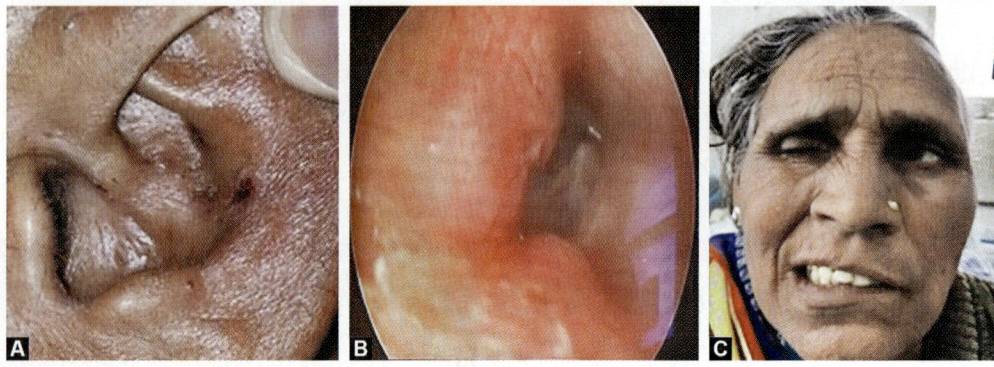

Ramsay Hunt syndrome (herpes zoster oticus)

Treatment
- Acyclovir
- Analgesics + steroids
- B_{12} + multivitamin supplements.
- Poor prognosis for facial nerve paralysis should be explained to the patient.

Tumors of EAC

Benign: Papilloma, adenoma, ceruminoma, fibroma, osteoma, exostosis.

Malignant: SCC and malignant tumors of sebaceous gland, basal cell carcinoma.

Exostosis of EAC: Multiple, usually bilateral, sessile bony swellings.
   Commonly found in swimmers.

Osteoma of EAC: Single, pedunculated bony swelling.

CHAPTER 5

Acute Suppurative Otitis Media

ACUTE SUPPURATIVE OTITIS MEDIA (ASOM)

Acute inflammation of middle ear cleft. Clinically has

1. Stage of retraction
2. Stage of congestion with cart wheel appearance of capillaries
3. Stage of suppuration
4. Stage of perforation with light house sign
5. Stage of healing or recovery
6. Stage of complications

Causative organisms are:
- *Streptococcus pneumoniae* 35%
- *Haemophilus influenzae* 23%
- Staphylococcus 3%
- *Streptococcus pyogenes* 3%
- *Moraxella catarrhalis* 14%

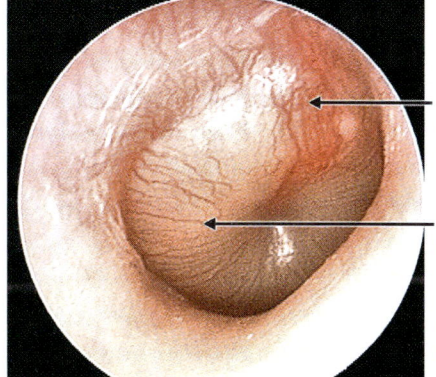

Congestion of tympanic membrane

Bulging tympanic membrane due to pus under pressure

Stage of suppuration

Antibiotic of choice: Amoxycillin + Clavulanic acid

Indications for myringotomy in ASOM
- Acute severe pain
- Very small perforation not adequate for drainage of pus
- No resolution after full course of antibiotics and
- Impending complications.

If the patient, even after 3 weeks of treatment, complains of hearing loss, otalgia with loss of cone of light and thick TM, then there is a chance that the patient has developed *masked otitis media or mastoiditis*. If these patients do not respond to routine treatment, may need complete blood investigations and X-ray. If there is increased ESR and lymphocytosis, it confirms masked otitis media or mastoiditis. Then the patient needs simple mastoidectomy which will relieve his symptoms. Hence, masked mastoiditis is a treacherous condition to deal with.

A suspicion of tuberculosis should be kept at the corner of mind if the patient is not responding well to regular treatment protocols for masked otitis media.

Acute Mastoiditis

It is diagnosed by persistence of pain behind the ear, otorrhea, fever and tenderness over the mastoid despite of adequate antibiotics.

Cortical mastoidectomy in cases of mastoiditis
- Deterioration of patient despite adequate treatment.
- Impending complication.
   Subperiosteal abscess following ASOM occurs due to erosion of the cortical mastoid bone and the pus is collected under the periosteum.

Acute necrotizing otitis media: It is preceded by viral fevers like measles with superadded bacterial infections causing complete necrosis of the middle ear mucosa and subtotal tympanic membrane perforation.

Caused by beta hemolytic *Streptococcus*

Common in children.

After initial phase, will either

A—heal completely

B—may present later-on as safe CSOM with subtotal perforation

C—with extensive necrosis of mucosa over promontory, squamous epithelium from the EAC migrates inside the middle ear along the necrosed annulus. This might present as a secondary cholesteatoma. In children, it may have finger like invasion into mastoid cellular system.

CHAPTER 6

Non-suppurative Middle Ear Diseases

OTITIS MEDIA WITH EFFUSION

Otitis media with effusion (OME) goes by other synonyms like glue ear, secretory otitis media, non-suppurative otitis media.

It is the collection of non-purulent fluid in middle ear cleft.

This is common in young children.

Diagnosis

Insularity, dual pain in ear, tinnitus, TM—looks dull, air fluid level, bluish.

PTA showing conductive hearing loss.

Impedance audiometry is the diagnostic test with Type B or C curve.

If fluid in middle ear is thin, then compliance will be between 0.20 and 0.40 ml and peak pressure will be between –50 and –250. If fluid is thick like glue, then compliance will be below 0.20 and peak pressure will be > –250.

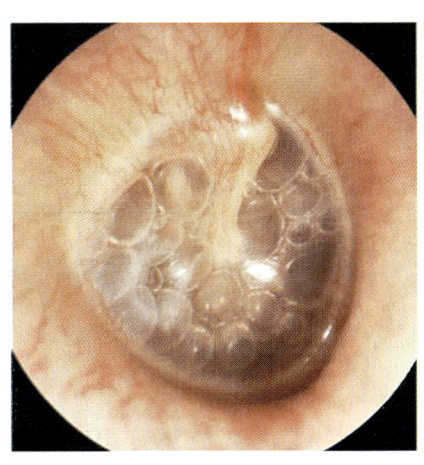

Treatment

- Conservative—mucolytics, anti-histaminics and nasal decongestants.
- Surgeries for the causes like adenoid, tonsil, DNS, etc.
- Grommet insertion, laser assisted tympanostomy.

Adults usually have acute SOM and have thin fluid while children usually have thick glue-like fluid and invariably need grommet insertion. Patients with thin fluids commonly respond to medical treatment.

Site of incision in myringotomy
1. Radial incision made in right SOM in the anteroinferior quadrant.

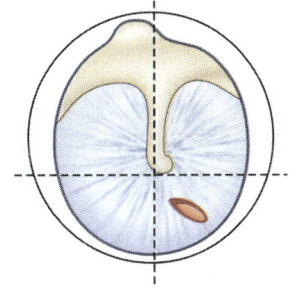
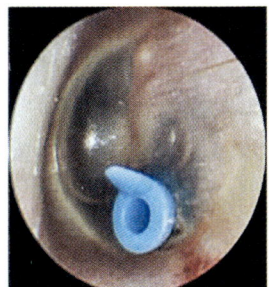

2. After placement of grommet.
  • Tympanoplasty with sialastic sheet or cartilage palisades in middle ear to prevent further retractions.
  • Hearing aid

TYPES OF GROMMET

Shepherd's, silicon T tube, Shah's tube, Goody's T tubes in recurrent cases, metal—titanium, gold tubes.

ATELECTASIS

Sade's grading for pars tensa retraction:

Grading	Nature
I	Mild retraction
II	Contact with incus or stapes
III	Contact with promontory
IV	Adhesion to promontory
V	Adhesion with perforation

Tos grading for pars flaccida retraction:

Grading	Nature
I	Mild retraction not touching the malleus head
II	Retraction pocket is in full view and adhesion to neck of malleus
III	Retraction is out of view and there is partial erosion of outer attic wall
IV	Complete erosion of outer attic wall (cholesteatoma)

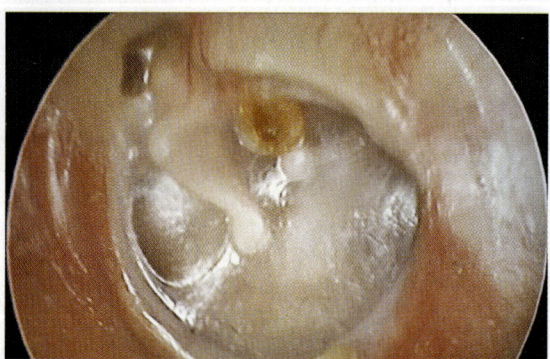

Tympanic membrane with grade III pars flaccida retraction

TYMPANOSCLEROSIS

It is the hyalinization and subsequent calcification of subepithelial tissue of tympanic membrane and middle ear. It occurs in healing tympanum following CSOM. There are 2 types:
1. Open type (tympanic membrane perforation)
2. Close type (without TM perforation)

Common sites: Incudostapedial joint, promontory, tympanic membrane, stapes footplate, malleus head, tegmen and round window.

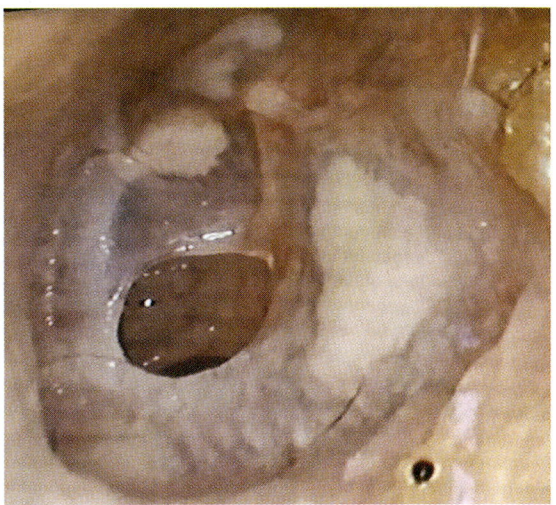

Tympanosclerosis (open type) of TM

CHAPTER 7

Chronic Suppurative Otitis Media

Classification of CSOM
- Tubotympanic/mucosal CSOM (safe ear)
- Atticoantral/squamosal CSOM (unsafe ear)

Perforation
- Small (one quadrant), medium (two quadrants), large (more than two quadrants), subtotal with only intact annulus and anterior and posterior malleolar folds.
- Total perforation: When annulus is involved all around or anterior and posterior malleolar are destroyed and perforation extends to attic.
- Attic perforation is perforation in pars flaccida.

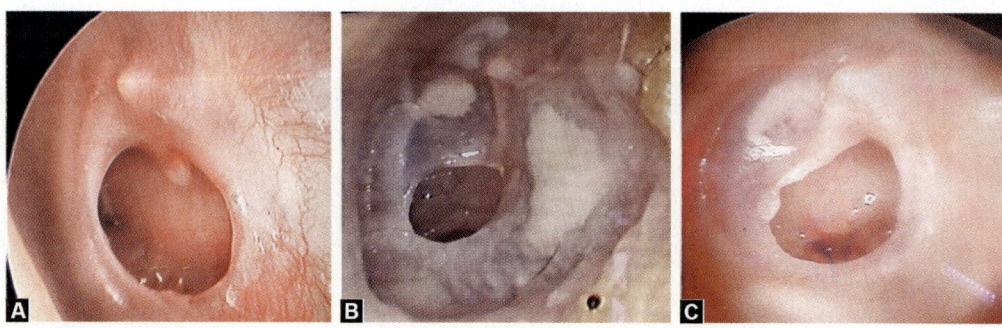

Various types of pars tensa perforations

Spread of Infection in CSOM
Destruction of bone due to hyperemic decalcification, thrombophlebitis, bony dehiscences and preformed pathways.

Causative Organisms in CSOM
Streptococcus pneumoniae, Staphylococcus aureus, Haemophilus influenzae, proteus, Pseudomonas, *E. coli*, anaerobes like *M. catarrhalis*.

Ear discharge: Mucoid (thread like on buds as in allergy), mucopurulent and profuse in tubotympanic type
Purulent, blood stained, scanty and foul smelling in atticoantral.

Dry perforation syndrome: Childhood CSOM turns inactive and the perforation remains till adulthood. This causes hearing loss but the patient might not remember ear discharge history. This might get reactivated at any point either due to entry of dirty infected water or where the host immunity decreases like febrile illness, pregnancy or other immunocompromised states like diabetes mellitus, etc.

Hearing loss: More in tubotympanic disease than atticoantral as pars tensa's role in hearing is more. In most cases of attic disease, there is auto type 3 tympanoplasty where remnant of TM is placed over stapes by erosion of incus. Ossicular erosion is commonly seen in unsafe CSOM.

Ossicular erosion in CSOM: Due to enzymatic osteoclastic overactivity. Incus (long process) > stapes > malleus is the order of frequency of involvement of ossicles in CSOM. Incus erosion is more common due to its shape, less blood supply and saw like cutting action of chorda tympani against the long process.

Factors preventing retraction of TM: Intact TM, annulus and malleolar folds, Intact ossicles, middle ear pressure, chorda tympani crossing the middle ear posteroanteriorly.

Foul smelling discharge in unsafe CSOM: It is because of decomposing squamous epithelium and keratin by saprophytic anaerobic bacteria and sequestered bone as seen commonly in cholesteatoma.

Foul smelling discharge in safe CSOM: It might occur due to anaerobic infection or presence of organic FB like dead flies which get attracted by the presence of pus.

Ear ache: In discharging ear, it is because of local inflammation and mastoiditis. In dry ear, it is because of isolated tip cell suppuration, foreign body reaction to tympano-sclerosis and mucous curtain in aditus with mastoid disease.

Differences between middle ear polyp and granulation

Middle ear polyps	Granulations
Usually arise from promontory	Usually from posterosuperior bony margins
Pedunculated	Sessile
Not painful to touch	Painful
Does not bleed on manipulation	Bleeds on manipulation
Probe can be passed all around	Probe gets arrested at posterosuperior aspect
Less vascular	Highly vascular
Histologically, it is mucosal layer with edematous lamina propria with non-existent nervous tissue	It is connective tissue with neo-vascularization and an attempt by the body for repair mechanism

Investigations for CSOM

Routine investigations

- Hb, TLC, DLC, blood sugar, renal function tests, coagulation assays
- Urine routine and microscopic examination
- Chest X-ray, ECG, 2D ECHO (if indicated), etc.

These routine investigations are done pre-operatively to have an idea about patient's baseline health and fitness for the surgery.

To confirm diagnosis

- *Microscopic examination of ear*

  To know about the disease, whether it is safe or unsafe

  To suck out pus and debris

  To evaluate the margin, ossicles, middle ear mucosa.

- *Pus culture and sensitivity:* In case of complication to start antibiotics accordingly.

- *Pure tone audiometry:* Base line hearing recording and cochlear reserve can be found.

  Type and degree of hearing loss.

  Medicolegal base line.

  – 20–30 dB in single perforation

  – > 45 dB in ossicular chain loss or associated tympanosclerosis.

- *X-ray:*

  Lateral oblique (Law's 15° or Schuller's 30° or *modified Mayer's* (BEST) or Owen's view)

  To see the pneumatization of mastoid bone

  To see the dural plate and sinus plate so that approach can be decided.

  To detect presence of cavities—smooth (cholesteatoma) or irregular (coalescent mastoiditis).

  To detect cloudiness of mastoid air cells or cell wall erosions.

  To detect homogenous haziness inside smooth cavity and evidence of rupture of cholesteatoma matrix and granulations.

- *Towne's view:* To compare the pneumatization of both sides.

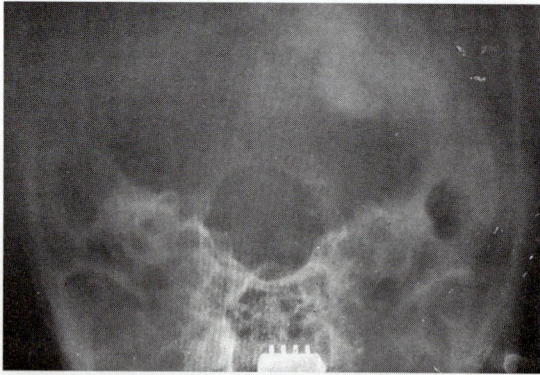

Bilateral mastoid shows cholesteatoma cavities (smooth walled cavities with sclerotic bony margin) [post operative cavity is smooth, coalescent mastoiditis cavity is irregular without sclerosis].

- *Contrast enhanced CT of temporal bone:* For suspected intracranial complication.

Complications of CSOM–More in Atticoantral CSOM

Classified into intracranial and temporal complications.

1. Temporal complications:

    I. Mastoiditis (acute or chronic),

    II. Mastoid abscess and postaural sinus

      - Classical postaural mastoid abscess

      - Zygomatic abscess

- Bezold's abscess (along the sterno-mastoid from mastoid tip)
- Citelli's abscess (along the digastric muscle through deep tip cells)
- Luc's abscess (erosion of perifacial cells presenting as a swelling in the postero-superior EAC wall—hanging posterior EAC can be confused with a polyp by a beginner)
- Postaural mastoid abscess in a young child is basically an extradural abscess with open skull sutures and lateral part of temporal bone lying within the abscess cavity.

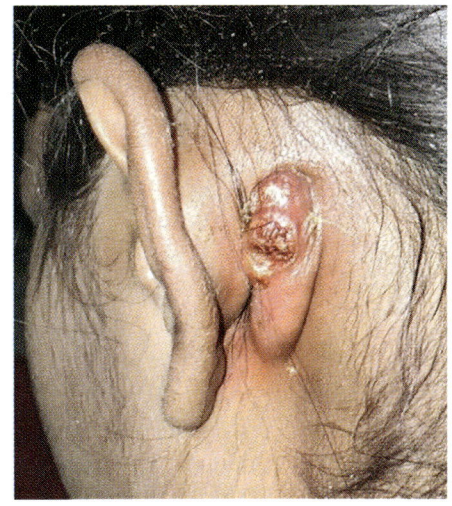

Mastoid abscess ruptured through skin forming a postaural sinus

III. Grieslinger's sign—oedema and tenderness over the mastoid emissary. It is an evidence of sigmoid sinus thrombophlebitis.

IV. Facial nerve paralysis either as a complication of ASOM in dehiscent horizontal portion or erosion by cholesteatoma commonly in horizontal portion. This is a lower motor neuron type paralysis.

V. Labyrinthitis—commonly it is chronic labyrinthine fistula with fistula sign positive with either normal bone conduction or sensorineural hearing loss. Complete cochlear loss is found if it is associated with acute suppurative labyrinthitis. Common sites of fistula are postampullary portion of LSCC. Sometimes it can involve pre-ampullary portion just above the horizontal portion of facial nerve. In pre-ampullary type, on pressing the tragus, nystagmus is seen towards the opposite side and in post-ampullary on dome of LSCC nystagmus is towards the same side.

VI. Petrositis—it is commonly seen with CSOM or postoperative mastoid cavity infections. When it has got a triad of retrobulbar pain (due to irritation of trigeminal ganglion in Meckel's cave on top of petrous apex; as sensory fibers of ophthalmic division or all three divisions are close to the petrous bone) or deep gnawing pain on the side of diseased ear, lateral rectus paralysis (diplopia on looking towards same side because of abducens nerve compression at Dorello's canal near petrous apex) and ear discharge, it is called **Gradenigo syndrome.** It is supposed to be caused by gram-positive bacteria almost always with added anaerobes like Bacillus fragilis and *Moraxella catarrhalis* and rarely by gram-negative bacteria.

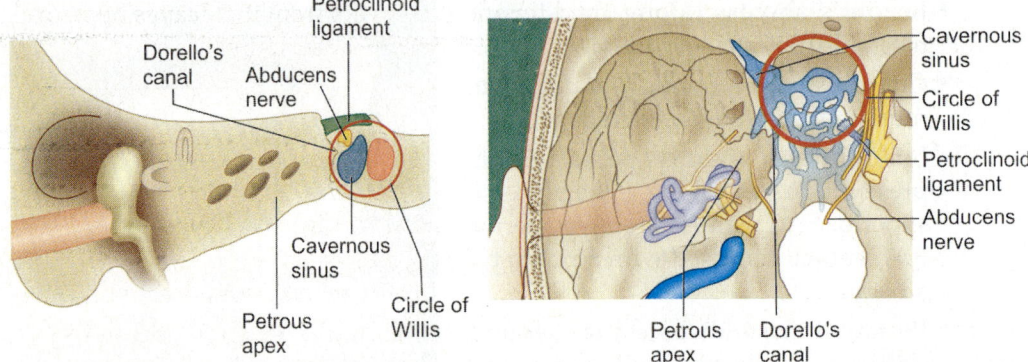

2. Intracranial complications

  a. *Lateral sinus thrombophlebitis*: Characterized by Picket-Fence fever with rigors, headache, nausea, vomiting (raised ICT). Griesinger sign is found, anemia due to infection with hemolytic streptococci as 6 L of blood flow through a sigmoid sinus in one minute along with chronic ear discharge which is most of the time foetid and foul smelling. Tober Ayre and Lillee Crow tests are of diagnostic value in this condition.

  b. *Brain abscess*: The spread of infection from middle ear to brain occurs commonly by thrombophlebitis of sigmoid sinus which in turn spreads to superior or inferior petrosal sinus and further into the sulci of brain via cerebellar or cerebral vein lying in Virchow-Robin's space and going deep up to the white matter of brain sparing grey matter. That is why brain abscess

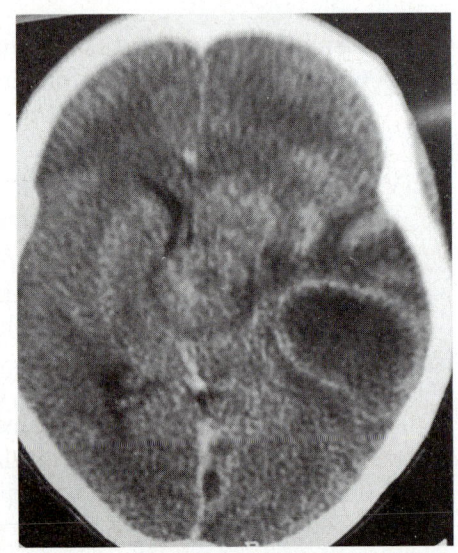

Temporal lobe abscess

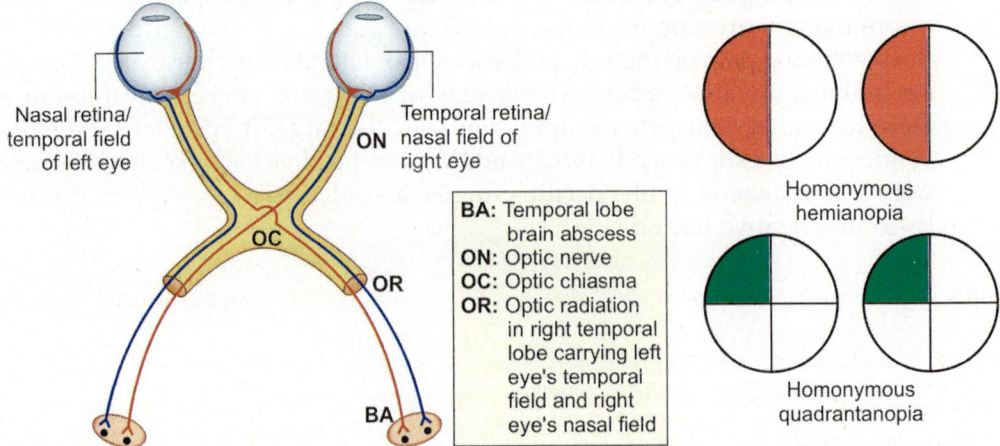

BA: Temporal lobe brain abscess
ON: Optic nerve
OC: Optic chiasma
OR: Optic radiation in right temporal lobe carrying left eye's temporal field and right eye's nasal field

occurs in white matter of brain and if patient recovers from it, it leaves no neural deficit because the gray matter is spared. It has 4 stages, namely

i. Encephalitis stage

ii. Latent/silent stage

iii. Expanding abscess stage

iv. Terminal stage—either due to rupture into ventricle or by coning of uncus (tentorium cerebri) or cerebellum (foramen magnum)

Temporal lobe abscess is common. Symptoms and signs are nominal aphasia, bradycardia, papilloedema, breathing irregularity, headache, nausea, vomiting, homonymous hemianopia/quadrantanopia are seen when optic radiation is affected.

Cerebellar abscess is not as common as temporal lobe abscess. Signs and symptoms apart from 4 stages of brain abscess are ataxia, spontaneous nystagmus, intentional tremors, dysdiadochokinesia and past pointing.

c. Meningitis

d. *Extradural abscess*—pus enters the epidural space through the eroded bone (near arcuate eminence or Trautman's triangle) and collects between the bone and meninges as dura is resistant to erosion. Ear discharge increases by occluding the jugular vein. Diagnosed by CT scan.

e. *Subdural abscess*—between dura and arachnoid.

f. *Otitic hydrocephalus*—in bilateral sigmoid sinus or superior sagittal sinus thrombophlebitis, if thrombus is not removed in initial phase, then 6th month onwards because of constant papilloedema due to increased ICT due to failure of absorption of CSF in occluded sinus, there is gradual loss of vision with headache, vomiting, cranial nerve paralysis and drowsiness. It is also known as Symond's syndrome.

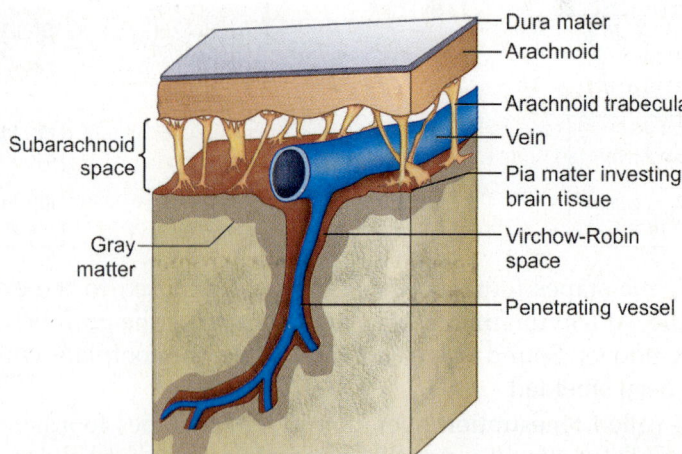

Virchow-Robin space—the commonest way of spread of infection from venous sinuses to brain

Cranial nerves involved in complications of CSOM:

II, III, IV: In cavernous sinus thrombosis

V: If petrous apex is involved

VI: Dorello's canal formed by petroclinoid ligament

VII: Erosion in mastoid

IX, X, XI and XIII: As jugular fossa is involved in cases of lateral sinus thrombosis.

Tympanoplasty (middle ear disease removal +/– reconstruction of hearing mechanism).

The fundamental principles of tympanoplasty were introduced by Wullstein and Zollner in 1956 and they classified tympanoplasty (modified Wullstein classification) in view of ossicular chain reconstruction (OCR) into the following types:

- **Type 1:** All the ossicles are present and mobile. OCR is not needed, and the TM graft is placed as an overlay (1-a) or underlay technique (1-b).
- **Type 2:** Malleus eroded and the TM graft is placed on intact incus and stapes.
- **Type 3:** Also called myringostapediopexy or columella tympanoplasty. This is done in cases where malleus and incus are absent or malleus is present with incus erosion sometimes. Subdivided into three different types based on the Nadol-Schuknecht modification of the original Wullstein classification: (3-A) Stapes columella tympanoplasty—placing a TM graft directly on the stapes head; (3-B) Minor columella tympanoplasty; (3-B₁) Placing a strut or prosthesis between the stapes head and the TM graft; (3-B₂) Incus interposition or transposition between intact malleus and head of stapes; (3-C) Major columella tympanoplasty—placing a strut or prosthesis between the stapes footplate and TM graft.

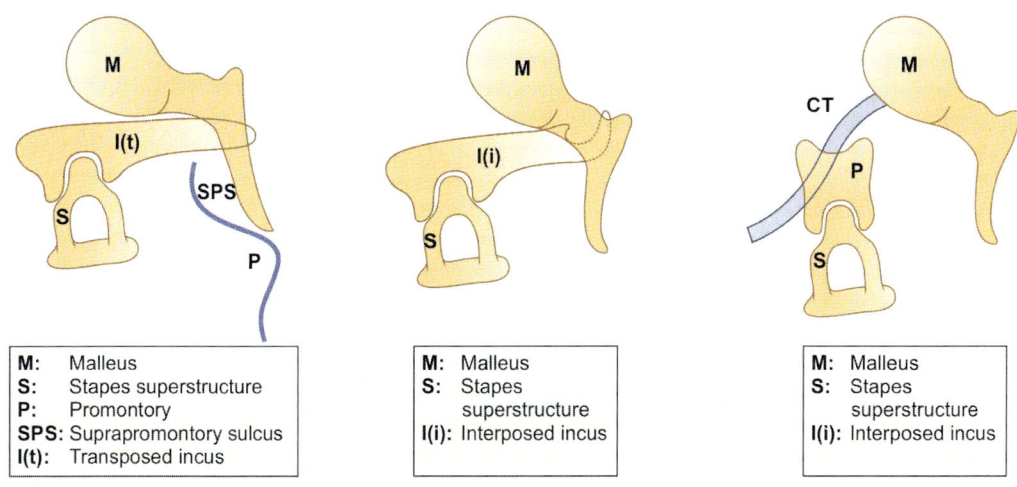

M:	Malleus
S:	Stapes superstructure
P:	Promontory
SPS:	Suprapromontory sulcus
I(t):	Transposed incus

M:	Malleus
S:	Stapes superstructure
I(i):	Interposed incus

M:	Malleus
S:	Stapes superstructure
I(i):	Interposed incus

- **Type 4:** Only the stapes footplate is present. It is exposed to the external ear. A narrow middle ear (cavum minor) is created by placing the graft between the oval and round windows. Sound waves act directly on the footplate while the round window has been shielded.
- **Type 5:** Also called fenestration operation in which stapes footplate is fixed, but round window is functioning. Another window is created on dome of horizontal semicircular canal and covered with a graft.
- **Type 6:** Sonoinversion—all sound waves enter through the round window keeping the oval window covered (reverse direction).

For performing the tympanoplasties, one should know the anatomical points like the following.

Suprapromontory sulcus:

- **Type 1:** Shallow sulcus—here incus transposition is possible (2b).
- **Type 2:** Moderate size—here incus transposition may or may not be possible.
- **Type 3:** Very deep sulcus—here incus transposition is not possible.

Pindborg classification of distance between head of stapes and malleus handle:

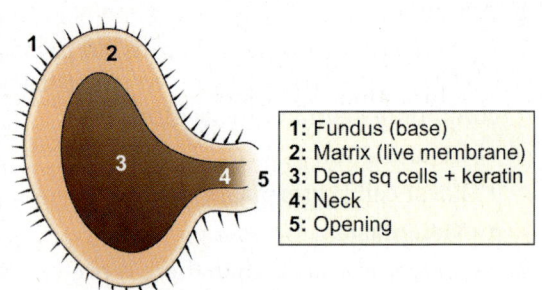

1: Fundus (base)
2: Matrix (live membrane)
3: Dead sq cells + keratin
4: Neck
5: Opening

- **Type 1:** Large gap between the two; transposition of incus is possible but interposition is not possible.
- **Type 2:** Moderate gap between the two; here both are possible.
- **Type 3:** Very small gap between the two; probe cannot be passed between them easily. Here only interposition of incus is possible.

PORP (Type 3 minor tympanoplasty) can be performed in all the Pindborg types (1–3).

CHOLESTEATOMA

Definition

Sac-like structure lined by keratinized squamous epithelium filled by debris and keratin. It is mentioned as skin in the wrong places.

Parts of a cholesteatoma sac are: Outer fibrous stroma, matrix, debris, neck and fundus.

Other names of cholesteatoma: Keratoma, epidermosis, cholesteoid.

Theories of Formation of Cholesteatoma

1. *Wittmack's theory:* Persistence of hyperplastic embryonic type of mucoperiosteum in epitympanum causes adhesions, creation of negative pressure inside middle ear and finally cholesteatoma.

2. *Migration theory-I (Haberman):* Migration of squamous epithelium from the deep external auditory meatus and remnant TM, through a perforation into middle ear leading to cholesteatoma formation.

   Migration theory-II (Tumarkin): Emphasizes the role of a preceding collapse of part or whole of the tympanic membrane (atelectasis) in the pars flaccida or postero-superior quadrant. Later keratin accumulates here and develops into a cholesteatoma.

3. *Metaplasia theory (Sade):* Under the influence of infection metaplasia of middle ear mucosa occurs (to stratified squamous epithelium) and cholesteatoma is formed.

4. *Papillary ingrowth (Ruedi):* Of epithelium through its own basement membrane.

Types of Cholesteatoma

A. Congenital

B. Acquired

1. *Primary acquired,* when there is no previous history of otitis media or perforation commonly seen in attic region.
   - Invagination
   - Basal cell hyperplasia
   - Metaplasia
2. *Secondary acquired,* when there is pre-existing perforation in pars tensa commonly seen in posterosuperior region.
   - Migration of epithelium
   - Metaplasia

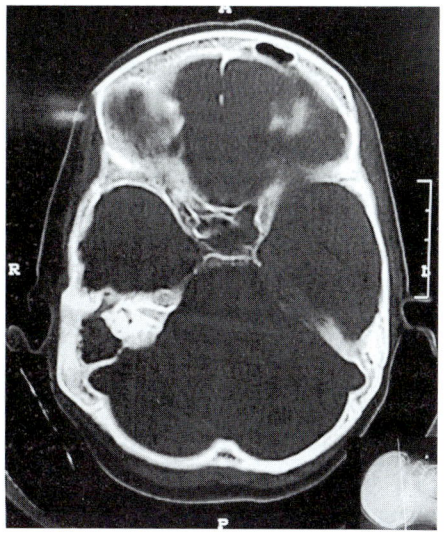

A large cavity seen in right mastoid caused by cholesteatoma is seen in CT mastoid axial section.

Destruction caused by cholesteatoma
- *Enzymatic theory*: Collagenase, acid phosphatase and other proteolytic enzymes liberated by osteoclasts.
- Pressure theory
- Pyogenic osteitis

Sites of congenital cholesteatoma: TM, petrous apex, CP angle and mesotympanum.

Presentation of congenital cholesteatoma: No ear discharge, no history of ear surgery, hearing loss, tinnitus, vertigo, headache, cranial nerve palsy depending on the site and intact TM.

Areas of hidden cholesteatoma: Sinus tympani, supra-pyramidal recess, facial recess, lateral tympanic sinus, petrous apex, sinodural angle, tip cells, anterior attic and inside a labyrinthine fistula. These areas should be made sure to be free of diseases during surgery. Failure will cause disease recurrence.

Options to close mastoid cavity: Sternomastoid flap, bone patty, temporalis muscle and fascia (Palva's flap), abdominal fat, osteocutaneous flap.

Closure of cavity gives results similar to a canal wall up procedure. Other than these techniques the cavity can be obliterated by keeping a shallow cavity by saucerization and exenterating every single air cell.

Canal Wall Down (CWD) Procedures

Modified radical mastoidectomy, radical mastoidectomy, atticotomy.

Advantages of CWD are: Easy to perform and less time consuming
- No risk residual disease
- Easy monitoring through meatoplasty

Disadvantages of CWD: Cavity problems like recurrent otomycosis
- No water sports
- Problems for hearing aid placement

Canal Wall Up (CWU) Procedures

Cortical mastoidectomy
- Combined approach tympanoplasty (CAT)
- Cavity obliteration procedures

Contraindications to CWU procedure: Only hearing ear
- Recurrent cholesteatoma
- Labyrinthine fistula
- Preoperative posterior canal wall destroyed

Advantages of CWU: Normal anatomy maintained
- Can swim (water sports)
- Can use hearing aid
- No cavity problem

Disadvantage of CWU: Higher chances of residual disease or recurrent disease up to 30%.
   Should be opened up again after 6 months.

Indications for radical mastoidectomy
A. Carcinoma of middle ear
B. Carcinoma of external ear, if involving bony external auditory canal
C. Unserviceable hearing with cholesteatoma
D. Malignant otitis externa
E. Others: Labyrinthectomy and glomus surgeries.

Modified radical mastoidectomy: A canal wall down procedure; the facial ridge is thinned and lowered adequately after taking down the posterior bony wall and communicating mastoid cavity with attic. The cavity produced is globular. Then this whole cavity is communicated into EAC via an adequate meatoplasty. The opening of the meatoplasty should be one finger width. Conchal and meatal cartilages should not be damaged as this will cause notorious perichondritis.

Causes of vertigo after MRM: Residual disease leading to erosion of SCC, perilymph fistula, irritative labyrinthitis due to drilling, separate vestibular or CNS pathology, brain abscess and delayed endolymphatic hydrops.

Causes of discharge after the mastoid surgery:
1. Residual or recurrent disease usually at the following sites:
   i. sino dural angle,
   ii. facial recess,
   iii. tip cells and
   iv. anterior attic.
2. Perichondritis
3. Granulation
4. Facial ridge inadequately lowered
5. Meatoplasty inadequate

Complications of large mastoid cavity (4Ds): Discharge, deafness, dizziness (Tullio's phenomenon) and disability.

CHAPTER 8

Diseases of Facial Nerve

It is the VII cranial nerve. It is composed of approximately 10,000 neurons out of which 7,000 are myelinated and supply the muscles of facial expression. 3,000 travels in nervus intermedius and are somatosensory and secretomotor.

Parts of Facial Nerve

A. Intracranial part (pontine segment) 23–24 mm. Brain stem to porus of internal auditory canal.

B. Meatal segment 7–8 mm long.

C. Labyrinthine segment 4 mm length and 0.68 mm diameter.

D. Tympanic or horizontal part 12–13 mm long; extends from from 1st to 2nd genu. 55% of cases fallopian canal is dehiscent.

E. Vertical mastoid segment 15–20 mm long. It extends from 2nd genu to stylomastoid segment.

F. Extracranial part.

Branches

1. Greater superficial petrosal nerve (at the level of 1st genu)
2. Chorda tympani
3. Nerve to stapedius
4. Sensory supply to part of EAC
5. Branches to post-auricular muscles
6. Nerve to posterior belly of digastric
7. Nerve to stylohyoid
8. Peripheral branches (Pes ansarinus just before or within the substance of parotid)
   - Temporal
   - Zygomatic (zygomatico orbital and zygomatico facial)
   - Buccal (upper buccal and lower buccal)—with maximum variations
   - Marginal mandibular (rima mandibularis)
   - Cervical

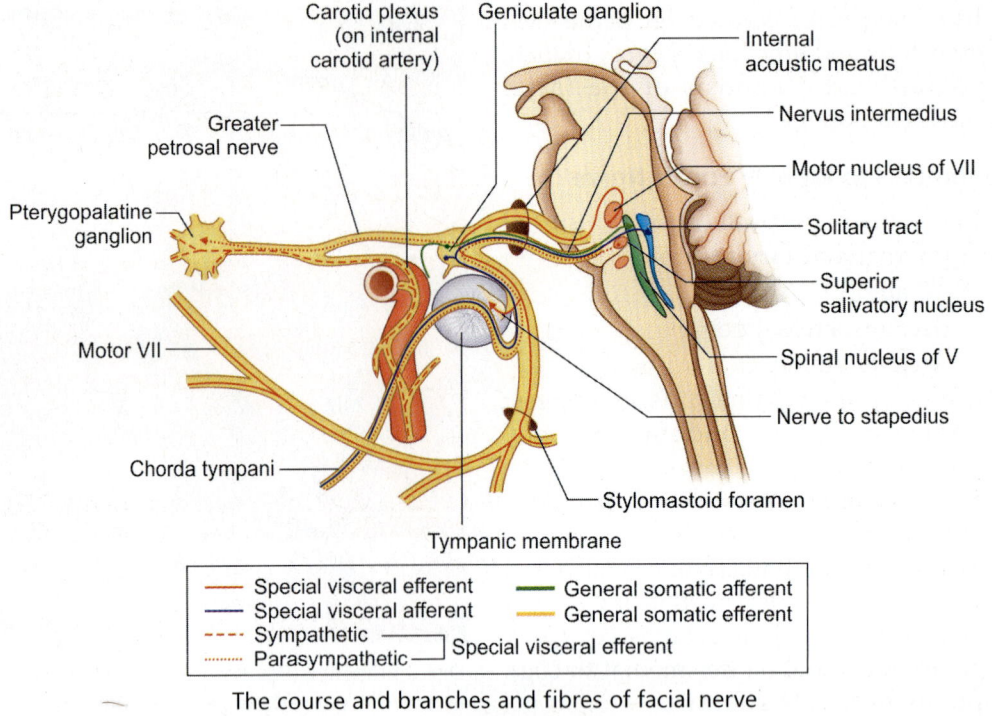

Carotid plexus (on internal carotid artery)

Geniculate ganglion

Internal acoustic meatus

Nervus intermedius

Motor nucleus of VII

Solitary tract

Superior salivatory nucleus

Spinal nucleus of V

Nerve to stapedius

Greater petrosal nerve

Pterygopalatine ganglion

Motor VII

Chorda tympani

Stylomastoid foramen

Tympanic membrane

—— Special visceral efferent	—— General somatic afferent
—— Special visceral afferent	—— General somatic efferent
---- Sympathetic	} Special visceral efferent
······ Parasympathetic	

The course and branches and fibres of facial nerve

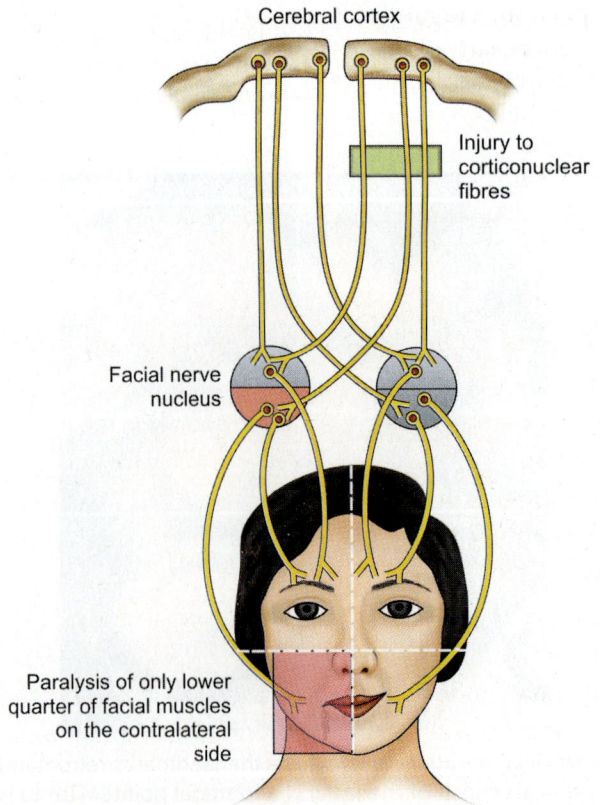

Cerebral cortex

Injury to corticonuclear fibres

Facial nerve nucleus

Paralysis of only lower quarter of facial muscles on the contralateral side

The difference between the facial muscle paralysis in LMN and UMN (supra-nuclear facial nerve lesions)

By having a clear knowledge of the level of branching and functions of every branch, topographical diagnosis of the facial paralysis is possible.

Landmarks to Identify Facial Nerve

- Intracranial approach
  - Internal auditory meatus
  - CP angle
  - Greater petrosal nerve
  - Arcuate eminence
- Intratemporal portion. It is the longest portion of the nerve and runs in a bony canal in body (28–37 mm).

  Tympanomastoid suture, digastric ridge, short process of incus, fossa incudis, lateral semicircular canal, blood vessels along vertical portion and second genu, chorda tympani, stapes, cog (pink geniculate ganglion lies medial to cog), processus cochleariformis.
- Extra tympanic portion. Tragal pointer, styloid process, in face—any of the distal branches and retromandibular vein crossing cervical branch.

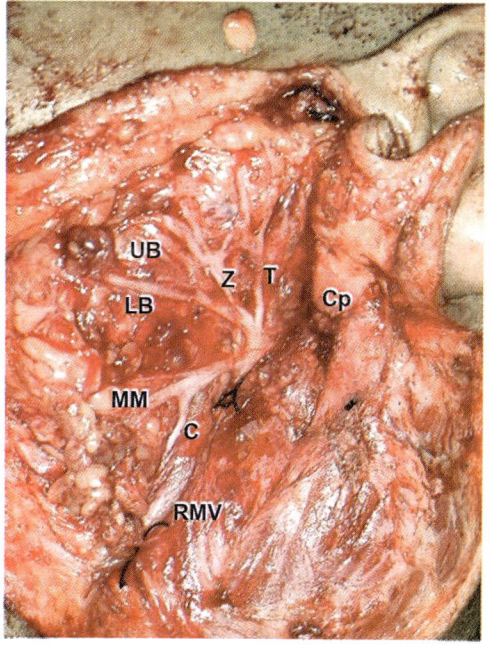

Distal branches (Pes ansarinus) of facial nerve as seen in parotid surgery; T—temporal, Z—zygomatic, UB—upper buccal, LB—lower buccal, MM—marginal mandibular, C—cervical, Cp—tragal cartilage pointer, RMV—retromandibular vein crossed by cervical branch.

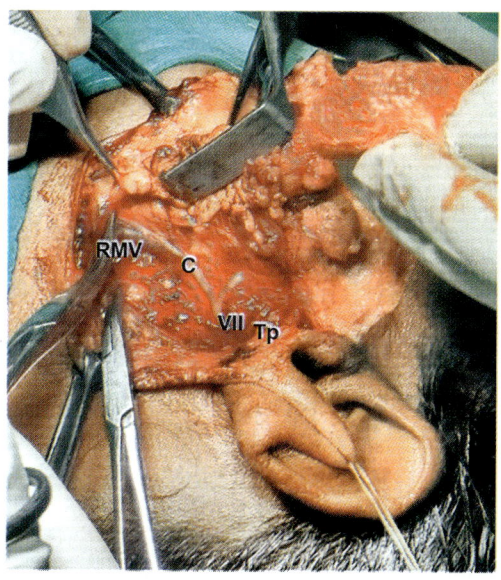

Photo taken during superficial parotidectomy where the landmarks retromandibular vein (RMV) is being crossed by the cervical branch of the facial N and tragal pointer (Tp) to which the main trunk of facial is seen 1 cm anteriorly and inferiorly.

Differences between supranuclear facial palsy (UMN) and infranuclear facial palsy (LMN): Upper part of face is spared in UMN facial palsy as the upper part of facial nucleus has inputs from bilateral cortex. Hence even when one side UMN fibers are damaged, the input from opposite side takes the role to innervate the upper face. This phenomenon is lacking in infranuclear paralysis and hence even upper part of face is paralyzed.

Causes of Facial Nerve Paralysis

1. At birth
   a. Forceps delivery
   b. Treacher Collins syndrome
   c. Möbius syndrome
2. Traumatic
   a. Skull base and temporal bone fractures (longitudinal and transverse fractures) with transverse fractures showing more chances of VII palsy
   b. Penetrating injury to middle ear and temporal bone
   c. Barotrauma
3. Infective
   a. Malignant otitis externa
   b. CSOM and cholesteatoma
   c. Ramsay Hunt syndrome, chickenpox, mumps, influenza
   d. Tuberculosis, leprosy, mucormycosis
   e. AIDS
4. Neoplastic conditions of parotid, 7th nerve, EAC, middle ear, glomus, meningioma carcinoma, sarcoma, acoustic neuroma.
5. Metabolic—diabetes, hyperthyroidism, vitamin A deficiency, acute porphyria, hypertension.
6. Toxic—tetanus, diphtheria, alcoholism.
7. Idiopathic—Bell's palsy, GB syndrome, multiple sclerosis, Melkersson-Rosenthal syndrome.
8. Iatrogenic—surgeries of parotid, mastoid, mandible, submandibular gland, embolization, antirabies vaccination.

Causes of Bilateral Lower Motor Neuron Facial Paralysis

Bilateral Bell's paralysis

- Sarcoidosis
- Skull base trauma
- Guillain-Barré syndrome
- Möbius syndrome
- Lyme's disease
- Cytomegalovirus

House-Brackmann Grading of Facial Paralysis

Grade	Description	Characteristics
I	Normal	Normal tactal function in all areas
II	Mild dysfunction	Slight weakness noticeable on close inspection; may have very slight synkinesis
III	Moderate dysfunction	Obvious, but not disfiguring difference between 2 sides; noticeable, but not severe, synkinesis, contracture, or hemifacial spasm, complete eye closure with effort
IV	Moderately severe dysfunction	Obvious weakness or disfiguring asymmetry; normal symmetry and tone at rest; incomplete eye closure
V	Severe dysfunction	Only barely perceptible motion; asymmetry at rest
VI	Total paralysis	No movement

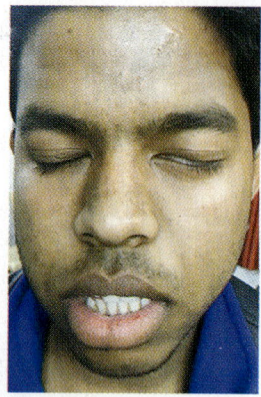

Grade III facial paralysis according to House-Brackmann grading as there is no complete closure of left eye.

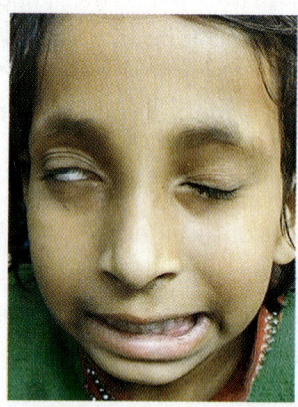

Grade IV facial paralysis according to House-Brackmann grading as there is deviation of mouth also.

Yanagihara Grading System for Facial Paralysis

This grading is useful in following up of a case of facial nerve paralysis. This is designed by Japanese doctors. The scores from 10 different actions are summed up to a total of 40 as mentioned below.

No.	Actions	Scale of 5 scores
1.	At rest	0, 1, 2, 3, 4
2.	Forehead wrinkling	0, 1, 2, 3, 4
3.	Blinking	0, 1, 2, 3, 4
4.	Light closure of eye	0, 1, 2, 3, 4
5.	Tight closure of eye	0, 1, 2, 3, 4
6.	Closure of eye on paralyzed side only	0, 1, 2, 3, 4
7.	Wrinkling of nose	0, 1, 2, 3, 4
8.	Whistle	0, 1, 2, 3, 4
9.	Grin	0, 1, 2, 3, 4
10.	Depress lower lip	0, 1, 2, 3, 4

Recurrent Facial Paralysis

Causes

- Bell's palsy—13% ipsilateral, 64% contralateral side
- Melkersson-Rosenthal syndrome
- Tumor
- Diabetes

BAD syndrome (notorious for corneal ulcers)

- Bell's phenomenon absent
- Anesthesia of cornea
- Dryness of eyes

Bell's Paralysis

Acute onset of LMN facial paralysis

- Diagnosis is always by exclusion
- 13% of cases it is recurrent.

Etiology

1. Viral infections like HSV1
2. Immunogenic
3. Ischemia
   Full recovery in 84% of cases

Treatment

Reassurance, physiotherapy, steroids and vasodilators, acyclovir, nerve decompression if on 14th day >90% degeneration present.

Tests for Facial Nerve

Topognosis	*Prognosis*	*Diagnostic assessment*
1. Schirmer's	EMG	Blink reflex
2. Stapedial reflex	NET	EMG
3. Salivary flow	Maximal stimulation	ENOG
4. Taste	ENOG	
5. CAP		
6. CT scan		

Schirmer's test: 50% difference between two sides is taken as positive. This means GSPN is gone and the level of paralysis is above the geniculate ganglion. These patients are poor candidates for facial nerve decompression.

Avoiding facial nerve injury during surgery:

- Knowledge of middle ear anatomy and facial nerve.
- Gentle handling of nerve when exposed
- Work along the nerve rather across with drill
- Use large diamond burr for drilling
- Irrigation with Ringer lactate when drilling near facial nerve.
- Facial nerve monitor should be used.

Facial Nerve Repair

1. Decompression
2. Neurorrhaphy 10–0 nylon used to repair end to end; tissue adhesives can also be used.
3. Nerve grafts—nerve grafts used to repair the end to end anastomosis.
   • Greater auricular nerve
   • Lateral femoral nerve
   • Sural nerve
4. 7th–12th nerve anastomosis—proximal stump of hypoglossal nerve is anastomosed to the distal stump of facial paralyzed nerve.
5. Rehabilitation of prolonged facial nerve paralysis when motor end plate is fibrosed, i.e. when in EMG polyphasic and fibrillation potentials are absent, we can do (a) dynamic muscle transfer, (b) static procedures like gold weight or tarsal spring of upper eyelid, sling procedure using fascia lata for angle of mouth, etc.

CHAPTER 9

Noise-Induced Hearing Loss

NOISE

It is any undesired and unpleasant sound within the hearing frequency range. White noise is a random sound with a spectrum of all frequencies. Pink noise is a fabricated sound.

NOISE-INDUCED HEARING LOSS (NIHL)

Hearing loss is due to exposure to noise for a prolonged term. The exposed can be in the form of steady state noise or short impact of noise. There are two types of NIHL, viz.

1. Noise-induced temporary threshold shift (NITTS) and
2. Noise-induced permanent threshold shift (NIPTS).

NITTS: This is a temporary increase in the hearing threshold in the higher frequency, commonly in 4000 Hz (acoustic dip in audiogram) when a person is exposed to heavy noise for a prolonged duration. The hearing in NITTS tends to improve after removal of exposure. This improvement occurs in a short duration if the noise intensity was low and longer if the noise intensity was greater.

NIPTS: Also called chronic acoustic trauma, occupational deafness, boiler maker's deafness, etc. 10–15 years of noise exposure is needed to term a hearing loss as NIPTS. For every 3 dB increase in the noise, the exposure time needed to cause hearing loss is halved. Safe noise exposure in industries is limited to 85 dB of noise for 8 hours/day × 5 days/week. NIPTS usually begins at 4000 Hz and then covers the nearby frequencies gradually. The process of involvement of other frequencies slows with years. It takes at least 30 years of noise exposure to affect hearing at 1000 Hz. But this duration can vary according to: (1) Noise level and (2) individual susceptibility.

How to diagnose NIPTS? Single test to diagnose noise-induced hearing instantly is not there. It can be diagnosed only with periodical audiometry of the exposed persons. This will show bilaterally symmetrical hearing loss with acoustic dip unless the patient was already having any unilateral hearing defects or if the patient is exposed to noise more in one ear (like firing rifle keeping it on one shoulder).

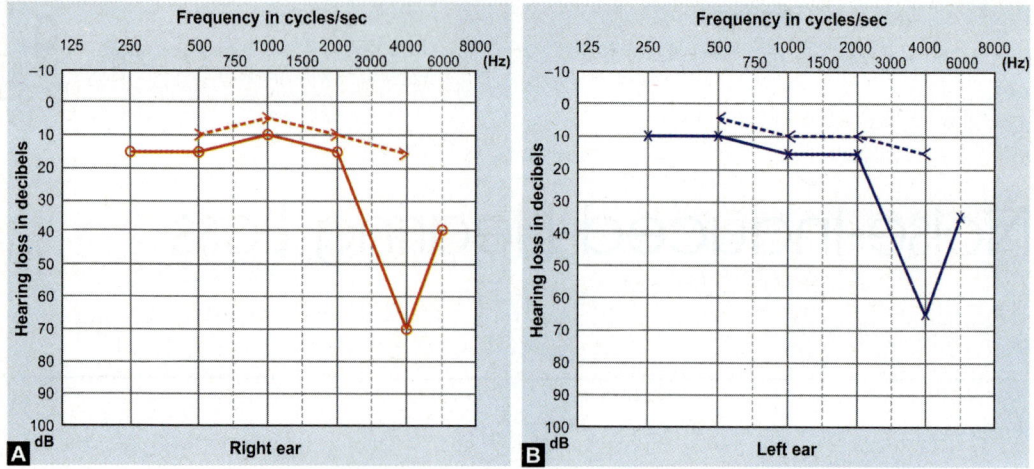

Audiogram showing bilateral symmetrical findings with dip at 4000 Hz in bone conduction

Treatment for NIHL

NIHL is totally a preventable illness, whereas it is totally incurable. Hearing aids can be used to some extent when the hearing impairment is severe. Personal protective aids like ear muff (best) and ear plugs should be always used by industrial workers.

Acoustic trauma: This is a hearing loss produced by a single impact of loud noise (like an explosion).

CHAPTER 10

Otosclerosis

Pathology

Active immature stage of vascularity and bone resorption followed by mature irregular bone formation stage causing fixation of stapes.

Inheritance—autosomal dominance.

Sites of Otospongiosis

Fissula ante fenestrum (anterior to oval window) followed by fibrocartilaginous slit in otic capsule, round window niche.

Other areas: Footplate, internal auditory canal, SCC, fissula postfenestrum, promontory, cochlear capsule and lateral SCC.

Theories

1. Localized venous congestion.
2. Osteogenesis imperfecta associated with otosclerosis, inherent defect in osteoclast causing fractures and otosclerosis.
3. Associated with Paget disease.
4. Enzymatic theory—imbalance in trypsin/antitrypsin in inner ear fluid initiate otosclerosis.

Types of Otosclerosis

1. Histological where no clinical symptoms are present.
2. Stapedial type causing conductive deafness.
3. Combined type with both conductive and sensory deafness as cochlea is also involved.

Clinical Features

Hereditary, usually bilateral (85%), 15–30 years of age, more in females especially during pregnancy, gradually increasing conductive deafness, tinnitus.

On Examination

Normal tympanic membrane: Flamingo pink sign may be seen in 10% cases due to increased vascularity over promontory during active phase of the disease. This is also known as Schwartz's sign.

Tuning fork test: Rinne is negative, Weber lateralized to same side of hearing loss and Gelle's test is negative.

Pure tone audiogram will show conductive hearing loss with characteristic Carhart notch in bone conduction due to ossicular inertia.

Tympanometry: Type As with compliance < 0.4 ml (diagnostic).

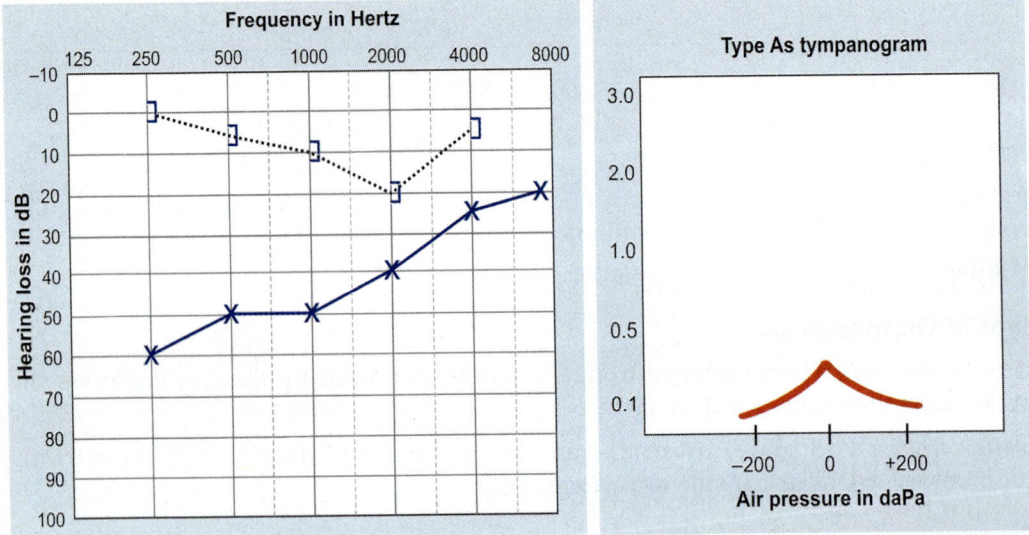

Carhart notch at 2000 Hz in bone conduction

Treatment

A. Medical management with sodium fluoride—20 mg BD for 2–3 years with vitamin D and calcium can be tried. But nowadays this is given for only for 3–4 months till the vascular focus gets matured.

B. Surgery to stapes, i.e. stapedotomy and piston placement.

Causes of sensorineural deafness after the stapedectomy: Labyrinthitis, perilymph fistula.

Measurement of Teflon piston
- Length 3.25–4 mm
- Diameter 0.5 mm

Measurement of length of piston: Distance from under surface of incus to stapes footplate + 0.5 mm.

Alternatives of Teflon piston: Gold wire, steel wire.

Indication of stapedotomy: Conductive loss to the extent of air-bone gap of 20 dB for speech frequencies.

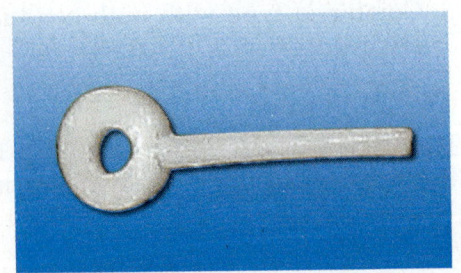

Contraindications for stapedotomy:
- Poor speech discrimination
- History of vertigo in recent months
- Only useful when hearing ear
- Active focus

Fenestra for stapedotomy: 0.6 mm will be piston diameter and hence 0.7 mm can be an fenestrum size. Hole is made at posterior part of footplate because of less postoperative vertigo due to lesser chances of perilymph leakage.
- Neostapedotomy (intact tendon stapedotomy)
- Preservation of tendon and incudostapedial joint

Instruction to patients after stapedectomy: Avoid nose blowing and keep mouth open while coughing and sneezing.
- Flying should be avoided for 10 days or when having URI.
- Diving and swimming should be avoided.
- Avoid lifting heavyweights.
- Hearing loss or vertigo or ear infection should be reported to concerned surgeon.

Reverse stapedotomy by Fisch: Insertion of piston before removal of stapes superstructure.

Advantages of LASER stapedotomy
1. Its hemostatic properties and precision to make correct size hole.
2. As it vaporizes the posterior crura chances of floating footplate are very less.
3. Minimal acoustic trauma during surgery.
4. Ability to fenestrate a floating footplate.
5. Useful in revision stapedotomy.

Laser stapedectomy minus prosthesis: It is done in limited anterior otosclerosis. Anterior crux is vaporized and anterior fixed portion of footplate is separated from the rest by laser. Now posterior crux acts like a piston as the posterior part of footplate is mobile.

Complications of stapes surgery:
1. Perforation
2. Infection
3. Perilymph fistula and chronic vertigo
4. 7th nerve paralysis
5. Granuloma
6. In 2% of cases total sensorineural deafness.

Causes of conductive deafness after the stapedectomy
- Dislocation of piston
- Necrosis of long process of incus
- Short piston
- Regrowth of focus

CHAPTER 11

Cerebellopontine Angle Tumors and Glomus Tumors

CEREBELLOPONTINE ANGLE (CPA)

Boundaries of CP angle
- *Anteriorly*: Middle cranial fossa.
- *Posteriorly*: Anterior surface of cerebellum.
- *Medially*: Edge of pons.
- *Laterally*: Medial portion of posterior temporal bone.
- *Superiorly*: Trigeminal nerve.
- *Inferiorly*: IX, X, XI and XII cranial nerves.

Contents: VIIth cranial nerve, VIIIth cranial nerve, anterior inferior cerebellar artery.

Internal auditory canal: Length—1 cm; Vertical diameter—2–8 mm.

Bill's bar: It is a vertical process which separates the superior portion of IAM.

Transverse crest (crista falciformis): It is a horizontal bar which divides the IAM into superior and inferior halves.

Contents can be remembered easily as "7 (Facial N) UP COKE (Cochlear N) DOWN" in the anterior half of the canal and posterior half contains superior and inferior vestibular nerves; facial nerve is accompanied by nervus intermedius in the medial portion of IAC.

Arcuate eminence: Bulging of superior semicircular canal can be seen on superior surface of temporal bone. It is used in middle cranial approach to acoustic neuroma as a landmark to identify facial nerve (geniculate ganglion).

Tumors of CPA: Vestibular neuroma (85%), meningioma, congenital cholesteatoma, arachnoid cyst, facial neuroma, glomus, lipoma.

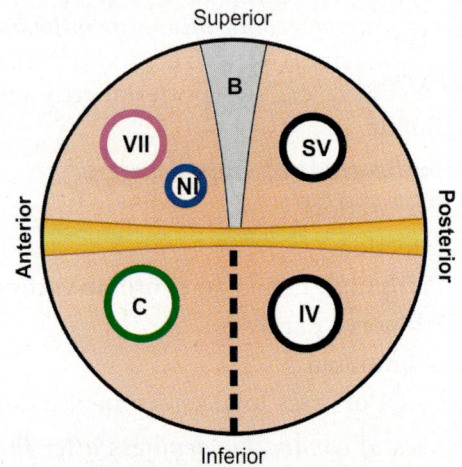

The orientation of facial nerve (VII), nervus intermedius (NI), cochlear nerve (C), superior vestibular (SV) nerve and inferior vestibular (IV) nerve within the internal auditory canal (IAC), B–Bill's bar, FC–falciparum crest.

Acoustic neuroma (vestibular schwannomas): 80% of CPA and 8% of all intracranial tumors.

Pathology

It originates from Schwann cells of superior or inferior vestibular nerve at transition zone of central and peripheral myelin. Vestibular schwannomas occur due to mutation in gene for tumor suppressor protein merlin, located on chromosome 22q12. Familial vestibular schwannoma occurs in neurofibromatosis 2-autosomal recessive trait.

Microscopic densely packed cells with spindle-shaped nucleus and fibrillar cytoplasm (Antony A areas) intermixed with hypocellular areas containing vacuolated, pleomorphic cells (Antony B areas).

Natural History

Tumor grows up to 1.8 mm/year. Rapid growth is due to either cystic degeneration or hemorrhage into tumor. Initial intracanalicular growth affects vestibulocochlear nerve, so hearing loss, tinnitus and vertigo occur. After reaching 3 cm, tumor abuts on CPA cranial nerves causing midface numbness, corneal numbness and facial weakness or spasm. Further compression causes Cushing CPA syndrome with ocular changes, headache, nausea, vomiting, mental changes and even death due to respiratory compromise.

Clinical Features of Acoustic Neuroma

Three stages
1. Otological stage
2. Neurological stage
3. Terminal or brain stem involvement

Otological stage: <2 cm intrameatal tumor
- Unilateral gradually increasing SN loss
- Tinnitus

Trigeminal nerve involvement > 2 cm and extrameatal:

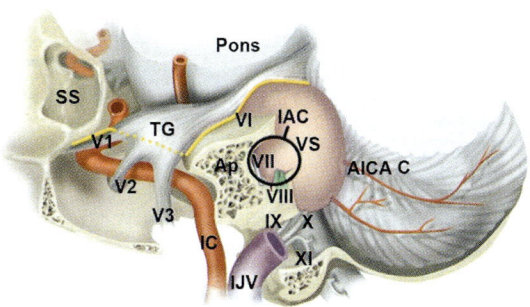

Diagram of spread of vestibular schwannoma (VS) in the CP angle; IAC: Eroded internal auditory canal, C: Cerebellum, AICA: Anterior Inferior cerebellar artery, Ap: Petrous apex, IC: Internal carotid artery, IJV: Internal jugular vein, TG: Trigeminal ganglion, VI: Abducens nerve, VII: Facial nerve, VIII: Vestibulocochlear nerve, V1, V2, V3: Branches of trigeminal nerve, X: Vagus nerve, XI: Accessory nerve, SS: Sphenoid sinus

Anatomy of CP angle

Pain and tingling along the trigeminal nerve distribution:
- Brain stem and cerebellar compression
- Increasing intracranial pressure headache and vomiting
- Terminal stage

On examination

TM normal:
- Corneal reflex absent
- Histelberger sign—loss of sensation—posterior external auditory canal
- Cranial nerve paralysis
- Nystagmus
- Cerebellar signs
- On an average patient takes 4 years from onset of symptoms to diagnosis

Investigation

PTA—unilateral high tone, low tone or flat audiogram:
- Canal paresis on caloric testing
- SDS is poor and rollover in high intensity
- Abnormal acoustic reflexes
- Contrast enhanced CT

MRI (Gadolinium enhanced): Gold standard and diagnostic
- BERA
- Increased interwave latency wave V > 0.2 ms
- Increased interpeak interval wave I–V > 4 ms

Important is interaural delay of wave V greater than 0.2 ms:
- ABR has >90% sensitivity
- CSF—raised protein level

Treatment

Surgery

Middle cranial fossa approach: For small tumor with serviceable hearing, i.e. <2 cm size.

Translabyrinthine approach:
- Suited for patients with poor hearing and larger tumors
- Hearing loss is the main disadvantage

Suboccipital approach:
- For bigger tumor
- Retrosigmoid approach for tumors <4 cm and good hearing

Combined approach

Latest: Gamma knife radiation is delivered by stereotactic technique.

Steps are pre-radiosurgery evaluation, dose planning (12–12.5 Gy by recent 192 Cobalt-60 source), dose delivery and postoperative management.

GLOMUS TUMORS

These tumors arise from the para-ganglian cells which are derived from neural crest.

Sites of Glomus Bodies

Jugular bulb, carotid, ciliary and vagal bodies, aorta and main branches, urinary bladder, adrenal medulla, larynx.

Histopathology

Epitheloid cells, veins and capillaries and connective tissue.

Glomus bodies in ear:
- Tympanic branch of glossopharyngeal
- Auricular branch of vagus

Glomus: More in females middle age
- May be multiple
- May show metastasis
- May secrete VMA
- Locally aggressive tumor

Clinical Features

- Pulsatile tinnitus
- Deafness
- Bleeding from ear
- VIIth, IXth, Xth, XIth nerve paralysis
- Polyp coming out of perforation and may present in external auditory canal.

On Examination

Ear:
- Pulsatile mass behind the TM
- Brown's sign bleeding mass blanching with positive pressure by Siegle speculum
- Rising sun sign, i.e. red mass behind TM
- Cerebellar signs.

Oldring and Fisch classification of glomus tumors:

Type A: Localized to middle ear (best prognosis).

Type B: Tumor of tympanomastoid region with no destruction of bone in infra-labyrinthine compartment.

Type C: Tumors involving the infralabyrinthine region with extension to petrous apex
- C_1: Limited involvement of vertical portion of carotid canal
- C_2: Tumor with extensive invasion of vertical portion of carotid canal
- C_3: Tumor with involvement of horizontal portion of carotid canal involvement.

Type D: Tumor with intracranial extension
- D_1: <2 cm intracranial extension
- D_2: >2 cm intracranial extension

Investigations
- Contrast CT of temporal bone and sometimes upper neck
- Urinary VMA (Vanillylmandelic acid)

Treatment

Radiotherapy, small tumor can be left as such.

Surgery:
- Transmeatal approach
- Extended facial recess approach
- Infratemporal approach

Phelps' sign: Erosion of crotch or bone between that ICA and jugular vein.

Meniere's Disease

It is a disease described by Dr Prosper Meniere in 1861. It is classically characterized by a triad of

1. Sudden fluctuant sensorineural hearing loss
2. Episodic vertigo
3. Roaring tinnitus

Lermoyez syndrome: It is a variant of Meniere's disease. Initially there is hearing loss and tinnitus and then vertigo develops with improvement in the other 2 symptoms.

Etiology:

1. Idiopathic
2. Disturbance in salt and water balance
3. Vascular disturbance in stria vascularis
4. Decreased absorption from endolymphatic sac
5. Disturbance in automatic regulation of endolymphatic system
6. Local allergy of inner ear
7. Manifestation of systemic disease like hypothyroidism or glucose metabolism, 8-autoimmune phenomenon
8. Saccin supposed to be a hormone released by dry endolymphatic sac which acts on stria vascularis to increase endolymph secretion and in blockage of endolymphatic duct due to any reason, the sac becomes dry and this leads to excessive secretion of saccin, thus causing endolymphatic hydrops.

Pathology: Earliest change is the dilatation of scala media of cochlea and saccule. This is followed by stretching of Reissner's membrane. Both these are due to accumulation of excess endolymph. The pressure causes degeneration of organ of Corti, loss of hair cell and long-standing pressure effect causes rupture of Reissner's membrane finally and proliferation of perilymphatic fibrous tissue.

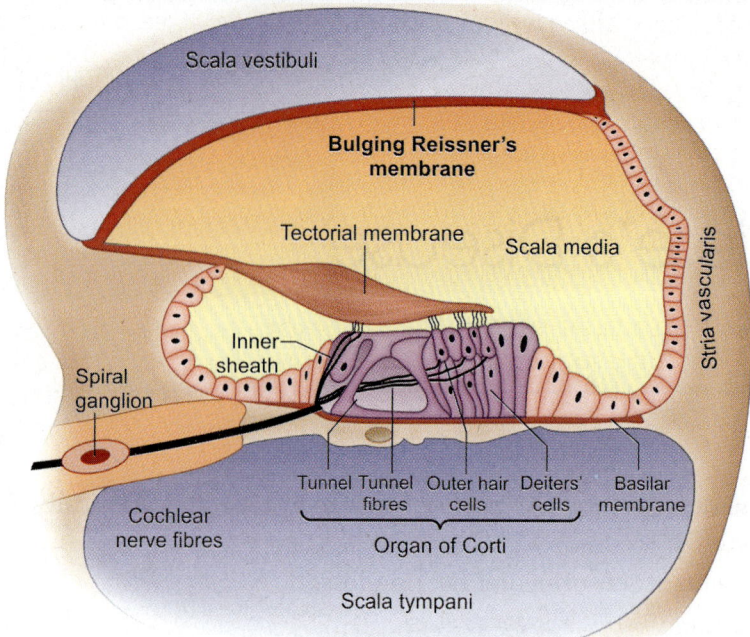

Clinical features: Age group of 40–50 years, men are more commonly affected and 85% of cases it is unilateral. Acute exacerbations and remissions are common. Vertigo is sudden, severe and episodic, to and fro or up and down movement can be felt. It is associated with nausea and vomiting with nystagmus. Nystagmus shows fast components towards affected side. Sometimes it is noise induced (Tullio phenomenon). This is due to fibrous band between footplate of stapes and distended saccule.

Hearing loss is of low frequency, fluctuating, sensorineural which recovers during initial episodes. Recruitment, diplacusis can be perceived.

Tinnitus is fluctuating, low pitched and may be of roaring or hissing type. Fullness in ear is present.

Investigations
- PTA
- Speech audiometry (discrimination score 40 to 70%)
- Bekesy audiometry
- Recruitment (ABLB)
- SISI

Inj. furosemide or oral glycerol test: After ½ hour in furosemide and 2 hours in glycerol, PTA shows 0 dB gain and this is taken as positive test and is good sign for endolymphatic sac surgery.

ECHOCHG: SP/AP ratio is >0.45.

AAO-HNS Classification of Meniere's Disease

1. *Possible Meniere's disease:* Episodic vertigo of Meniere type without documented hearing loss, or sensorineural hearing loss, fluctuating or fixed, with disequilibrium but without definitive episodes. Other causes excluded.

2. *Probable Meniere's disease*: One definitive episode of vertigo, audiometrically documented hearing loss on at least one occasion, tinnitus or aural fullness in the treated ear. Other causes excluded.
3. *Definite Meniere's disease*: Two or more definitive spontaneous episodes of vertigo of 20 mins or longer, audiometrically documented hearing loss on at least one occasion, tinnitus or aural fullness in the treated ear, other causes excluded.
4. *Certain Meniere's disease*: Definitive Meniere with histological confirmation.

Treatment

Medical management: Diuretics, vasodilators, cinnarizine, promethazine can be given. Meniett device can be used after performing a myringotomy and ventilation tube placement.

Surgical treatment: Conservative procedures like repeated intratympanic dexamethasone injection, endolymphatic sac decompression, endolymphatic sac shunt procedures and superior vestibular neurectomy are hearing preservation surgery.

Destructive surgeries like surgical, LASER, chemical (intratympanic gentamicin) or ultrasonic labyrinthectomy are preferred when hearing is poor.

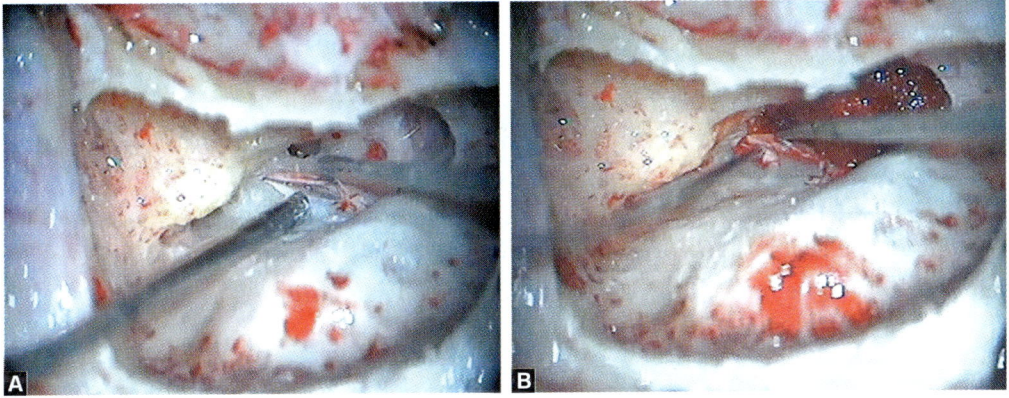

Endolymphatic sac surgery: (A) The sac being opened up with sharp instrument; (B) A silastic stent being placed to keep the stoma patent

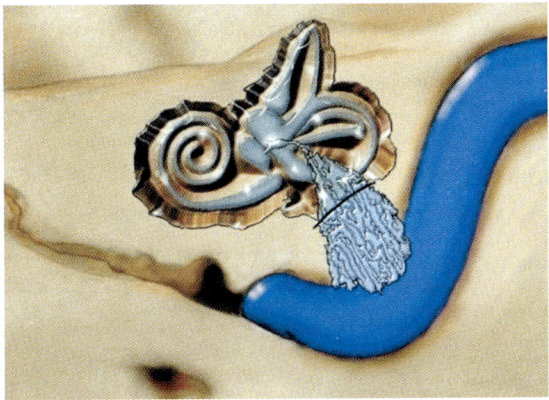

Black line divides endolymphatic sac into osseus and extraosseus part or dural part. Dural part sometime overlaps sigmoid sinus.

CHAPTER 13

Hearing Aids, Cochlear Implant, Middle Ear Implants, BAHA

HEARING AIDS

It is an electromechanical device that amplifies the sound.

Parts of Hearing Aids

- *Microphone:* It collects the sound stimulus and transduce into electrical energy by Piezoelectric effect.
- *Amplifier:* Increases the electric signals.
- *Receiver:* Transduce the electric energy to sound energy.
- Battery.

Feedback problem in hearing aid: It happens when the microphone picks up amplified sound and that disturbs the original sound.

Requirements to be fulfilled before prescribing a hearing aid:
- Cochlear pathology
- Good discrimination score
- Less recruitment
- Peak clipping to avoid Tullio's phenomenon

Types of Hearing Aids

1. Body worn
   Advantages
   - No feedback problem
   - Amplification can be increased
   - Relatively cheap
   Disadvantages
   - Size big
   - Conspicuous
   - Rubbing clothes might give added sound
2. Behind the ear (BTE)
3. All in ear (ITE, CIC)
   - Small size can be fitted inside the concha or ear canal.
   - Only disadvantage is feedback problem and cost factor.

4. Bone transducers: These are used when bilateral ears are discharging.
   Contralateral routing of signals (CROS)
   Microphone is placed on one side and ear phone (receiver) on the other side. It reduces the problem of feedback. This is preferred when high gain is required.
5. Spectacle
6. Implantable hearing aids: Cochlear implants, active middle ear implants and bone anchored hearing aids.

COCHLEAR IMPLANTS

Approved by US-FDA in 1985 for postlingual deafness. They replace the sensorineural epithelium of the cochlea.

Ideal candidates for cochlear implant are: Postlingual deafness because of ototoxicity, meningitis and trauma or children of 1 year of age or above (current US-FDA advice).

Patient selection: Bilateral deafness with average hearing threshold >95 dB in speech frequency.

- No improvement with hearing aid.
- Physically and mentally normal.

Patient should be present in the same geographic area so that postoperative rehabilitation program can be carried out successfully.

Should be speaking same language as of speech therapist.

Surgical techniques: Placement of stimulator in a well made post-aurally and the electrode is introduced either through facial recess approach or transcanal tunnel creation by varia technique.

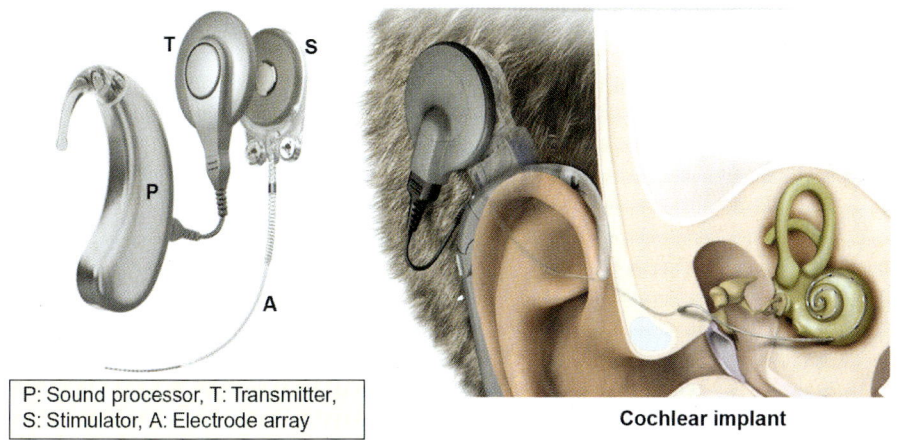

P: Sound processor, T: Transmitter,
S: Stimulator, A: Electrode array

Cochlear implant

Cochlear implant

Active Middle Ear Implants

Active middle ear implants, e.g. vibrant sound bridge and middle ear transducer.

They just amplify the remnant hearing functions by augmenting the middle ear coupling mechanism. They are better than classical hearing aids by their invisibility, no or minimal feedback, no meatal occlusion effect and superior gain.

Bone Anchored Hearing Aids (BAHA)

They are bone conduction hearing aids developed to bypass the conductive hearing mechanisms. Titanium screw is implanted and the external apparatus is connected through abutment after screw is osteo-integrated. This will directly stimulate the cochlea.

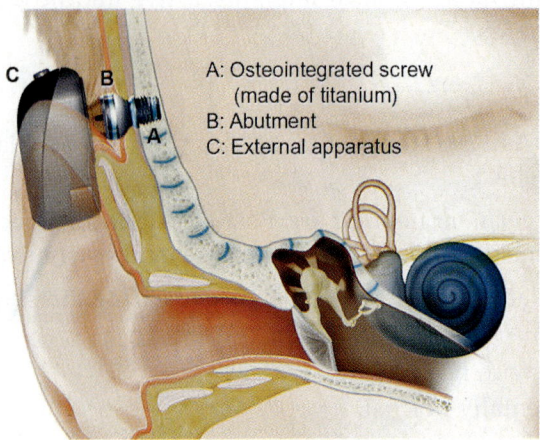

A: Osteointegrated screw
    (made of titanium)
B: Abutment
C: External apparatus

Bone anchored hearing aids

CHAPTER 14

Vertigo and Tinnitus

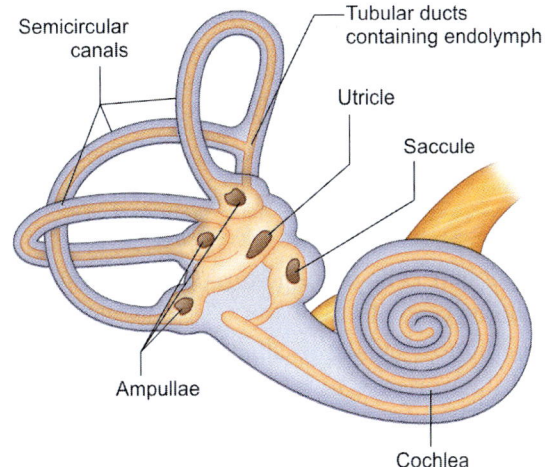

Semicircular canals
Tubular ducts containing endolymph
Utricle
Saccule
Ampullae
Cochlea

The outline of vestibular system

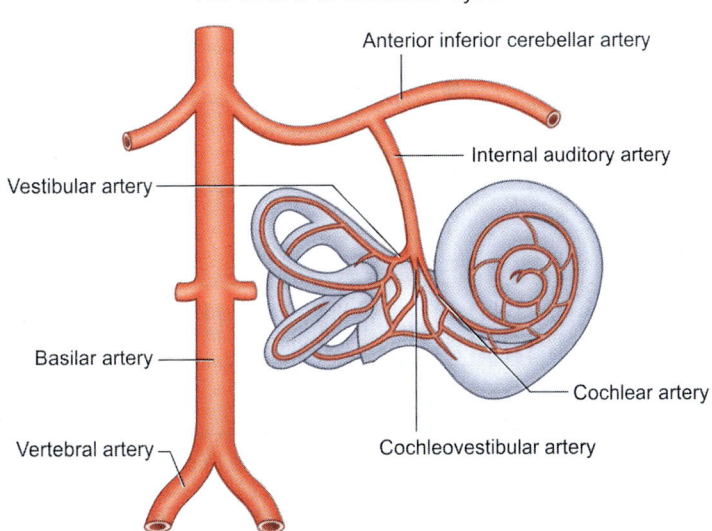

Anterior inferior cerebellar artery
Internal auditory artery
Vestibular artery
Basilar artery
Cochlear artery
Vertebral artery
Cochleovestibular artery

Blood supply to the inner ear

Vertigo: Central and peripheral; associated with nystagmus due to defective **vestibulo-ocular reflex**.

Other reflexes in relation to the balance and equilibrium are:
- Vestibulospinal reflex
- Vestibulocolic reflex (used in VEMP)
- Cervico-ocular reflex
- Cervicospinal reflex

Differences between central and peripheral origin nystagmus

Characters	Central	Peripheral
Intensity	Less severe	Severe vertigo
Direction	Direction changing	Unidirectional
Fatigability	Absent	Present
Latency	Not seen	Present (2–20 seconds)
Duration	No fixed duration	Usually <1 minute

Physiology of Peripheral Vertigo

Vestibular apparatus consists of:
- Semicircular canal
- Utricle
- Saccule

  All these have sensory hair cells having stereocilia arranged in ascending fashion. The longest stereocilia is kinocilia.

  Movement of stereocilia towards kinocilia: Stimulation/depolarization.

  Movement of stereocilia opposite to kinocilia: Inhibition/hyperpolarization.

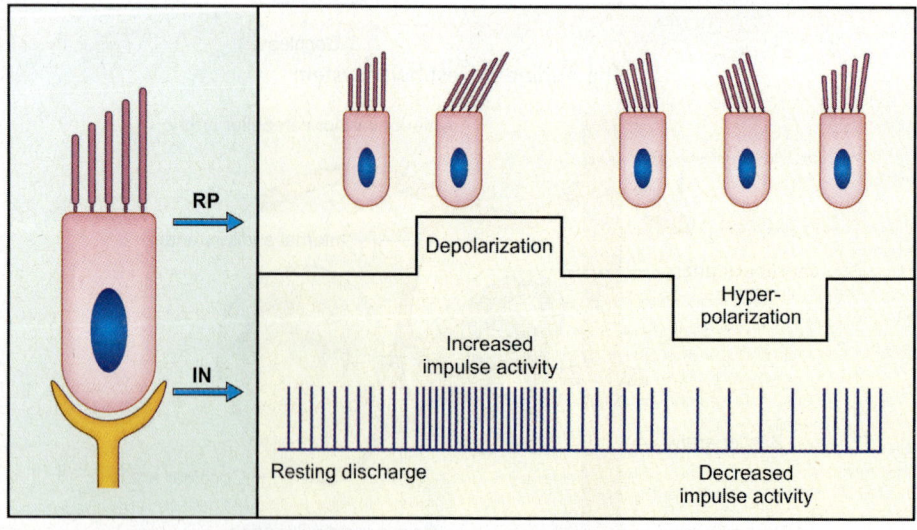

RP: Receptor potential; NI: Nerve impulse

Conditions resulting in stimulation of only one labyrinth results in unequal impulses reaching the brain leading to a state of disequilibrium and manifests as vertigo or dizziness.

Central projection of peripheral vestibular system

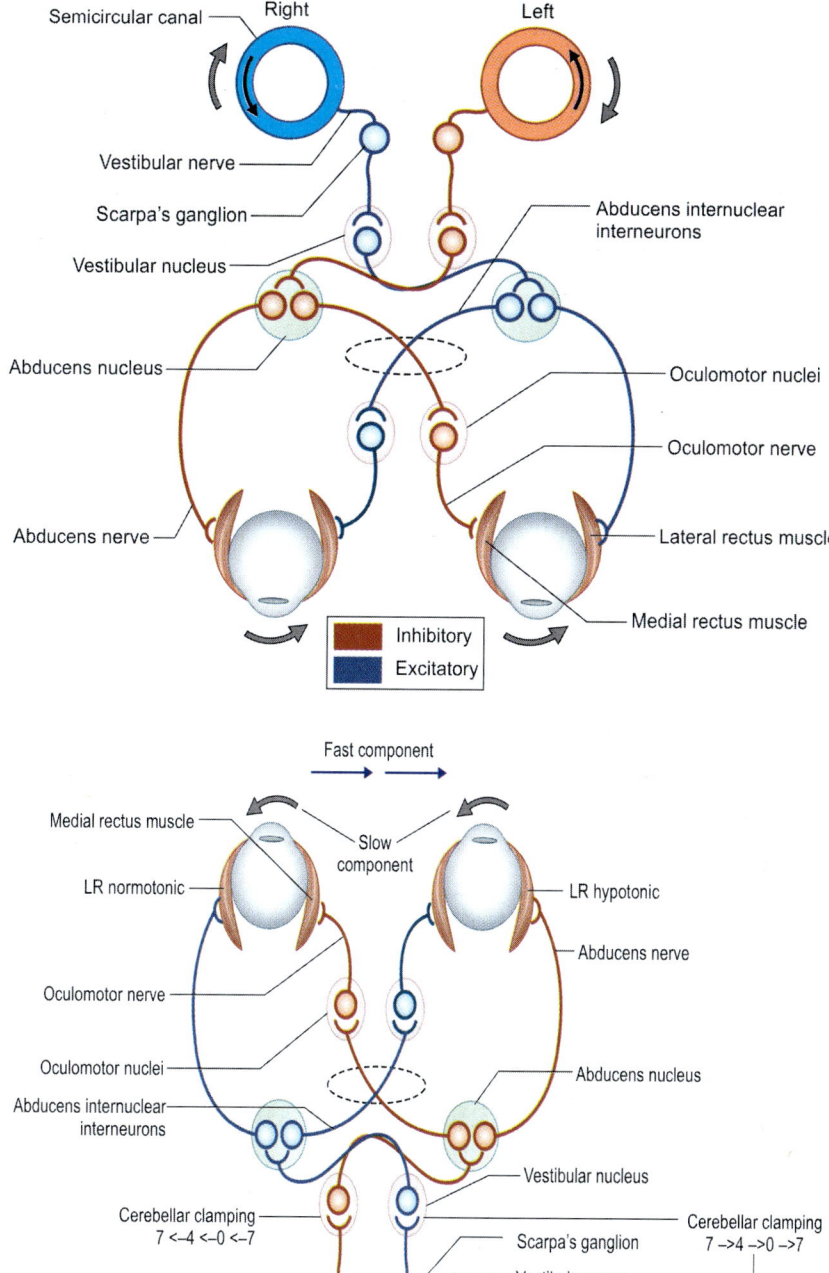

Diagram showing what happens when left labyrinth (with resting discharge of say 7) is damaged or left ear is irrigated with cold water (thus reducing the resting discharge from 7 to 0 in that labyrinth and vestibular nucleus leading to hypotonia and slow phase to left side and fast component to right side). The diagram also shows the central correction by cerebellar clamping and declamping.

Subjective sense of imbalance
- Vertigo isolated
- Vestibular neuronitis
- Drugs
- Disseminated sclerosis
- Others

Vertigo associated with position
- Ageing
- BPPV
- Central malignant positional vertigo

Vertigo + Deafness + Tinnitus
- Meniere's disease
- Acoustic tumors
- Syphilis

Labyrinthitis
- Trauma

Vertigo with central lesions
- Intracranial neoplasm
- Arterial thrombosis

Nystagmus
Involuntary movement of eyes: Horizontal, vertical, rotatory, pendular. Nystagmus has two components:
1. Slow component is because of imbalance of inputs from vestibular nuclei.
2. Fast component is central corrective process.
   Direction of nystagmus is decided by direction of fast component.

Intensity of nystagmus
- *First degree*: Visible only when patient looks in direction of fast component.
- *Second degree*: When patient looks straight.
- *Third degree*: Nystagmus is present in all directions even when patient looks in the direction of slow component.

Benign Paroxysmal Positional Vertigo

Commonest peripheral vertigo; associated with past head injury even trivial. Caused by dislodged otoconia ($CaCO_3$) which floats freely in the endolymph (canalolithisis) or deposited in cupula (cupulolithiasis). This can happen with any of the three semi-circular canals with posterior canal being commonly involved.

The clinical picture is sudden, disarming positional vertigo lasting for seconds. Patients can clearly outline the position that causes them vertigo and it creates a fear in assuming those positions. Hearing is normal. No cerebellar disorders. Diagnosed by neck movement tests and Dix Hallpike test. It is done by rapidly changing the position of patient from sitting to head hanging position (at least 10 degrees). DHT stimulates ipsilateral (down ear) lateral and posterior canals and contralateral (up) lateral and superior canals. DHT is diagnostic of BPPV when the patient develops torsional nystagmus (vertical canals) or horizontal nystagmus (lateral canals). The BPP nystagmus shows following characters, namely (1) Latency of at least 20 seconds; (2) Short duration; (3) Reversal of direction while sitting up with head turned; (4) Fatiguability and (5) Habituation. In cases where nystagmus is absent but patients experience vertigo, DHT is taken as negative only. Here tests can be repeated after tapping or vibrating the ipsilateral mastoid.

In canalolithiasis, otoconia takes time to travel and hence latency is longer and when they settle down nystagmus subsides. Whereas in cupulolithiasis, there is no latency and the peak of nystagmus is longer. Cupulolithiasis is more symptomatic than canalolithiasis. In cupulolithiasis, the nystagmus subsides due to central adaptation. But even after nystagmus subsides, there are micro eye movements which are not seen in canalolithiasis. Cupulolithiasis nystagmus is less fatiguable than canalolithiasis. Usually a self-limiting condition. Absolute management is canalolith repositioning (CRP) methods. CRP should be provided only if diagnosis of BPPV is established and not in all vertigo.

- *Semont*: Posterior cupulolithiasis.
- *Epley*: Posterior canalolithisis.
- *Hamid*: Horizontal cupulolithiasis.
- *Lempert*: Horizontal canalolithiasis.

Epley's maneuver for right PSCC canalolithiasis

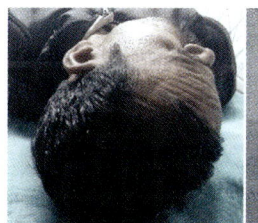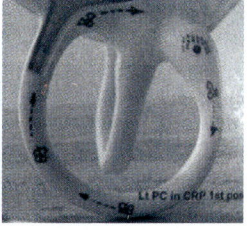

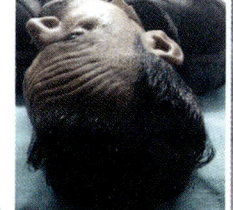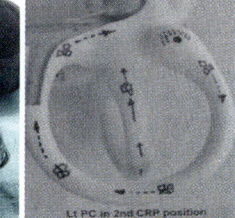

Position 1: Supine with neck turned to same side 45° and head hanging at 15°

→ Position 2: Neck turned 90° to face the opposite side

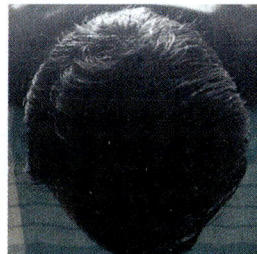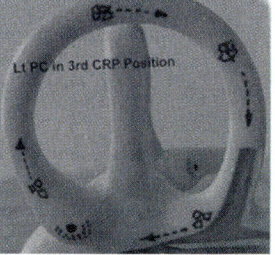

Position 3: Patient is kept in this position for 2 mins for the otoconia to settle down

Semont maneuver (right side posterior SCC cupulolithiasis)

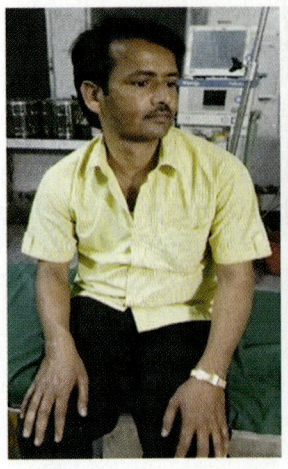
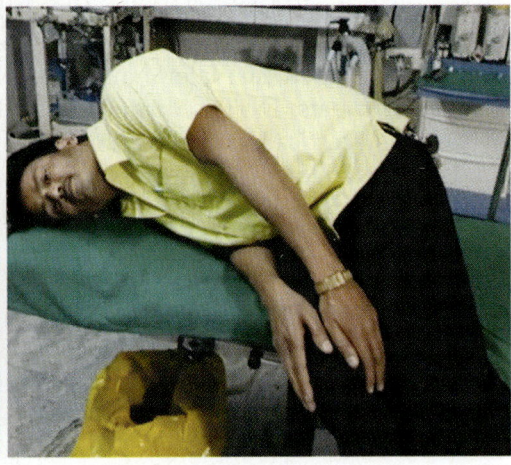

Position 1: Head is turned to opposite side

Position 2: Suddenly laid laterally to right

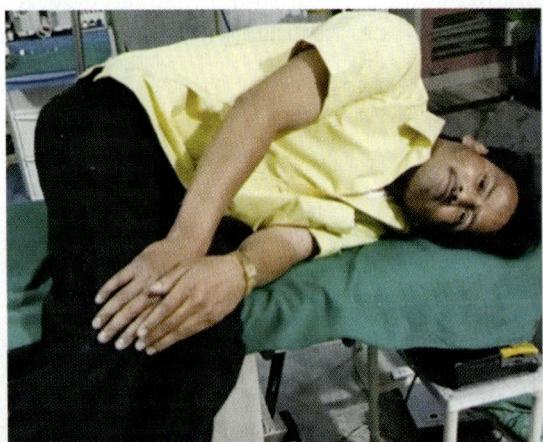
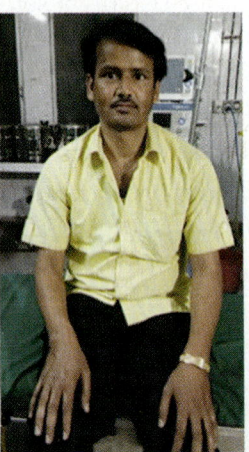

Position 3: Change of position to left lateral position with head in same tilt after 1 minute

Position 4: After waiting for 1 minute the patient is made to sit up with neutral head position

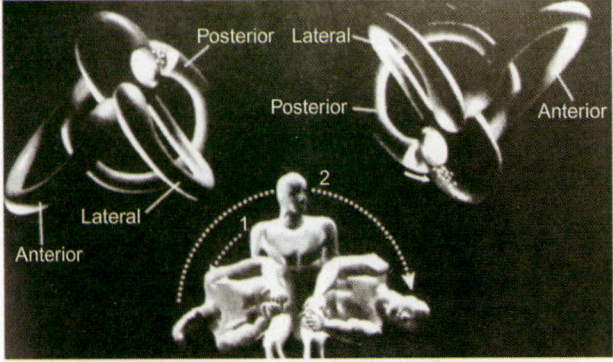

Movement of otoconia in Semont's maneuver

Hamid's maneuver (for any sided lateral cupulolithiasis)

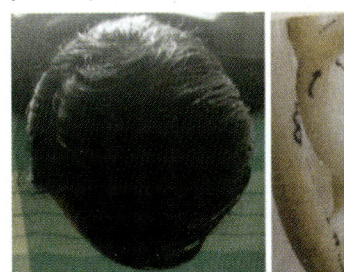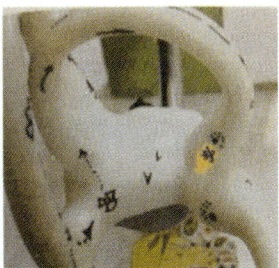

In prone position mastoid massage is done to bring the otoconia into vestibule (yellow color)

Lempert's maneuver (for left lateral SCC canalolithiasis

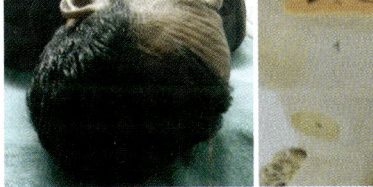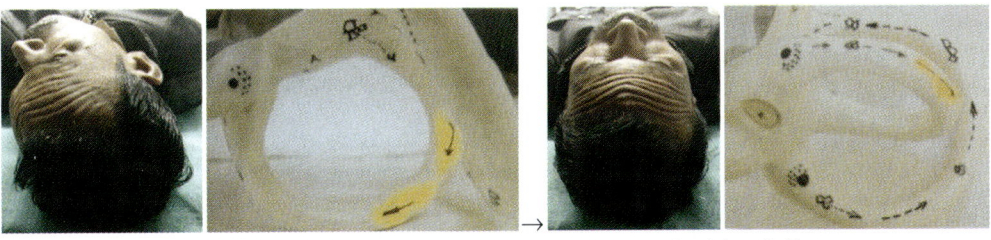

Position 1: Supine with face to left   Position 2: Face up

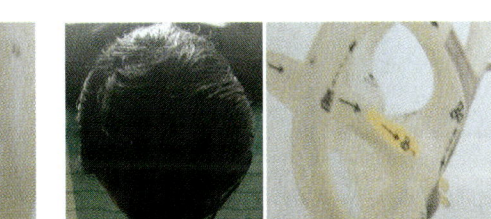

Position 3: Supine with face to right   Position 4: Prone

Each position should be maintained for at least 1 minute

BPPV of superior semi-circular canal is extremely rare due to its superior position. This can happen incidentally during treatment of posterior canal BPPV CRP.

Vestibular Neuronitis

Peripheral vestibular disorder characterized by acute attacks of vertigo with nausea and vomiting. Hearing and central nervous system are normal. There is almost always a preceding history of viral upper respiratory tract or gastrointestinal infection. It occurs due to degenerative changes to Scarpa's ganglia.

Treatment is done with anti-emetics and vestibular sedatives. Symptoms resolve within 10 days. But residual positional dizziness is found in significant number of patients.

Common differential diagnoses are BPPV, transient ischemic attack, posterior vestibular artery infarcts, cerebellar stroke and brain stem infarcts. BPPV can be confirmed with Dix Hallpike test. Other diagnoses are challenging for a young surgeon to make. To differentiate them from true vestibular nystagmus is by HINT battery.

1. Head impulse test
2. Nystagmus
3. Test of skew deviation

Head impulse	Nystagmus	Skew	Diagnosis
Abnormal	Unidirectional	Absent	Vestibular neuritis
Abnormal	Unidirectional	Present	Stroke
Abnormal	Bidirectional	Absent	Stroke
Abnormal	Bidirectional	Present	Stroke
Normal	Unidirectional	Absent	Stroke
Normal	Unidirectional	Present	Stroke
Normal	Bidirectional	Absent	Stroke
Normal	Bidirectional	Present	Stroke

TINNITUS

Treatment for tinnitus has been found recorded in the ancient Egyptian literatures under the name "treatment for bewitched ear". They have also described it as worms in the ear or humming ear.

Rene Laennec invented the stethoscope and he used it to examine tinnitus. He could not hear anything, thus he concluded that tinnitus is an auditory hallucination. EP Fowler found out in 20th century that presence of tinnitus is always associated with hearing impairment, pathology is related to neurophysiological source and all the tinnitus were easily masked by similar frequency sounds.

Tinnitus is broadly classified into—subjective (heard only by patient) and objective (heard by both patient and examiner).

Subjective tinnitus is found to be because of neuronal excitatory and inhibitory imbalance. Recently it is postulated that because of ageing and ischemia there is loss of subcortical filter in auditory tract which leads to trapping of sound impulse between two damaged subcortical filters causing tinnitus.

Treatment

By pharmacological therapy, psychological support, biofeedback mechanisms, sound therapies and neuromodulatory treatments.

1. Pharmacological therapy by systemic or intratympanic *steroids, vasoactive drugs* like pentoxifylline and isoxuprine, nootropics—improves cognitive functions, e.g. piracetam, *local anesthetics* like lidocaine, betahistine, antidepressants like amitryptyline, anticonvulsants like carbamazepine, NMDA antagonists like caroverine, etc.
2. Hyperbaric oxygen therapy.
3. Sound therapy with hearing aids—increases patient's hearing, thus the gained sound will act as masking.
4. Cognitive behavior therapy—by educating the patient to tolerate the symptom.
5. Magnetic and electrical brain stimulation.
6. Music therapy.

Rhinology

CHAPTER 15

Facial Pain and Headache

Physiology of Pain

When thick fibers are damaged as in herpes zoster and postherpetic neuralgia, diabetes or B_1, B_6, B_{12} deficiency pain travels in posterior column of spinal cord. Even touch is experienced as pain due to GATE Control theory. Thalamus receives 50% of thin fibers (pain fibers) and 50% thick fibers (touch fibers). So, in case of above mentioned diseases, touch fibers are lost, so touch goes through pain fibers and is felt as a pain.

When thin fibers are damaged as in leprosy, pain is not perceived by the patient in response to heat and his fingers start to get ulcerated because thermal pain is felt as touch by him.

$$50\% \text{ Input of thick fibers} \longrightarrow \text{Gate control of pain}$$
$$50\% \text{ Input of thin fibers} \longrightarrow \text{In thalamus}$$

Pain Pathophysiology

This is explained in the following flowchart.

Headache: It is the most common medical complaint; rarely caused by organic cause. Classification is as follows:

1. Vascular, e.g. migraine, giant cell temporal arteritis, postcoital headache.
2. Cluster headache
3. Cervicogenic headache
4. Tension headache
5. Chronic daily headache or daily headache, e.g. myofacial pain
6. Specific headache with organic cause like meningitis, sinusitis, dental infections, cranial neuralgias, increased ICT, TMJ dysfunction, toxic (CO), thyroid diseases, stroke, TIA, ocular pain, uncontrolled HTN, post-traumatic, etc.

Migraine: Types are:

1. Migraine without aura
2. Migraine with aura (typical, prolonged aura, hemiplegic, basilar, without headache, vestibular, etc.)
3. Ophthalmoplegic migraine
4. Retinal migraine

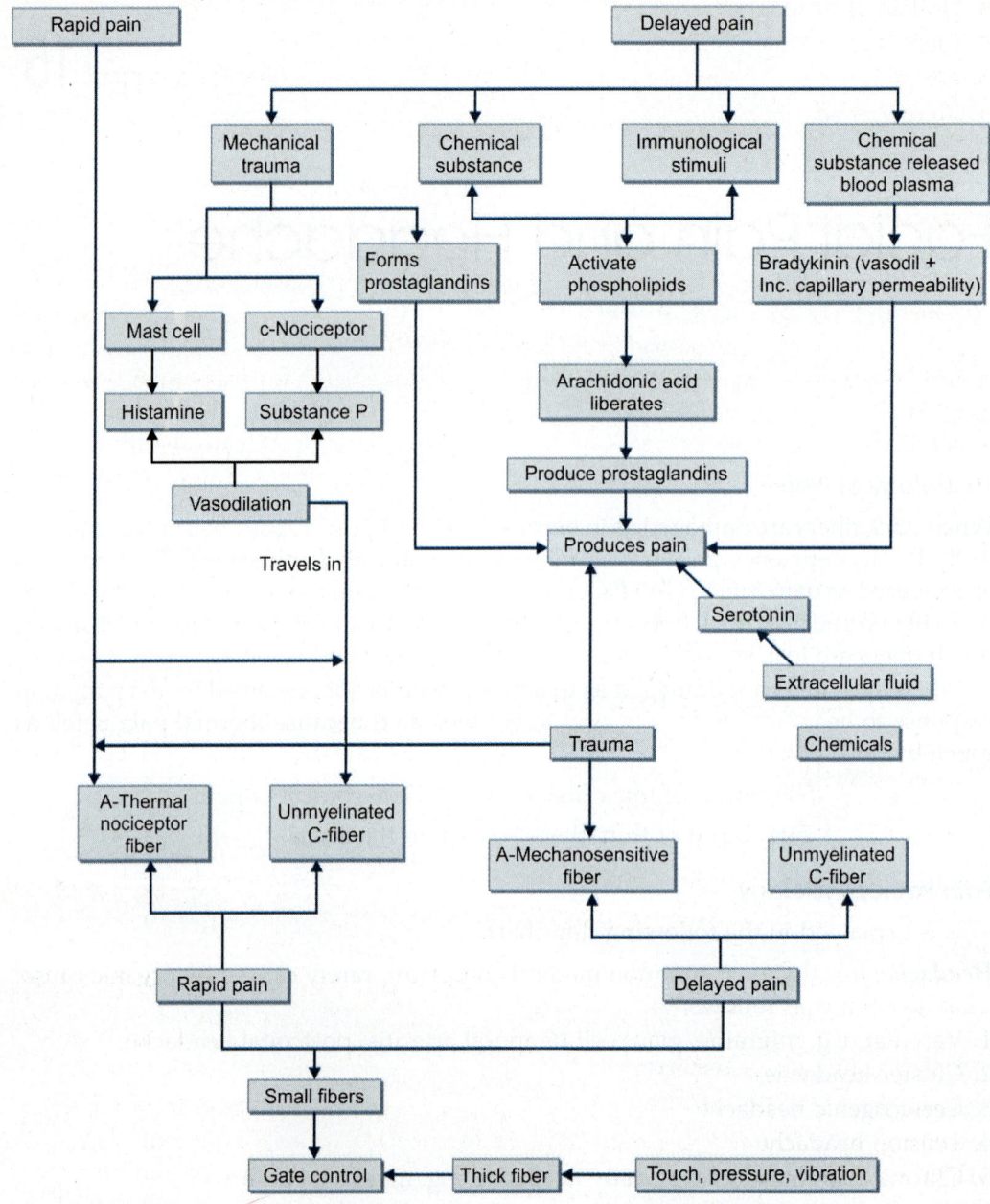

5. Complicated migraine (status migrainous, migrainous infarct)

6. Migraine not fulfilling above criteria

Clinical features: Unilateral headache, episodic, aggravates with light, nausea and vomiting, visual defects, etc. Each variant will have different presentation. More in females.

Diagnostic criteria:

1. History for 5–6 attacks

2. Attack lasts for 4 hours

3. Unilateral headache
4. Elicit able prodromal symptoms not necessarily visual aura
5. No underlying organic pathology

Treatment: Cognitive, ergotamine, beta blockers, sibelium and triptans.

Cluster Headache

Also called red migraine, sphenopalatine neuralgia, erythromelalgia, histaminic headache, etc.

Common in males (5:1). Comes in clusters (1–2 episodes per year) and lasts for 2–3 months. No aura. Usually unilateral but can interchange sides with every attack. Headache is sudden and peaks in 10 minutes; lasts for 1 hour. Pain is in the region of 1 and 2 division of trigeminal nerve. There can be associated parasympathetic over-activity.

Variants are: Cluster tic (along with trigeminal neuralgia), cluster vertigo, cluster migraine (h/o migraine), cluster headache wih organic lesion, cluster following trauma, cluster with infections.

Treatment: Similar to migraine attack with some differences. Oxygen inhalation, ergotamine, local anesthetic agents to nasal mucosa, steroids, etc. play a role. Prophylaxis can be done with lithium, histamine de-sensitizaion, beta-blockers and calcium channel blockers.

Trigeminal Neuralgia (Tic Douloureax)

Severe facial pain in the territory of trigeminal nerve occurring after the age of 30 years. Strictly unilateral with midline demarcation of trigger zones. Pain aggravates with mild touch also (diagnostic). Pain is stabbing in nature lasting for 20–30 seconds followed by several seconds of relief and then another stabbing attack.

Treatment: Carbamazepine 100–200 mg BD for weeks to months. It can treat acute episode and can also act as prophylaxis. Other drugs are baclofen, diphenylhydantoin, etc.

Surgical treatment is radio ablation or chemical ablation (glycerol or absolute alcohol) of trigeminal nerve. Recurrence is 25%.

Glossopharyngeal Neuralgia

Presentation is similar to trigeminal neuralgia. Pain is aggravated by swallowing, yawning, etc. Unilateral in presentation. Medical treatment is also the same like trigeminal neuralgia. If the cause is found to be elongated styloid, a styloidectomy can help.

CHAPTER 16

Applied Anatomy and Physiology of Nose

Embryology

External nose: Nasal placodes appear in fourth week intrauterine life, cranial to stomatodeum.

Septum: Septum develops from frontonasal process, a part of mesoderm which slowly gets narrower.

Nasal cavity: Ectoderm overlying the frontonasal process forms two thickening known as nasal placodes, which sink below the surface forming nasal pits giving rise to nasal cavities.

Paranasal sinuses: Diverticula from nasal cavity ultimately invading the surrounding bones (mesoderm) based on which these are named.

Palate: Palatine process of maxillary mesoderm which ultimately fuse in midline.

Dangerous area of face: Lower part of external nose and upper lip—infection of these areas may reach cavernous via anterior facial vein, which has no valves, and can lead to thrombosis which is life-threatening condition.

Olfactory area of nose: Upper 1/3 of nasal cavity with surface area of about 2–5 cm^2

Boundaries of olfactory area are
- *Superiorly*: Cribriform plate
- *Laterally*: Superior turbinate
- *Medially*: Upper part of septum

Infection of this area can lead to meningitis as it is continuous with the intracranial cavity directly through the nerve endings.

Anterior group of sinuses are maxillary sinus, frontal sinus and anterior ethmoidal cells.

Posterior group of sinuses are posterior ethmoidal cells and sphenoid sinus.

Sinuses present at birth:
- *Maxillary*: Maximum development till 25 years.
- Ethmoid
- *Sphenoid*: First to reach full development.

Sinus which is absent at birth: Frontal sinus; it appears at the age of 6 years, radiologically.

External nose:

1. *Bony pyramid:* Formed by two nasal bone, two frontal process of maxilla and nasal process of frontal bone

2. *Upper cartilaginous vault:* Formed by two upper lateral cartilage and cartilaginous nasal septum.

3. *Lower cartilaginous vault:* Formed by lower lateral cartilage (alar). Alar cartilage has a medial crus and a lateral crus and both meet at dome. Between alar cartilage and maxillary margin are 2 to 3 small sesamoid cartilages.

Length of nasal cavity: 7–8 cm; usually the length of the commonly used Tilley's nasal forceps.

Dome of nose: Highest point of lower lateral cartilage usually at the junction of medial and lateral crus.

Columella: Formed by medial crus of lower lateral cartilage.

Septal angle: Anteriorly the junction of dorsal and caudal border of septal cartilage. Posteriorly the junction of inferior border and caudal border septal cartilage.

Nasolabial angle: Angle between columella and upper lip:

- 90°–95° in males and
- 100°–110° in females.

Nasofrontal angle: Angle between frontal and nasal bone 135°.

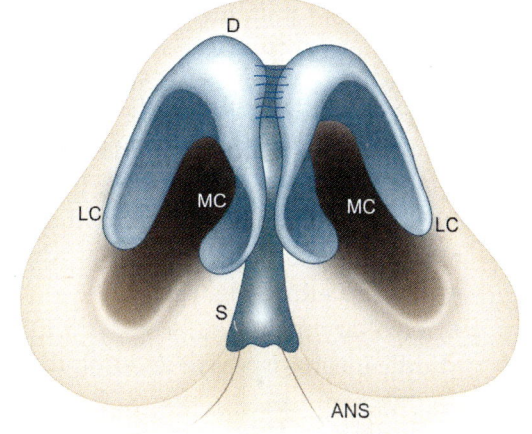

D—dome, MC—medial crus of alar cartilage, LC—lateral crus, S—nasal septum, ANS—anterior nasal spine.

Soft triangle: Facet between the columella and lateral rim of nostril.

There is no cartilage here. Any surgical interference should be avoided, as deformity in this area is difficult to correct.

Empty triangle: Fibrofatty tissues between lateral end of upper lateral cartilage and pyriform aperture.

Angle of nasal projection: N 23°–38°.

Nasal index (N) = (Width/Height of nose) × 100

Leptorrhine = Caucasian = 42–47

Plateyrrhine = Negro = 53–58

Weak triangle: Connective tissue between septal cartilage and upper lateral cartilage border above septal angle.

Nasal Cavity

Parts:

1. Vestibule contains vibrissae, sebaceous gland, hair follicle and covered by skin.
2. Respiratory epithelium low 2/3 of nasal cavity lined by ciliated columnar epithelium and erectile tissue.
3. Olfactory region roof of nasal cavity level above superior turbinate and corresponding septum.
4. Floor anterior ¾ by palatine process of maxilla, and posterior ¼ by horizontal process of palatine bone.
5. Medial wall or septum. Septum has 3 parts—membranous, cartilaginous and bony parts.
   Bony septum has major and minor components: (a) Major includes vomer perpendicular ethmoid, (b) minor includes anterior nasal spine of premaxilla, crest of maxillae and palatine bone. Rostrum and crest of sphenoid postnasal spine of frontal bone and crest of nasal bone superiorly.
6. Lateral wall. Anatomy of lateral wall of nasal cavity is discussed in various coming chapters.
   a. Inferior turbinate and inferior meatus with Hasner valve inside.
   b. Middle turbinate and meatus: It has bulla ethmoidalis, hiatus semilunaris and ethmoid infundibulum. Ethmoid infundibulum receives drainage from
      • frontal recess
      • anterior ethmoidal cells
      • maxillary ostium
   Middle meatus do have anterior and posterior fontanelles in relation to uncinate process
   c. Atrium present between vestibule and anterior end of middle turbinate
   d. Agger nasi. The anterior most ethmoidal cell near attachment of middle turbinate
   e. Superior turbinate and meatus. Here open the posterior ethmoidal cell
   f. Sphenoethmoidal recess and receives drainage from sphenoid sinus.

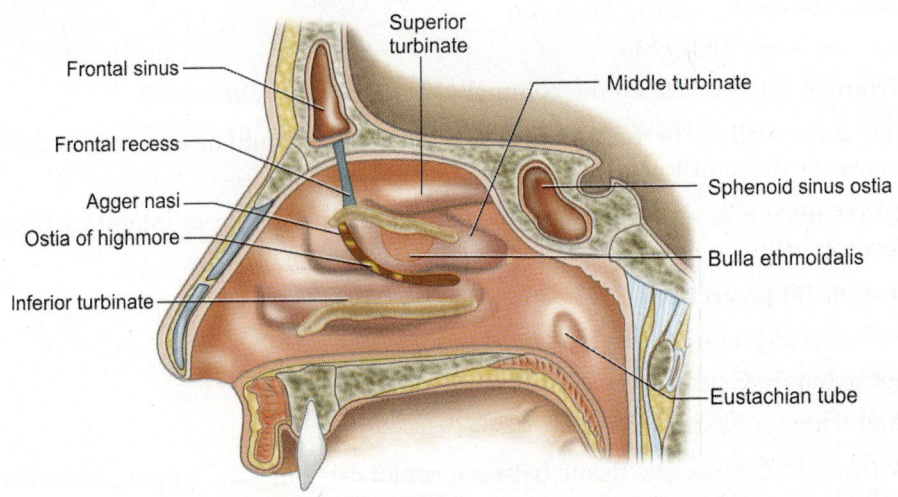

Lateral wall of nose

Thinnest wall of maxillary sinus: Medial wall; that's why we do antral puncture through this wall.

Thinnest wall of frontal sinus: Floor superior to medial canthus

Thinnest wall of ethmoid sinus: Lamina papyracea

Thinnest wall of sphenoid sinus: Superior

Fourth turbinate: Supreme turbinate

Fifth turbinate: Agger nasi

Biometric index of face

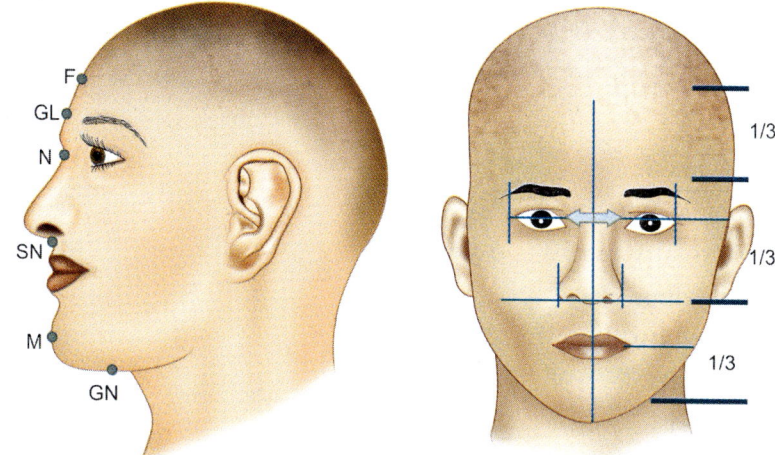

F: Frontale
GL: Glabella
N: Nasion
SN: Sub-nasion
M: Mental point
GN:Gnathion

Biometric angles of face
- Naso-frontal angle at point N is normally 135 degrees
- Nasolabial angle is:
  - Male—90–95 degrees
  - Female—100–110 degrees
- Angle of nasal projection/naso-facial angle—23–38 degrees. Protection of lower airway.

Physiology of nose and paranasal sinuses
1. Olfaction
2. Passage for respiration
3. Filtration of inspired air
4. Air conditioning of inspired air
5. Protection of lower airway
6. Vocal resonance
7. Nasal reflexes (nasogastric, sneezing and nasobronchial)
8. Drainage of tears
9. Ventilation of sinuses and eustachian tube.

CHAPTER 17

Nasal Septum and Epistaxis

Formation:

- Cuticular part
  - Fibrofatty tissues and skin
- Cartilaginous
  - Septal cartilage
- Bony parts
  - Vomer
  - Perpendicular plate of ethmoid
  - Nasal spine of frontal bone and maxillary spine
  - Rostrum of sphenoid
  - Crest of maxilla and crest of palatine bone

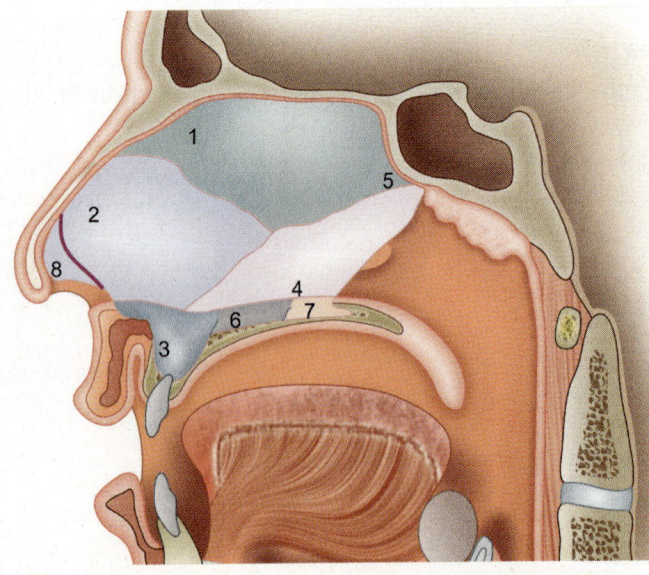

1. Perpendicular plate of ethmoid
2. Quadrangular cartilage
3. Anterior nasal spine
4. Vomer
5. Rostrum of sphenoid
6. Maxillary crest
7. Palatine crest
8. Membranous septum

Vessels supplying the septum
- Septal branch of sphenopalatine artery (the artery of epistaxis)
- Septal branch of superior labial artery
- Anterior ethmoidal artery
- Greater palatine artery

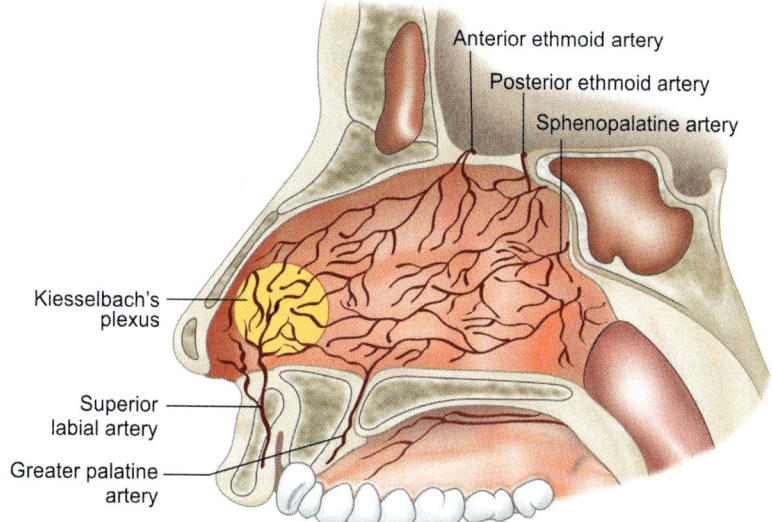

Demarcation between external carotid (ECA)/internal carotid (ICA) system: Middle turbinate on lateral wall and its corresponding area on septum roughly demarcates the division. If bleeding is above the middle turbinate, then internal carotid system is responsible, otherwise external carotid system.

Little's area: Situated on anteroinferior portion of septum

Blood supply
- Anterior ethmoidal artery
- Septal branch of sphenopalatine artery
- Greater palatine artery
- Septal branch of superior labial artery
  These vessels form a plexus called Kiesselbach's plexus.
  Airflow is directed to this point and causes drying up of mucosa and crust formation. Children tend to pick these crusts and such a minor trauma causes significant nasal bleeding.

Woodruff's plexus (nasopharyngeal plexus): It is a collection of large blood vessels in lateral wall of inferior meatus in its posterior end. Bleeding from this plexus is common in elderly patients with hypertension and usually the epistaxis is posterior. Pathological studies showed the blood vessels to be of veins and they lack muscle layers.

Sites of epistaxis
- Little's area
- Woodruff's area
- From above the middle turbinate (origin—anterior and posterior ethmoidal vessels)

- From below the level of middle turbinate (branches of sphenopalatine artery)
- Nasopharynx
- Roof of nasal cavity when fractured
- Posterior part of nasal septum (Brown's area)
- Diffuse nasal bleed

Causes of epistaxis are:

Local causes: They constitute to the most common causes

1. Congenital: Multiple telangiectasiasis (Osler-Rendu-Weber syndrome)
2. Traumatic
   Digital trauma
   Nasal fractures
   Fractures of the anterior cranial fossa
   Surgical trauma
   Chemical trauma, e.g. arsenic
   Traumatic septal perforation
   Forceful blowing of the nose and sneezing
3. Foreign body: Maggots, rhinolith, neglected foreign body
4. Inflammations
   Acute non-specific rhinosinusitis
   Acute specific inflammations—nasal diphtheria
   Chronic non-specific inflammations like
   - Atrophic rhinitis
   - Rhinitis sicca
   - Rhinitis caseosa
   - Chronic rhinitis
   Chronic specific, e.g.
   - Rhinosporidiosis
   - Tuberculosis, lupus
   - Syphilis
   - Rhinoscleroma
5. Neoplasms: Benign growths like bleeding polyps of the septum (hemangiomas), angiofibromas, inverted papillomas, etc.
   Malignant tumors of nose, paranasal sinuses and nasopharynx.
6. Miscellaneous:
   Deviated nasal septum and spurs
   Vicarious menstruation
   Barotrauma of paranasal sinuses

Systemic:

1. Congenital: Coagulation disorders like hemophilia, von Willebrand disease, functional platelet disorders, etc.

2. Infective:

Acute exanthematous fevers like
- Measles
- Varicella
- Influenza

Malaria

Typhoid

Kala-azar

Pertussis

Rheumatic fever

Dengue fever

Infectious mononucleosis

3. Disorder of blood and blood vessels: Purpuras, leukemias, hemophilias, aplastic and pernicious anemias, vitamin K deficiency, DIC.
4. Systemic diseases: Hypertension, atherosclerosis, mitral stenosis, cirrhosis chronic nephritis.
5. Drugs: Anticoagulants, aspirin, phenytoin.
6. Mediastinal compression by tumors of the lower neck, mediastinal growth, puberty.

Idiopathic

Management

1. Assessment of general condition: Investigation like CBC, coagulation profile, X-rays of nose and paranasal sinuses, CT scan, etc. are done.

Epistaxis

Anterior: If blood flows from front of nose in sitting position

Posterior: If blood flows into throat in sitting position

Fluid replacement and oxygen supplement in case of massive bleeding

Blood transfusion in epistaxis
- Blood loss > 300 ml
- Markedly decreased Hb levels, i.e. less than 10 gm Hb
- Epistaxis needing repeated nasal packing and if every time bleeding is severe.
- Platelet count less than 1 lakh.

2. Local management: Pinching of nose, ice cubes around nose, patient head kept upright.

Trotter's method with patient upright and leaned forward with open mouth until patient becomes hypotensive but this carries risk of coronary thrombosis.

Suction clearance and endoscopy to locate the bleeding site and cauterize bleeding point.

If bleeding is diffuse then do anterior nasal packing with BIPP or soframycin ointment.

If still bleeding present then it is supplemented with posterior nasal packing

Posterior nasal packing can be done with Foley's catheter.

As a last resort external carotid or internal maxillary artery ligation or sphenopalatine artery cauterization can be done.

Specific cause can be treated with either septoplasty, removal of NPA, or tumor or treat the hypertension.

Deviated Nasal Septum

Aetiology

1. Trauma—birth or accidental trauma
2. Developmental or birth moulding theory like where abnormal pressure of amniotic fluid in LOA position of foetus in uterus lead right DNS commonly.
   Cleft palate and high arch palate leading to buckling of septum to one side.

Classification of septal deformity

1. C- or S-shaped deviation
2. Spur at either cartilage premaxilla junction (anterior) or cartilage and vomer junction (posterior spur). Anterior lead nasal blockage and posterior leads sinus infection due to blockage at middle meatus level.
3. Fracture involving both bone and cartilage.
4. Dislocation—where caudal end of cartilage gets displaced from its groove.
   Symptoms are nasal obstruction, headache, epistaxis, anterior ethmoidal nerve syndrome, snoring, deformity of nose and ear problems.
   Obstruction of nasal cavity may be vestibular, valvular, attic, turbinal or choanal k/a Cottle's areas of nasal cavity. Obstruction may be only for 12 hours of day or may be 24 hours of day due to physiological nasal cycle. When there is compensatory hypertrophy of opposite inferior turbinate then obstruction is for 24 hours and worse for patients.
   Often in old injury of septum leading to fracture of cartilaginous portion and overlapping of two fractures end the picture will be of very peculiar type of DNS shown in one of the diagrams.

Septal Surgeries

Killian's incision: Given in submucous resection of septum. It is given 5 mm behind the caudal border of septal cartilage.

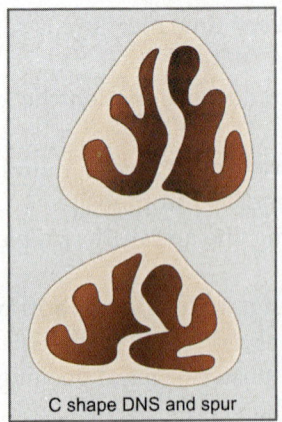
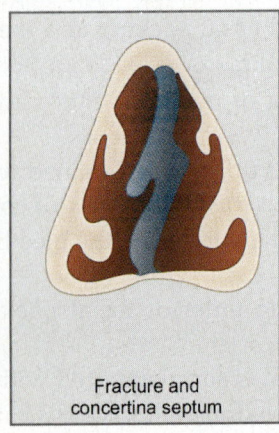
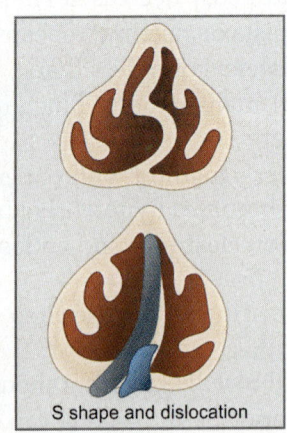

| C shape DNS and spur | Fracture and concertina septum | S shape and dislocation |

Left-sided septal spur impinging against inferior turbinate (IT) and middle meatus (MM) causing headache and epistaxis.

Freer's incision: Hemitransfixation incision. Given at lower border of septal cartilage.

Advantages:
- Avascular plane
- Easy access to whole septum
- Can be combined with rhinoplasty incision

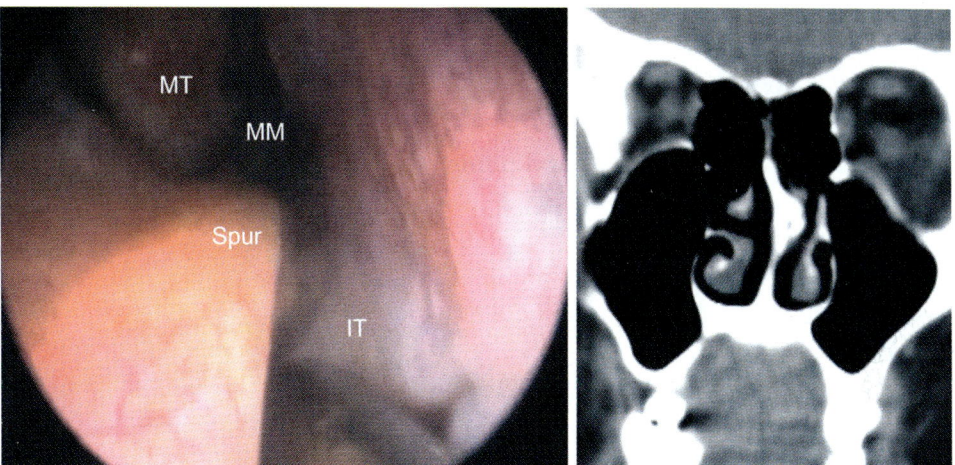

Hemitransfixation incision means incision on only one side of septum.

Transfixation incision means incision on both sides of septum, e.g. rhinoplasty and degloving approach.

Anterior tunnel: Making a pocket above the chondrovomerine junction.

Inferior tunnel: Making a pocket below the chondrovomerine junction.

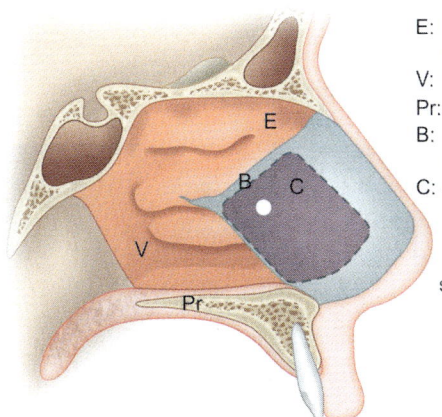

E: Perpendicular plate of ethmoid
V: Vomer
Pr: Premaxilla
B: Septal bone removed all around the cartilage
C: Septal cartilage with convex deviation corrected by removing multiple wedge-shaped full thickness

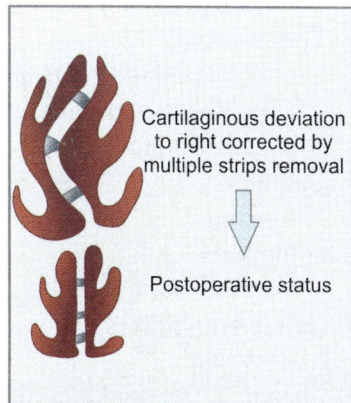

Cartilaginous deviation to right corrected by multiple strips removal

Postoperative status

Morselization of septum: Deviated septum is broken/incised at one or multiple sites after raising the mucoperichondrium to small pieces. This helps to break the swing of the cartilage (due to elasticity) and hence the deviation gets corrected.

Differences between septoplasty and submucous resection (SMR)

Submucous resection	Septoplasty
Not done in children	Can be done in children
Flaps elevated on both sides of septum	Flap is raised on one side only
Most of the cartilage is removed	Cartilage preserving surgery
Caudal dislocation cannot be corrected	Can be corrected
Perforation chances are high	Low risk
Revision surgery is difficult	Can be done

Indications for SMR
- DNS (symptomatic)
- Trans-septal access to sphenoid and pituitary gland
- Taking septal cartilage for graft
- Vidian neurectomy

Complications of SMR
- Septal hematoma and abscess
- Septal perforation
- Floppy septum
- Saddle nose
- Synechia

Toxic shock syndrome: The nasal pack acts as a hygroscopic material in the nasal cavity which also acts as a medium for the growth of *Staph. aureus*. The toxins released by the *Staph. aureus* enter the blood stream and causes toxemia and life-threatening complications. This can be prevented by avoiding long standing (>48 hours) nasal packs.

Septal Perforation

Causes
- Cosmetic perforation to wear ornaments
- Traumatic
  - Surgeries like SMR, septoplasty
  - Repeated cauterization of septal mucosa
  - Digital trauma
- Chemical
  - Cocaine
  - Steroids
  - Decongestant
- Industrial workers exposed to dry heat, e.g. oven worker
- Chronic inflammations like
  - Wegener's granuloma
  - Tuberculosis—cartilaginous septum
  - Syphilis—bony septum
  - Lupus
  - Malignancy

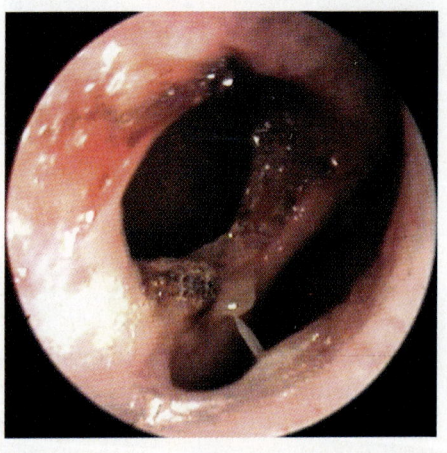

Simplest treatment of septal perforation
- Keep the nose clean
- Silastic buttons

Cauterizing agents used
- 15% $AgNO_3$
- 50% TCA (Trichloroacetic acid)
- Chromic sulfate, carbolic acid

Inferior Turbinate Procedures

Reduction of bulk of inferior turbinate: Cautery, submucous diathermy, cryo surgery, radio scalpel, laser turbinectomy—partial or complete; nowadays microdebriders are used.

CHAPTER 18

Rhinitis

Etiological classification of rhinitis infective
- Bacterial
- Viral
- Fungal

Allergic: Seasonal/perennial

Chronic non-allergic
- Non-atopic eosinophilic
- Infant bronchial asthma

Hyperplastic: Nasal polyposis
   Turbinate hypertrophy

Chronic non-specific
- Atrophic
- Rhinitis caseosa
- Rhinitis sicca
- Medicamentosa rhinitis
- Vasomotor

Metabolic/endocrine
- Hypothyroidism
- Pregnancy
- Alcohol
- Honeymoon

Systemic disorder: Cystic fibrosis
- Secondary to structural abnormality
  - Septal deviation
  - Adenoid hypertrophy
  - Choanal atresia
  - Post total laryngectomy

Common Cold

Viruses: Rhinovirus adenovirus, respiratory—syncytial influenzae A, B (variant of influenza 1. Chikungunya from monkey, swine flu from pig and birds flu from chicken), parainfluenza type I, II, III, corona and coxsackie.

Predisposing factors: Malnutrition, cold climatic condition, fatigue, poor hygiene and drop of nasal or pharyngeal temperature below 30° due to chilled cold drinks or drying one under a/c or fan after getting drenched in rain water.

Vasoconstriction followed by vasodilation and 3rd day onward bacterial invasion by streptococci commonly but other bacteria can infect secondarily.

Clinically:
1. Prodromal, i.e. tickling for hours
2. Irritation watery discharge with redness and sneezing and blockage for 4 days
3. Secondary infection for 2 days with mucopurulent discharge
4. Resolution stage: Takes 5–10 days.

Treatment: Isolation, vaccine (for influenza), paracetamol, antihistaminic, steam inhalation, bedrest, and plenty of fluid intake.

Atrophic Rhinitis

Chronic inflammatory disease leading to progressive atrophy of nasal mucosa and underlying bones of nasal cavity. Crust formation is characteristic of this disease.

Causes

Primary atrophic rhinitis: Hormonal imbalance, nutritional and autoimmune.

Secondary atrophic rhinitis: Excessive tissue removal from nose during surgeries, e.g.
- Turbinectomy
- Leprosy
- Syphilis
- Tuberculosis
- Chronic rhinosinusitis

Bacteria involved: Coccobacillus, *Klebsiella ozaenae, Bacillus mucillus* and diphtheroid bacillus.

Primary atrophic rhinitis has 2 types:
Type I: Underlying pathology is endarteritis
Type II: Vasodilatation under influence of estrogen.

Ozaena: Bad smell emanating from the nasal cavity of the patient of atrophic rhinitis.

Treatment of Atrophic Rhinitis

1. *25% glucose in glycerin nasal drops:* After careful removal of crusts, nasal cavity is painted with solution of 25% glucose in glycerin. Glucose inhibits the proteolytic organisms, which causes foul smell. Glycerin has hygroscopic action and helps in loosening up of the crusts.
2. *Alkaline nasal douche:* 1/2 pint (280 ml) of water is mixed with the following and is used to give douching.

Sodium biborate 28.4 gm—antiseptic

Sodium bicarbonate 28.4 gm—loosens the crusts

Sodium chloride 56.8 gm—provides isotonicity.

3. *Kemicetine antiozaena solution:* Chloramphenicol, estradiol, vitamin D_2.

4. *Surgical options for atrophic rhinitis:* Basic principle is to reduce the size of nasal cavity.

    A. Lautenslager's operation for medialization of lateral wall by cartilage, bone chips, silicon, teflon, etc.

    B. Young's operation

    C. Modified Young's operation

    D. Stenson's duct transplantation (in maxillary sinus).

Rhinoscleroma

Chronic granulomatous inflammation of upper respiratory tract of bacterial aetiology. Woody nose.

Caused by *Klebsiella rhinoscleromatis* (Frisch bacillus). It is a diplobacillus. Histologically a large foam cell with a central nucleus and vacuolated cytoplasm containing bacilli known as Mikulicz cells.

On examination, the soft palate has gothic arch appearance with uvula pulled towards the nasopharynx. OSMF also shows gothic arch palate with uvula pulled anteriorly towards oral cavity.

Russell bodies and Mikulicz cells are diagnostic findings on histopathology. Plasma cell with eosinophilic inclusion bodies are called Russel bodies.

Stages

• Atrophic, nonspecific rhinitis and fishy smell

• Granulomatous or nodular, rubbery feeling at mucocutaneus junction initially

• Cicatrizing stage with disfigurement of nose called Hebra nose

Treatment: Streptomycin, tetracycline, rifampicin and steroid and local 2% acriflavine solution for a prolonged duration in stenosis excision of tissue and recanalization.

Rhinosporidiosis

Rhinosporidium seeberi, a fungus.

Irregular mass with mulberry appearance with recurrent bleeding.

Sporangia on the surface of the mass are diagnostic.

May involve lips, palate, uvula, larynx, conjunctiva, skin, penis and vulva.

Treatment: Local excision with cautery of the base.

Long-term dapsone.

CHAPTER 19

Nasal Polyposis and Fungal Rhinosinisitis

Polyp: Polyp is prolapsed, pedunculated and edematous mucosa of nasal or paranasal sinuses.

Etilogy of nasal polyposis includes:

- Allergy
- Infection
- Bernoulli's phenomenon
- Vasomotor imbalances

Cystic fibrosis: Bilateral polyposis in children should arouse the suspicion of cystic fibrosis.

Other conditions

- Asthma, aspirin sensitivity, nasal polyposis forms **Samter's triad**.
- Kartagener's syndrome—bronchiectasis, sinusitis, situs inversus and ciliary dyskinesia.
- NARE syndrome—non-allergic rhinitis with eosinophilia.
- Allergic fungal sinusitis—is the commonest cause of polyposis.
- Young's syndrome—nasal polyps, bronchiectasis, sinusitis and azoospermia.

Polyposis Nasi Classification

  I. Antrochoanal polyp

 II. Large isolated choanal polyp

III. Polyps with chronic rhinosinusitis (non-eosinophil dominant)

IV. Polyps with chronic rhinosinusitis (eosinophil dominant)

 V. Polyp with specific diseases (cranio-facial malignancies, e.g. olfactory neuroblastoma).

Differences between antrochoanal polyp and ethmoidal polyp

Antrochoanal polyp	Ethmoidal polyp
Single	Multiple
Unilateral	Bilateral
Recurrence rate low	Recurrence is high
From maxillary sinus	From ethmoidal cells
Extends posteriorly	Grows anteriorly
Dumb-bell shaped or three lobed	Grape-like clustered
Common in younger age group	Common in adults

Etiology: Infection allergy.

Antrochoanal polyp can arise from:
1. Floor or postwall of maximum antrum.
2. From accessory ostia of maximum antrum.
3. From margin of true ostia.
4. From uncinate process (in this case uncinate is highly pneumatized and blocking the infundibulum).
5. From bulla ethmoidalis.
6. From middle turbinate (when it arises from middle turbinate or bulla or uncinate, then the cause is Bernoulli phenomenon and usually on the side of DNS and from maxillary sinus when arising from opposite to the DNS side, again the cause is sinusitis or infection).

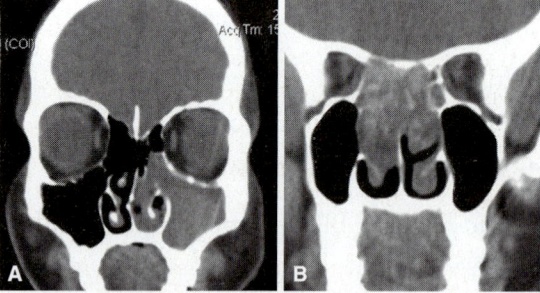

(A) CT of left antrochoanal polyp; (B) Bilateral ethmoidal polyp

Why AC polyp grows posteriorly?
• More space to grow posteriorly
• Direction of mucous flow because of ciliary activity
• Direction of ostium

Topical steroids used to reduce recurrence of ethmoidal polyps: Hydrocortisone, beclomethasone, budesonide, fluticasone, mometasone, etc.

Common sites of origin of nasal polyps: Uncinate process, turbinates, infundibulum, face of bulla, hiatus semilunaris, frontal recess.

FUNGAL RHINOSINUSITIS

3 types
1. Invasive form (serious)
   • Acute (fulminant),
   • Chronic indolent (aspergilloma, mycetomas, etc.)

2. Non-invasive
   - Saprophytic
   - Fungal ball (sinolith)
   - Eosinophilic mediated form (systemic reactions)
     I. Eosinophil fungal rhinosinusitis (EFRS)
     II. Allergic fungal rhinosinusitis (AFRS)
3. Transitional form: Like fungal meningitis.

Allergic fungal rhinosinusitis and fungal ball

- Aspergillosis (commonest) by *Aspergillus fumigatus*, *Aspergillus niger*.
- Blastomycosis by *Blastomyces dermatitidis*.

Organisms for mucormycosis

- *Mucor circinelloides*
- *Mucor javanicus*
- *Basidia corynybacteria*
- Cryptomycosis by *Crypto neoformans*
- Actinomycosis by *Actinomyces israelii*
- Histoplasmosis by *Histoplasma capsulatum*
- Candida infection by *Candida albicans*.

Most allergic rhinosinusitis is initiated by immunologic reaction by the eosinophils to fungi which are considered as foreign body and they de-granulate and release eosinophilic major basic proteins (EMBP) which is very toxic to the nasal mucosa.

Fungal debris in the sinuses look like *peanut butter*.

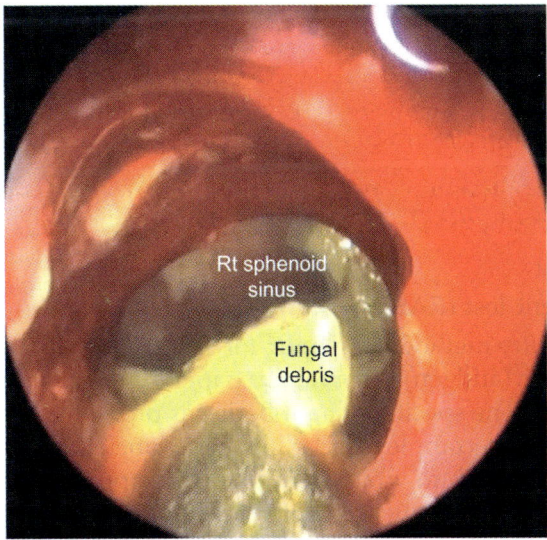

Peanut butter fungal debris in sphenoid sinus being removed

Conditions predisposing to fungal infections of nose: Immunocompromised patient, diabetic ketoacidosis, uremic acidosis, malnutrition, antimetabolite or antibiotic therapy, leukemia, warm and moist environments like sea coasts.

CHAPTER 20

Allergic Rhinitis

IgE mediated nasal hypersensitivity to allergens.

Signs of allergic rhinitis

Horizontal crease above the tip of nose—Darier's line conjunctival congestion.

Periorbital puffiness and watering from eye

Dark circles around eyes—allergic shiners

Allergic salute (the child pushes the tip of his nose up with base of his palm in an attempt to control itching).

Crease in the lower eyelids due to spasm of Muller's muscle—Dennie Morgan sign.

Diagnosis:

1. History
2. Nasal smears
3. Blood eosinophilia
4. Skin tests
   - Prick test
   - Scratch test
   - Intradermal test
5. Radioallergosorbent test (RAST)

   It was the first *in vitro* method developed for detection of IgE. It is done as follows: The specific allergen (antigen) is bound to a paper disc. The test serum is then added to it and incubated. The specific IgE antibodies if present in the serum will bind to the allergens and form complexes. Radioisotope labeled anti-IgE antibody is then introduced into the medium which will bind to the pre-existing complexes on the paper disk. The resultant "allergen IgE–anti-IgE" is then measured in a gamma counter and the amount of antibody is calculated.
6. Paper radioimmunosorbent test (PRIST): It is based on incubating the IgE containing serum with radioactively labelled anti-IgE. The total concentration of IgE is then proportional to measured radioactivity.
7. Nasal provocation tests (nasal challenge tests).

Classification of antihistamines

First generation (highly sedative)	Second generation (non-sedative)
Pyrilamine	Loratadine
Diphenhydramine	Terfenadine
Clemastine	Fexofenadine
Chlorpheniramine, Phenramine	Cetrizine (sedating than the rest)
Cyclizine	Levocetrizine
Promethazine	Azelastine
Cyproheptadine	Olopatadine
Cinnarizine	Astemizole
	Ebastine
	Bepotastine

Comparison of allergic and vasomotor rhinitis

Allergic rhinitis	Vasomotor rhinitis
1. Usually starts from teenage	Starts at 3rd or 4th decade
2. History of exposure to allergens	No such history
3. Itching and sneezing are prominent	Itching and sneezing less prominent
4. Conjunctival itching and lacrimation are common	No conjunctival itching
5. Skin tests are positive	Skin tests are negative
6. Etiology is type I reaction	Vasomotor instability is the cause
7. Nasal smears show increased eosinophils	No increase in eosinophils
8. Blood eosinophil count is raised	Blood eosinophils are normal
9. Blood IgE levels are increased	IgE levels are not increased
10. Vidian neurectomy is not helpful	Vidian neurectomy helps transiently
11. Rhinorrhea comes later on	Rhinorrhea is the first symptom

CHAPTER 21

Choanal Atresia and Oroantral Fistula

Etiology: Postnatal persistence of bucconasal membrane.

Types
- Membranous/bony
- Complete/incomplete
- Unilateral/bilateral

Newborns are obligatory nose breathers, so if a neonate is having bilateral complete choanal atresia, death might occur if immediate attention is not given. When a newborn is presenting with frothing from mouth, cyanosis and respiratory failure, then a rubber or silicone feeding tube can be passed through nasal cavity and failure of the tube to pass into nasopharynx is diagnostic of the disease.

Investigations
- Cold spatula test
- Catheter cannot be passed through the nose into nasopharynx
- CT nose and paranasal sinuses

Treatment
- Transnasal perforation, transpalatal excision, laser excision
- Endoscopic endonasal perforation.

Oroantral Fistula

A communication between maxillary antrum and oral cavity.

Causes
- Upper dental extraction, malignancy, Caldwell-Luc's operation
- Penetrating trauma

Treatment
- Primary closure by taking local tissue
- Rotation flap of mucosa from cheek
- Nasolabial flap.

CHAPTER 22

CSF Rhinorrhea

Cerebrospinal fluid: CSF is secreted by choroid plexus. This is mediated by osmotic gradient produced by unidirectional ionic transport in the ventricles. The component of CSF is similar to perilymph. CSF is drained by arachnoid villae present in the dural venous sinuses.

CSF leaks through the nasal cavity occurs at the following sites:
- Medial to middle turbinate
- Lateral to middle turbinate

Based on the cause CSF rhinorrhea is divided into the following:
1. Congenital
2. Traumatic
3. Iatrogenic
4. Neoplasia related
5. Idiopathic or spontaneous.

CSF otorhinorrhea: When CSF comes from ear through the nasopharynx into nasal cavity.

Causes

Traumatic
- Accidental fracture of cribriform plate
- Iatrogenic FESS

Spontaneous
- High pressure tumor, hydrocephalus
- Normal pressure idiopathic congenital anomalies, focal atrophy osteomyelitis.

Tests:
1. *Clinical testing*: History and physical examination; nasal endoscopy; handkerchief test; halo sign +ve (when done immediately after trauma).
2. *Biochemical testing*: β_2 transferrin estimation which is specific to CSF; glucose estimation of collected CSF >30 mg % (at least 1/3rd of serum glucose).
3. *Sinus CT scan*: Non-contrast and contrast enhanced to detect any meningo-encephalocoeles and traumatic etiologies. Metrizamide CT cisternography is done to localize the site of leak.

4. MRI/MR cisternography

5. *Intrathecal fluorescein injection* is done when there is high suspicion of leak even after multiple negative work-ups.

Treatment

I. Conservative management as most of the traumatic cases subsides spontaneously with 7–10 days. Head end elevation is advised. Good antibiotic coverage should be used to avoid intracranial infections.

II. Surgical management by endoscopic endonasal approach to remove the encephalocoeles and neoplastic growths and closure of the defects with fascia/ osteoplastic flap/fat/cartilages give good result in most of the cases, thus making the need for intracranial surgery almost obsolete.

CHAPTER 23

Cosmetic Surgeries of Nose

Rhinoplasty

Bony pyramid: Also called pyriform aperture; bounded by nasal bones, frontal processes of maxilla, anterior nasal spine. In midline it is divided by the bony nasal septum. Common clinical problems associated with bony pyramid are bony hump, thick frontal process of maxilla, malunited nasal bone fractures, etc.

Cartilaginous pyramid: Formed by cartilaginous nasal septum, upper and lower lateral (alar) cartilage. Junction of upper and lower cartilages has the cranial end of alar cartilage overlapping the upper

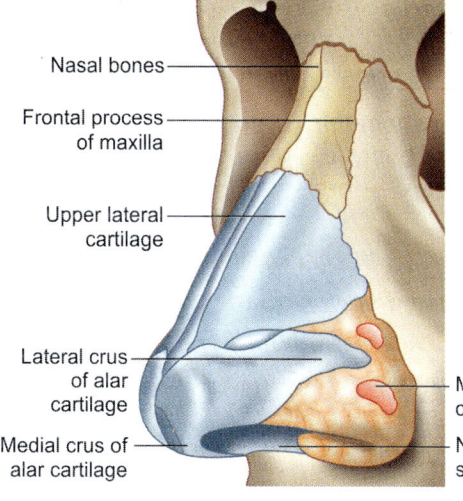

lateral cartilage to form nasal valve. Clinical abnormalities are deviated nose, hump, saddle nose, tension nose, alar collapse and tip deformities. These conditions can be treated with procedures like cartilage reshaping (morselizing, spreader grafts, suture techniques and tongue in groove technique) and cartilage reconstruction (extra corporeal resection with or without polydioxanone foil, use of conchal or rib cartilage). These can be done in most cases by closed approach but cases with severe deformities should be approached with open technique.

Supports To Nose

Portion	Central	Lateral
Upper 1/3rd	Bony septum	Nasal bone and frontal process
Middle 1/3rd	Cartilaginous septum	Upper lateral cartilage and frontal process
Lower 1/3rd	Caudal septum and columellar complex	Alar cartilage, alar soft tissue and frontal process

Rhinoplasty is many a times done in combination with nasal septal correction and the procedure is called septorhinoplasty.

Terminologies in Rhinoplasty

Alar base: Lower most portion of nose. Ideally it should be equal to the inter-canthal distance. It is the central 1/5th of the vertical divisions of face biometry.

Alar rim: It is the outer edge of the external nares.

Alar retraction: Also called notched ala. It is a cephalic malpositioning of the alar rim occurring either due to iatrogenic cause (cephalic trimming of the lateral crus of LLC) or congenitally.

Bony vault: Upper 1/3rd of the nose.

Closed rhinoplasty: Endonasal rhinoplasty. It avoids visible columellar scarring.

Columellar show: Part of the columella visible from lateral profile through the alar rim.

Columellar strut: Type of autologous septal cartilaginous graft used to increase tip projection and upward rotation.

Excisional rhinoplasty: Type of reduction rhinoplasty where no spreader graft or osteotomies are used. This method has more contour defects in postoperative period.

Hanging columella: Tip ptosis.

Nasal valve: Anatomical bottleneck of nasal airflow. Regulates nasal cycles.

Naso-frontal angle: Between the nasal bridge and forehead.

Naso-labial angle: Between columella and upper lip.

Open book deformity: Gap between the nasal bones following median osteotomy.

Percutaneous osteotomy: Type of lateral osteotomy where the incision is just a stab.

Rhinion: Junction between upper and middle third of the nasal framework.

Secondary rhinoplasty: Also called revision rhinoplasty.

Spreader graft: Middle vault augmentation graft placed between the septal cartilage and the ULCs.

Step-ladder deformity: Formed by high lateral osteotomy.

Tip projection: Distance between facial plane and nasal tip at sagittal plane.

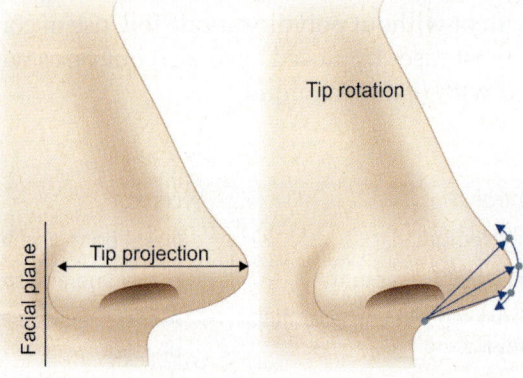

Tip rotation: Movement of tip at a circular arc with radius formed by the distance from centre of nasolabial angle to tip defining point.

Tongue in groove technique: A procedure to correct caudal dislocation by suturing the caudal end of septum to the medial crura after creating a pocket.

Intra- and inter-domal sutures: Suturing techniques between the medial and lateral crura and between medial crura of lower lateral cartilages respectively used in tip-plasties.

Key-stone area: Junction of perpendicular plate of ethmoid with the dorsal septum.

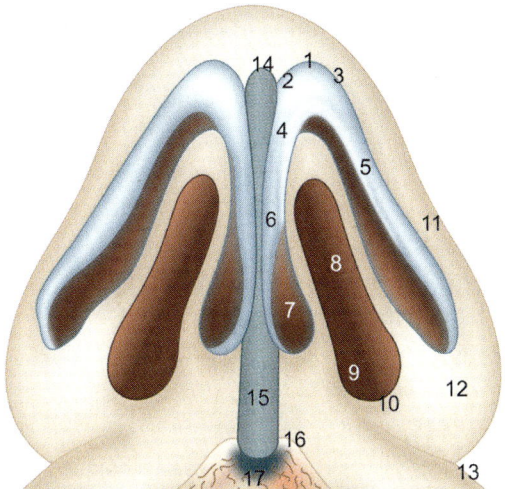

(1) Apex of ala; (2) Medial dome angle; (3) Lateral dome angle; (4) Middle crus; (5) Lateral crus; (6) Medial crus; (7) Medial crura footplate; (8) Nostril/external nasal valve; (9) Nostril floor; (10) Nostril side wall; (11) Lateral alar sidewall; (12) Alar lobule; (13) Alar-facial junction; (14) Anterior septal angle; (15) Caudal septum; (16) Maxillary crest; (17) Anterior nasal spine.

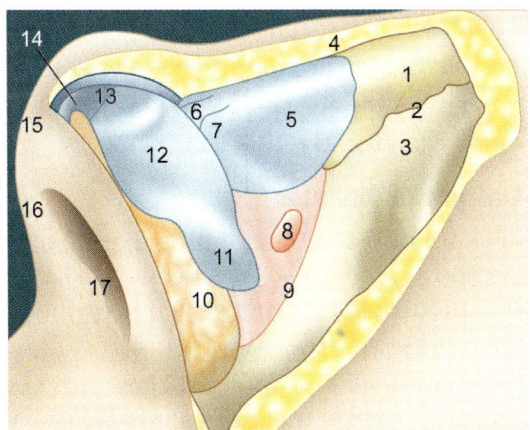

(1) Nasal bone; (2) Nasomaxillary suture; (3) Frontal process of maxilla; (4) Rhinion; (5) Upper lateral cartilage; (6) Anterior septal angle; (7) Caudal free edge of ULC; (8) Sesamoid cartilage; (9) Pyriform margin; (10) Alar lobule; (11) Lateral crus of alar cartilage (lateral portion); (12) Lateral crus of alar cartilage (central portion); (13) Tip defining point; (14) Middle crus; (15) Infra-tip lobule; (16) Columella; (17) Medial crura footplate.

Photographs Before Rhinoplasty

Common and necessary views of photos
1. Right and left lateral
2. Right and left lateral oblique
3. Frontal
4. Skyline (Helicopter) and
5. Basal view

Anesthesia for rhinoplastic surgeries
A. Local anesthesia with intravenous mild sedation
B. Monitored anesthesia care (moderate sedation)
C. Unconscious or deep sedation
D. General anesthesia

Various incisions used in rhinoplasty
Inverted—V-shaped columellar incision—placed at the junction of upper 2/3rd and lower 1/3rd of the columella. The lateral ends of the V are connected to transfixation incisions by horizontal incisions.

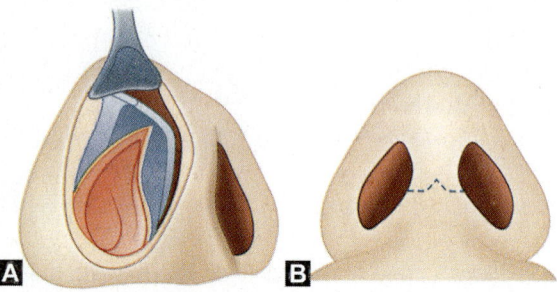

Transfixation/hemitransfixation incisions: Placed 1–2 mm above the caudal end of the septum. Exposes septum, anterior nasal spine and medial crura. Hemi is unilateral incision.

(A) Endonasal technique via combined hemitransfixation and intercartilaginous incision. (B) Transcolumellar inverted V incision that will join with bilateral A incision for external rhinoplasty.

Inter-cartilaginous incision: Completes the incision from the upper end of transfixation incision into the lateral wall to expose the middle vault and tip. It is placed between the ULC and LLC. Care should be taken not to cut the caudal end of ULC.

Intra-cartilaginous incision: Similar to inter-cartilaginous incision but it is 3–4 mm caudal to it; cutting through the LLC. Avoids nasal valve stricture postoperatively.

Rim incisions: Made at the caudal end of LLC.

Postoperative Nasal Support Techniques

Taping of the nose from supra tip to nasion with paper tape; this avoids hematoma formation under the flap and altered expected outcome. Usually this taping is kept till 7 days in postoperative period. Some surgeons even keep them till 3 weeks.

Splinting: Both internal and external are kept. External splints are usually made of aluminium, plaster of Paris or dental compound. They provide support to the nasal framework and are kept for 3 weeks. Internal splints are mainly for septal support and they are made of silicone, plastic or X-ray plates. They can be kept for 4–5 days.

Septal Surgery

Septoplasty is done to correct both nasal obstruction and external deviation. Hence it is both functional and aesthetic. There are two approaches to correct deviated septum—

open (extra-corporeal) and endonasal approaches. Endonasal approaches are classical and endoscopic.

Incision. Hemitransfixation incision 1–2 mm behind the caudal end of the septum by which the whole of the cartilaginous and bony septum can be reached.

Mobilization of the deviated part of nasal septum is done by making upper and lower tunnels which are ultimately connected with each other. The *cartilaginous swinging door* is created by making lower horizontal and posterior vertical chondrotomies and making the quadrangular septum free from anterior nasal spine, pre-maxilla and the maxillary crest and the posterior bony septum. Severely deviated part of the cartilage/spurs can be removed preserving at least 1 cm of the dorsal septum. The cartilaginous elasticity is broken by making multiple full thickness incisions on the concave side of the septum or removing a wedge of cartilage (again partial thickness) from the convex side of the septum. Bony deviations need to be removed after raising a bilateral posterior tunnel.

If there is caudal dislocation, the caudal end of the septal cartilage should be fixed between the medial crura of the alar cartilage by making a pocket in the columellar septum. If the length of the caudal end is more than required, minimal resection of the septal cartilage at the caudal end can be done taking care not to reduce the nasal projection. If the height of the caudal end is less due to previous trauma, it can be grafted with cartilage graft from the posterior end of the septal cartilage and this graft can be fixed to it by guide sutures. After correcting the deviation, the remaining of the septum needs to be fixed at the midline. Fixation can be done by septal splinting, nasal packing and sutures (figure of eight).

In cases of severe septal deviations, we might have to do extra-corporeal septoplasty.

Correcting the nasal septum is most of the times the first step in rhinoplasty as septum acts as the anchor for the whole nasal framework. Septoplasty can also be the first step to do endoscopic sinus surgery or beyond.

Management of Dorsum of Nose

Dorsum can have deformities like dorsal hump (cartilaginous or bony) and saddle nose deformity.

Humps can be corrected by reduction rhinoplasty. Both cartilaginous part as well as bony part need correction to maintain the smooth contour even if there is hump in only one part. Bony humps are removed by either rasping or midline osteotomy to remove the protruding segment. After midline osteotomy, the open book deformity of the nasal bone is corrected by either lateral or intermediate osteotomies. Cartilaginous protrusions are resected accordingly. Hump correction might lead to internal nasal valve incompetence and inverted-V deformity.

Saddle nose deformity is a depression in the middle 1/3rd of the nasal dorsum in comparison to the bony vault and the tip. Causes of saddle nose deformity are over resection of septal cartilage during septoplasty, trauma or infections like leprosy. This is corrected by augmentation rhinoplasty with autologous cartilaginous spreader grafts (best) or sometimes even bone grafts. Spreader grafts are placed between the dorsal septum and the upper lateral cartilages in submucosal plane. Usual size is 6–12 mm in length, 3–5 mm in height and 2–4 mm in width. Cephalic end of the graft should be wider. Unilateral spreader graft is needed in cases of dorsal asymmetry.

Other uses of spreader grafts are to correct internal nasal valve collapse. Other techniques to correct dorsal depression are onlay of crushed cartilage, autologous rib graft, flaring sutures, etc.

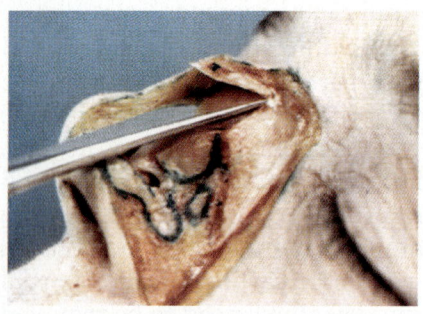 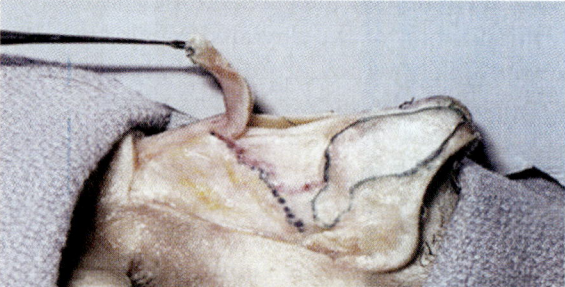

Osteotomies in Rhinoplasty

1. Lateral (low to low) osteotomy
2. Median osteotomy
3. Intermediate osteotomy with guarded curved osteotome

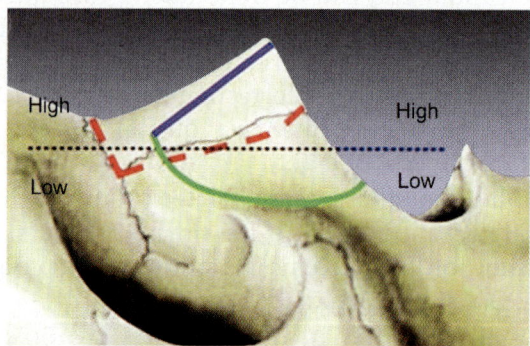

4. Cross root or transverse root osteotomy

Complications can be step ladder deformity in lateral and intermediate types. Open book deformity in the median type.

Three-point fixation: In cases of extra-corporeal external rhinoplasty, the septum can be constructed and remodelled with the help of perpendicular plate of ethmoid and straightened septal cartilage sutured together at multiple places and fixed at three points, i.e. (1) Nasal bone, (2) Anterior nasal spine and (3) Upper lateral cartilages using with or without spreader graft. Usually the suturing is done with PDS (polydiaxone) but in that place vicryl can also be used.

Crooked Nose Deformity

Commonest cause for which the patient seeks rhinoplasty. This usually follows a trauma to nose. Crooked nose can result from abnormalities in any of the thirds of nasal vaults, i.e. lower third (tip), middle third or upper third.

Lower vault techniques include correcting the caudal deviation by minimal resection and suturing, columellar supporting graft, etc. following this symmetry of the lower lateral cartilages should be done. Middle third techniques include correcting the septal deviation and aligning upper lateral cartilages. Upper bony third needs various osteotomies to bring the nose in midline.

Sequence of corrections in rhinoplasty:

1. Septum correction.
2. Dorsum correction, osteotomies and spreader grafts if needed.
3. Securing the upper lateral cartilage to prevent internal nasal valve collapse.
4. Tip correction.

Role of Glabellar Flap

In cases of nasal mutilation after trauma or surgeries for cancers, large tissue loss the skin over the external nose can be reconstructed with glabellar flap (based on supratrochlear and supraorbital arteries). In cases of minimal loss, it can be managed with full thickness skin graft.

The following diagrams show pre- and postoperative photos of a patient with right alar defect (post-traumatic) reconstructed with glabellar flap.

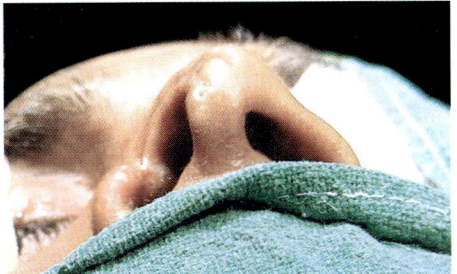
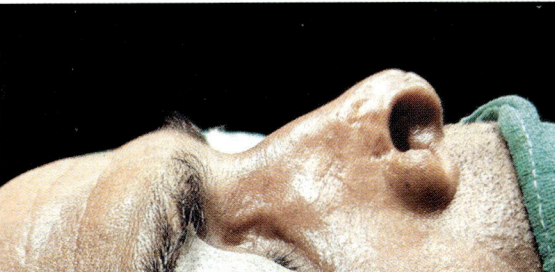
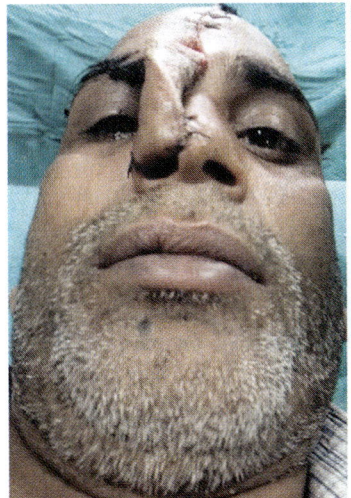
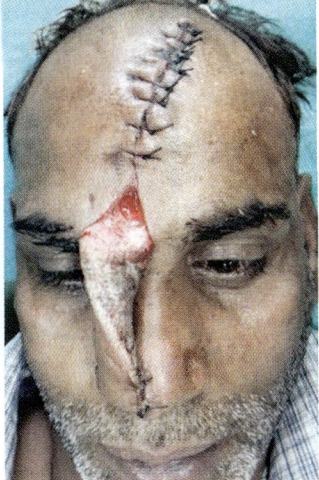
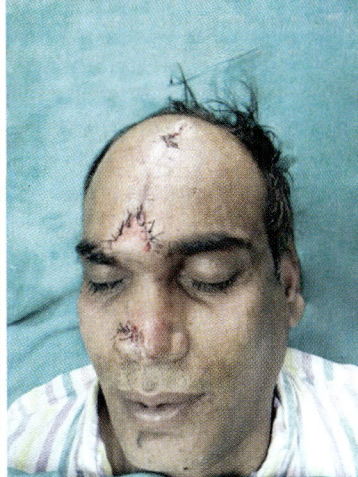

CHAPTER 24

Endoscopic Sinus Surgery

Limen nasi: It is the junction between upper and lower lateral cartilage of nose where inter-cartilaginous incision is given.

Hasner's valve: Mucosal flap present where nasolacrimal duct opens into inferior meatus.

Ethmoid sinus: Number of anterior ethmoid cells is 12–15; posterior 3–5.

Ground lamella of middle turbinate divides in anterior and posterior cells. Anterior cells drain into middle meatus and posterior cells drain into sphenoethmoidal recess via superior meatus.

Uncinate process: It is boomerang shaped, sagittally oriented bony leaflet running anterosuperior to postero-inferior direction. The posterior margin of uncinate is sharp, concave and free. It lies parallel to anterior face of bulla ethmoidalis. It is mobile as compared to frontal process of maxilla which is immobile. It can get attached anteriorly to lateral wall or skull base or medially to middle turbinate.

Hiatus Semilunaris

Inferior: The two-dimensional sickle shape cleft between posterior free margin of uncinate and anterior surface of bulla ethmoidalis.

1–2 mm wide.

It leads to infundibulum.

Endoscopic picture of right nasal cavity showing pneumatized uncinate getting attached medially to the middle turbinate (MT) giving a double middle turbinate (DMT) appearance.

Superior: Superior and retrobulbar recesses open into the infundibulum through this.

Infundibulum: Hiatus semilunaris inferioris (2D structure) leads into a three-dimensional space lateral to uncinate process called infundibulum where frontal, maxillary and anterior ethmoidal cells drain.

Ethmoidal bulla: Largest, most constant and easily demonstrable anterior ethmoidal air cell. Forms posterior boundary of frontal recess. This may or may not extend superiorly up to skull base.

Suprabullar cell: This is a cell above bulla ethmoidalis; roof is skull base; its anterior wall does not bulge into frontal sinus. If present this can show anterior ethmoidal artery near its roof.

Frontal bullar cell: This is also a cell above bulla. Its roof is skull base; anterior wall protrudes into frontal sinus.

Sinus lateralis of Grunwald (lateral sinus): It is a space bounded laterally by

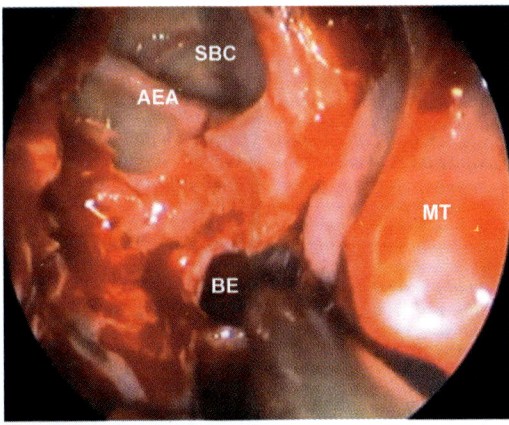

Anterior ethmoidal artery (AEN) is seen in the suprabullar cell (SBC); Bulla ethmoidalis (BE) is seen below this. MT—middle turbinate

lamina papyracea, superiorly by the roof of the ethmoid, inferiorly by roof of bulla, posteriorly by ground lamella and medially by middle turbinate.

Anterior and posterior fontanelles: These are defects in the bony lateral wall of nose between the uncinate process and inferior turbinate covered by connective tissue. These are also known as membranous area of lateral wall of nose. There is sometimes an opening in this membranous fontanelle known as accessory ostium.

These open into maxillary sinus, so should not be confused with natural ostium. Anterior fontanelle is anterior to uncinate insertion and posterior is behind it.

Frontal Recess

Infundibulum opens anterosuperiorly into the frontal recess which is an hour-glass shaped space that acts as a conduit for frontal sinus.

Cells anterior to frontal recess	Cells posterior to frontal recess
Agger nasi—anterolateral	Bulla ethmoidalis—posterior
Kuhn's frontal cells—type 1, 2, 3 and 4—anterior	Suprabullar cells—posteromedial
	Supra-orbital ethmoidal cells—posterolateral
	Frontal bullar cell—posterior

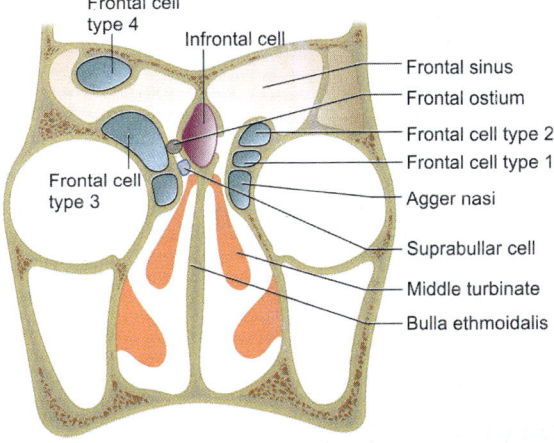

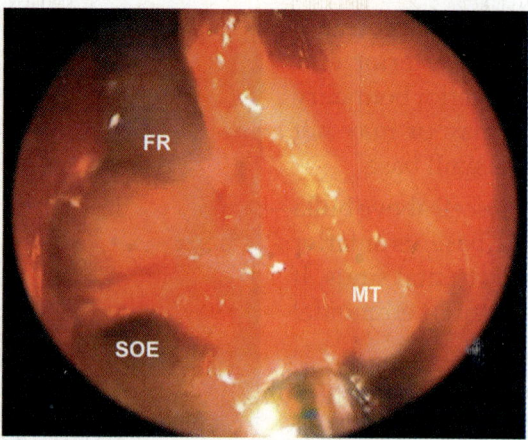

Frontal recess (FR) is seen along with its posteroinferior relation to supraorbital ethmoidal (SOE) cell; vertical lamella of middle turbinate (MT) is also seen medially

Agger nasi: It is a key to frontal recess along with bulla and is the anterior most ethmoidal air cell on lateral wall of nose just anterior to the attachment of middle turbinate.

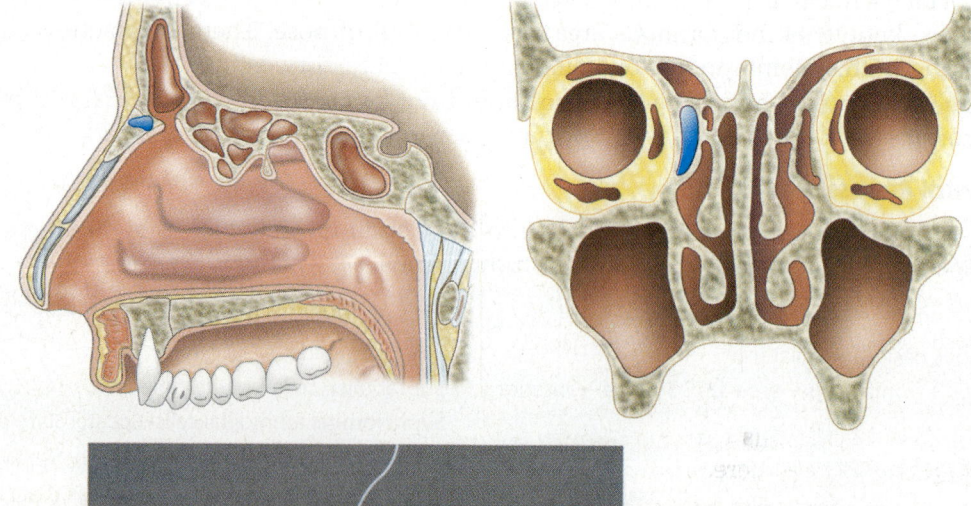

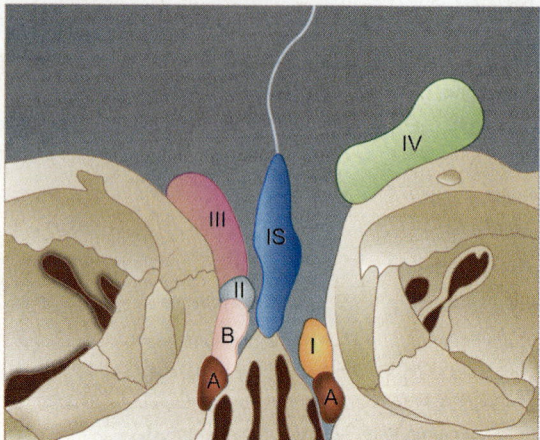

A and B: Agger nasi
I: Type I Frontal cell
II: Type II Frontal cell
III: Type III Frontal cell
IV: Type IV Frontal cell
IS: Interfrontal septal cell

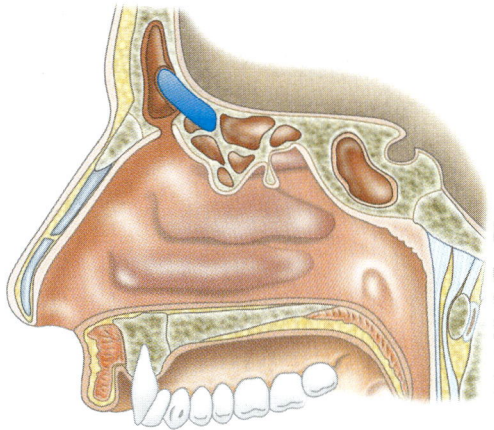 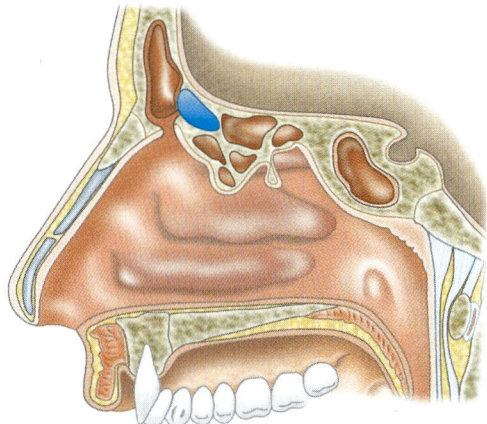

Osteomeatal complex: The uncinate process, the bulla ethmoidalis and infundibulum form the key area of osteomeatal complex and into it drain the frontal, maxillary and anterior ethmoidal sinuses drain.

It consists of: Maxillary ostium, hiatus semilunaris, infundibulum, uncinate process, bulla ethmoidalis, frontal recess.

Attachments of middle turbinate
- *Vertical (anterior 1/3)*: Inserts in sagittal direction on the lateral border of lamina cribrosa.
- *Oblique (Middle 1/3)*: Attached to lamina papyracea.
- *Horizontal (posterior 1/3)*: Attached to lamina papyracea or maxilla.

Concha bullosa: Pneumatized middle turbinate. When very large can cause symptoms like nasal obstruction, headache and sinusitis.

Haller's cells: Ethmoid cells that develop into the floor of the orbit adjacent to and above the maxillary sinus ostium. When missed during surgery can cause recurrent sinusitis.

Onodi cell: It is the pyramidal extension of posterior most ethmoid cell in supero-lateral direction of the sphenoid sinus (at least >1.5 cm), usually optic nerve is found within this cell and injury should be avoided here.

Rigid nasal endoscopes: 0°, 30°, 70° and latest is 45°
- 4 mm in diameter in adults
- 2.7 mm in children

Best for beginners: 0° as it gives direct vision.

Advantages of rigid endoscopes
- Better optics
- Easy to pass

Instrument can be rotated along its axis.

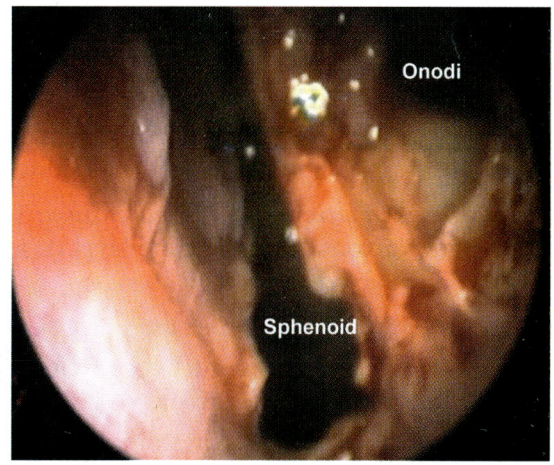

Endoscopic intraoperative picture showing left sphenoid sinus with Onodi cell.

Indications of endoscopic endonasal surgeries

- Chronic sinusitis
- Nasal polyposis
- Epistaxis
- Optic nerve decompression
- Orbital decompression
- Chronic dacryocystitis
- Benign nasal tumors
- CSF leaks
- Hypophysectomy
- Mucocele and pyocele of ethmoid
- Nasal encephalocoeles
- Craniopharyngioma
- Biopsy of nasal mass
- Vidian neurectomy, etc.

Contraindication of FESS

- Sinus infections with intracranial complications
- Osteomyelitis
- Aggressive fungal disease
- Disease involving primarily anterior and lateral wall of frontal sinus
- Malignancy

Tips for identification of site of incision of uncinate process: Usually anterior free end of middle turbinate corresponds with uncinate process. Sulcus is at the insertion of uncinate to lateral wall, so posterior to it incision can be given. Uncinate process is mobile compared with frontal process of maxilla which is immobile. Posterior free margin can also be felt and removed with back biting punch forceps.

Tips for identification of maxillary ostium: It can only be seen after resection of uncinate process. It can be palpated along the bony insertion of inferior turbinate into lateral nasal wall. Pressure against the fontanelles may lead to appearance of air bubbles and ostium can be identified. The bone anterior to ostium is thick and hard. Nasolacrimal duct can get injured if extensive enlargement of ostium is done anteriorly. Haller cell if present should not be missed to achieve good results.

Tips for identification of sphenoid ostium: The upper margin of maxillary ostium is in straight horizontal line with the level of sphenoid sinus ostium. Sphenoid ostia is 1.35 to 1.5 cm above posterior choanae.

Prevention of injuries to orbit: Incision of uncinate should be done in sagittal plane.

Earliest identification of the periorbital fat if there is lamina papyracea erosion or injury. It looks yellowish in color.

Put every tissue removed in saline; only fat and brain tissue float.

Pain and hematoma in the eye under local anesthesia means possible entry to orbit.

Common complications of FESS

Intranasal complications	Orbital complications	Intracranial complications
Bleeding	Periorbital hematoma	CSF leaks
Synechiae	Orbital emphysema	Pneumoencephalus
Crusting	NLD injury	Bleeding
Osteitis	Intraorbital hematoma	Meningitis
	Extraocular muscle entrapment	Brain abscess
	Optic nerve injury	Encephalocoele
		Frontal lobe damage
		Anosmia

Keros' classification of olfactory fossa

Type I: Low lateral lamella

Type II: Higher.

Type III: Most dangerous to surgeon because of high chances of injury to cranial fossa.

Draf Frontal Recess Surgery

Type 1: Obstruction to frontal recess are removed like uncinate, agger nasi, frontal cells, etc.

Type 2: Type 1 + removal of frontal floor

Type 3: Bilateral frontal floor, lower interfrontal septum, upper nasal septum and anterior end of middle turbinate are removed. Similar to modified Lothrop procedure.

Indications of Caldwell-Luc's operation: With the arrival of FESS, the role of CWL operation has declined significantly but it is still done in the following conditions like
- Recurrent AC polyp
- Foreign body in antrum, e.g. amalgum or tooth
- Dentigerous cyst
- Oroantral fistula
- For biopsy in suspected cancer of maxilla
- As an approach to

Sphenoid
- Pterygopalatine fossa
- Transantral ethmoidectomy
- Orbital decompression
- Elevation of orbital floor fracture.

Sphenoid Sinus

The most posteriorly located paranasal sinuses. Pneumatization starts rapidly between 5 and 7 years of age and gets completed by 20 years.

Hamberger's classification: This is done based on its pneumatization
- Sellar (60%) is the commonest; pneumatization extends below the pituitary fossa.
- Presellar (40%)—pneumatization extends to anterior wall of the pituitary fossa.
- Conchal (1%)—minimal pneumatization.

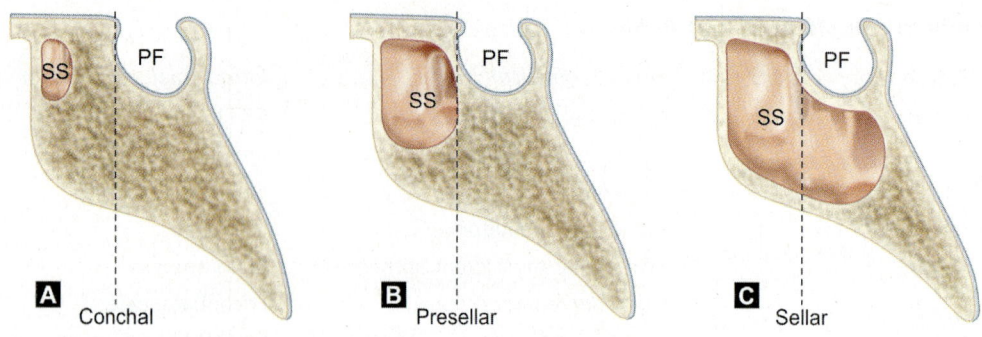

Parasellar Anatomy

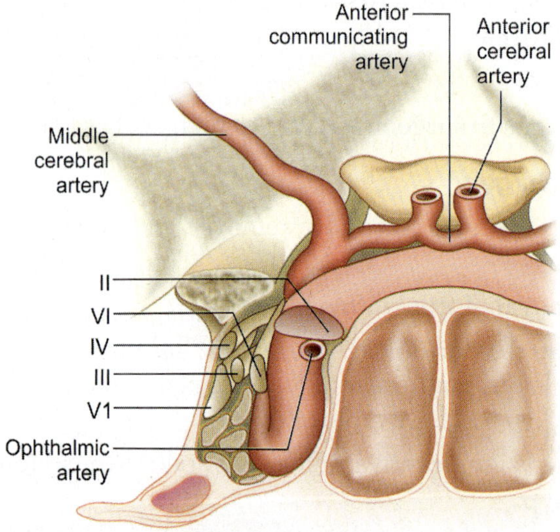

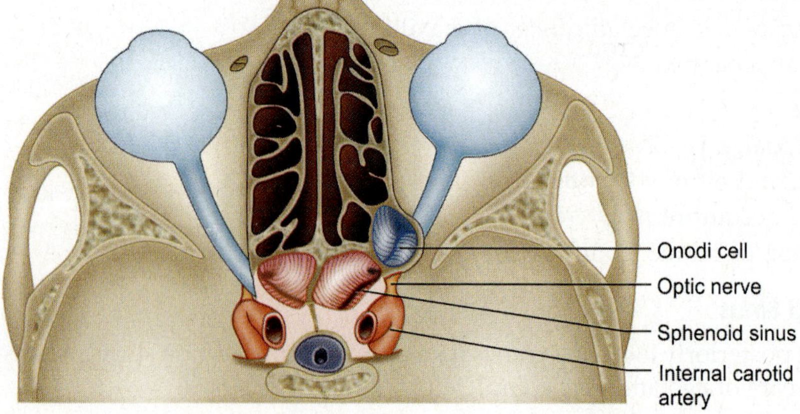

Axial section showing sphenoid sinus, posterior ethmoidal and Onodi cell and their relationship with optic nerve and ICA.

Prominences on the Lateral Wall of Sphenoid Sinus

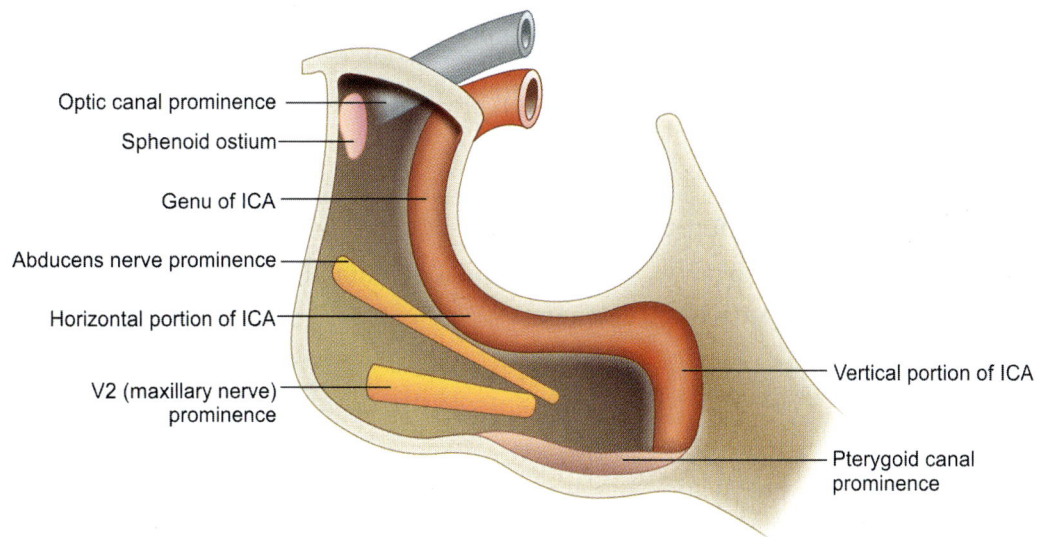

Optic canal prominence
Sphenoid ostium
Genu of ICA
Abducens nerve prominence
Horizontal portion of ICA
V2 (maxillary nerve) prominence
Vertical portion of ICA
Pterygoid canal prominence

Maxillary Sinus

- Antrum of Highmore
  Pyramidal shaped with apex downwards; Present at birth.
  Capacity   15–30 ml
  Dimensions   33 mm height
                    23 mm mediolateral
                    34 mm anterioposterior

Complications of Sinusitis

- Orbital
  - Subperiosteal abscess
  - Orbital cellulites
  - Orbital abscess
  - Orbital apex syndrome
- Osteomyelitis
  - Maxilla—more common in children
  - Forntal—more common in adults
- Intracranial
  - Meningitis
  - Extradural abscess
  - Subdural abscess
  - Brain abscess
  - Cavernous sinus thrombosi
- Descending infections
  - Pharyngitis
  - Otitis media
  - Laryngitis

- Superior orbital syndrome
  - Deep orbital pain
  - Frontal headache
  - Progressive palsy of cranial nerves with decreasing frequency VI > III > IV
- Orbital apex syndrome: All of the above + optic nerve and maxillary division of 5th nerve.

Risk Factor for Sinonasal Tumors

- Hardwood dust (Mahogany): Adenocarcinoma of ethmoid
- Softwood dust: Squamous cell carcinoma
- Nickel
- Boot, shoe and textile workers
- Snuff

Ohngren's line: It is an imaginary plane extending from medical canthus of eye to angle of mandible thus dividing the structures above it as superstructures and below it as infrastructures. Malignancies of suprastructures have the worst prognosis compared to the malignancies involving infrastructures.

Lines of Sebileau and Lederman's classification: In Lederman's classification using two imaginary lines, sinonasal malignancies are divided into suprastructure, mesostructure and infrastructure. Superior line passes through the inferior orbital margin and inferior line passes through the floor of antrum.

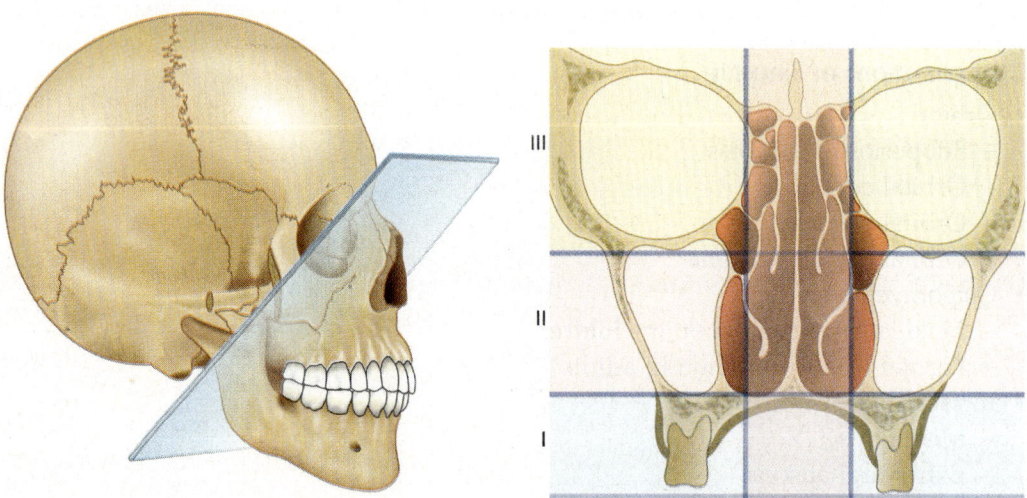

Based on these vertical lines each of the supra, meso and infrastructure has medial and lateral protions.

Benign sinonasal mucosal tumors: Inverted papilloma—it arises from Schneiderian membrane from lateral wall of nose mainly ethmoids. It has been linked to HPV infection in some literatures. It has got 13% chances of conversion into transitional cell carcinoma. In incomplete removal, the recurrence rate is very high. As the name suggests the clinical presentation is usually a papuliferous polypoidal growth arising from the lateral wall of nose. Treatment of this tumor is either endoscopic removal or lateral rhinotomy.

Malignant tumors of maxilla: Squamous cell carcinoma, adenocarcinoma, adenoid cystic carcinoma, mucoepidermoid carcinoma, malignant melanoma and rhabdomyosarcoma.

Malignancy of nose and PNS constitute to 3% of head and neck malignancies. 60–90% of malignant sinonasal tumors are squamous cell carcinoma. Common stage at which the disease is diagnosed is usually IV a (50%). 5 years survival rate in best centers of the world is 30–40%. Local recurrence rate is 40% and distant metastasis is 6% within 12 months. Incidence of lymph node metastasis is 20%. Presentation of sinonasal malignancy could be: (1) Nasal, (2) Orbital, (3) Facial, (4) Palatal, (5) Dental, (6) Infratemporal fossa and (7) Intracranial. CT is the mainstay of investigation and MRI is needed for cranial and orbital invasion. Biopsy can be done by intranasal or Caldwell-Luc approaches and in cases of fungating tumors by simple punch biopsy. Accepted mode of treatment is combination of surgery and radiation therapy.

Incisions for sinonasal malignancy surgeries are: Lateral rhinotomy, Denker's sublabial approach, Weber-Fergusson and facial degloving approach.

Procedures done are: Partial medial maxillectomy (specially for malignant inverted papilloma), total maxillectomy with or without orbital bony floor removal, radical maxillectomy (when pterygoid plates and muscles are involved), radical maxillectomy with orbital exenteration (peri-orbita invasion), inferior partial maxillectomy (inferior palatal/floor of maxillary antrum tumors). Important 4 steps are: (1) Orbital floor involvement, (2) Zygomatic involvement laterally, (3) Anterior facial invasion and (4) Posterior involvement of pterygoid plates and muscles which may change the course of the surgery like removal of bony orbital floor (periosteum left intact), body of zygoma, facial cheek skin, pterygoid muscles and plates. To reduce the bleeding intraoperatively ligation of internal maxillary artery is must.

Deformity produced during maxillectomy are: (1) Orbital floor defect and diplopia (can be reconstructed by rotating septal mucoperichondrium/middle turbinate by fixing to zygoma), (2) Epiphora due to nasolacrimal system injury (DCR is needed), (3) Palatal defect (dental obturator is used to close the defect).

CT and MRI every 6 months postoperatively for 2 years is must for follow-up.

X-ray PNS of a patient with left maxillary carcinoma; note the opacity and surrounding bony erosion (orbital floor).

Lymph nodes involved in carcinoma of maxilla: Retropharyngeal nodes are the first to get involved, however, these are not palpable.

Upper deep cervical then level I submandibular node when jaw, cheek or skin is involved.

Contraindications to maxillectomy: Distant metastasis, contralateral involvement, skull base involvement.

Osteotomies in maxillectomy: Ipsilateral side of hard palate at midline, zygoma/zygomatic process of maxilla, nasal bones/nasal process of maxilla, pterygoid plates.

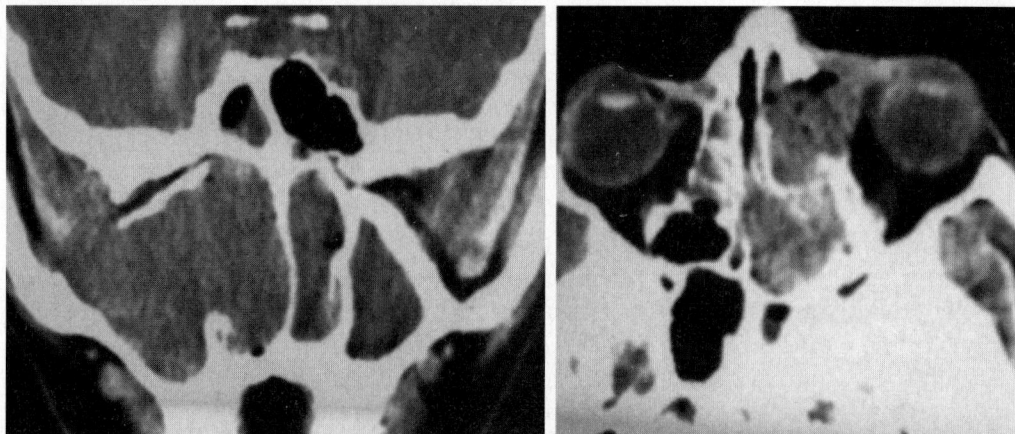

CT PNS of patient with maxillary sinus carcinoma; first picture is a coronal view showing erosion of medial and lateral wall of maxillary sinus; second picture is an axial view showing erosion of medial orbital wall.

Sequelae of maxillectomy: Crusting (because of atrophic changes), change of voice, epiphora, diplopia, lid edema.

CHAPTER 25

Trauma of Face

PRIMARY CARE OF INJURIES TO THE MIDFACE

The basic principles to adhere are A, B, C, D, E = A (airway maintenance—intubation or tracheostomy), B (breathing establishment—aspiration of blood due to severe bleeding—stop bleeding and suction of aspirated blood), C (circulation maintenance—blood transfusion in massive bleeding), D (deficits of neurological and consciousness—head injury assessment), E (exposure of patient to locate polyorgan injuries).

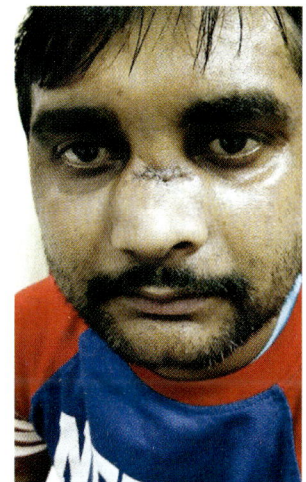

Deformity Following Trauma

Fracture of Nasal Bones and Septum

1. According to direction of impact: (a) Frontal or depressed fractures—splaying of nasal bones, collapse of septum or open book fracture, (b) lateral or angulated fracture: Due to blow from side—one-sided depression and angulation.
2. According to severity of injury:
   Class I: Involves nasal bones and cartilaginous septum, no gross deformity.
   Class II: Involves nasal bones, septum , frontal process of maxilla ethmoid and orbital structure normal.
   Class III: All of the above and fracture extends to ethmoid and orbit. It is further divided into two subtypes—(a) Anterior skull base, posterior wall of frontal sinus and optic canal remain intact; (b) Another type where above are involved.
   Symptoms and signs are bleeding per nose, nasal obstruction, pain, deformity, tenderness, crepitation and periorbital ecchymosis.

Treatment: Under GA nasal bones are disimpacted with Walsham's forceps septum is reduced with Ash's forcep. POP splint is applied over nose.
   Delayed fractures need septorhinoplasty.

Complication of fracture nasal bone: (1) Saddle nose, (2) septal hematoma, (3) septal abscess, (4) septal deviation, (5) CSF rhinorrhea, (6) disorder of smell.

Special nasal fracture: (1) Chevallet, here trauma is because of blow below the nose and septum is fractured in horizontally just below dorsum of nose. (2) Jarjavay fracture, here blow is directly from front with crescentric fracture involving lower cartilaginous septum vomer and perpendicular ethmoid.

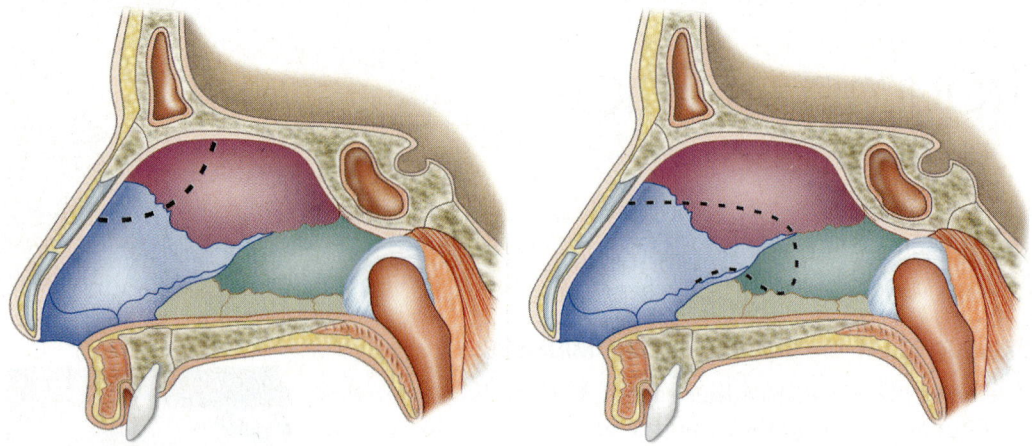

Face is divided into three parts
- *Upper third*: From hair line to superciliary arch
- *Middle third*: From superciliary arch to upper law
- *Lower third*: From hard palate to chin

Nasal bone is the commonest to get fractured due to its prominent position in the face. X-ray shows fractured nasal bone in lateral view of nose.

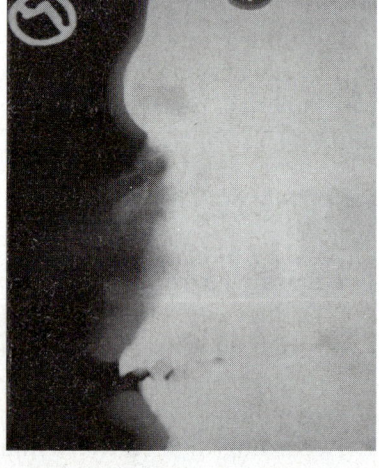

Fractures of Maxilla

Three types:
- *Type I Guérin (Le Fort I)*: Fracture line passes above the floor of nasal cavity through the nasal septum, maxillary sinus and inferior part of medial and lateral pterygoid plates.
- *Type II (Le Fort II)*: Fracture runs from floor of maxillary sinus superiorly to infraorbital margin of lacrimal bone to nasion.
- *Type III (Le Fort III)*: Craniofacial disjunction of facial skeleton from cranial base. The fracture runs from medial wall of orbit to superior orbital fissure and exits across the greater wing of sphenoid and zygomatic bone to zygomatico frontal suture, exact posteriorly it runs under optic foramen to pterygomaxillary fissure and sphenopalatine foramen.

Clinically, there is epistaxis, nasal obstruction, dental malocclusion, periorbital swelling and ecchymosis also k/a raccon eyes, elongation of midface and CSF rhinorrhea. CT scan is very helpful.

Treatment: Manage ABCDE and interdental wiring, intermaxillary fixation, arch bar, plaster head cap and frontal traction in Le Fort II arch bar can be fixed with wire to zygomatic arch both sides for upward traction, all types of Le Fort need upward and frontal traction.

Nowadays use of absorbable miniplates in open reduction have started. For frontal traction, halo frame, box frame, Levant frame, Plaster of Paris head cap all are used. When there is defect in the bone, bone grafts can be used.

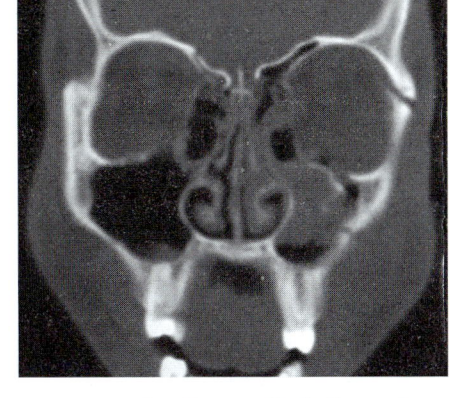

Tripod fracture in the lateral middle third face
Fracture of zygomatic bone at three places:
- Frontozygomatic suture
- Infraorbital rim
- Zygomatic buttress

This can be treated with conservative management when the fracture is undisplaced and mouth opening is normal, Gelle's reduction or open reduction and plating when there is displacement.

MANDIBLE

Develops from second branchial arch
- Angle between body and ascending ramus 110°–120°
- Changes with age in mandible
- Ascending ramus, body angle 140°
- Tooth sockets get resorbed
- Height of body is shortened.

Fracture of mandible with decreasing frequency: Body 29% > condyle 26% > angle 25% > symphysis 17% > ramus 4% > coronoid process 1% > alveolar process.

Most of the fractures are due to direct trauma, however, condylar fracture could be due to indirect trauma, e.g. trauma of chin or opposite side.

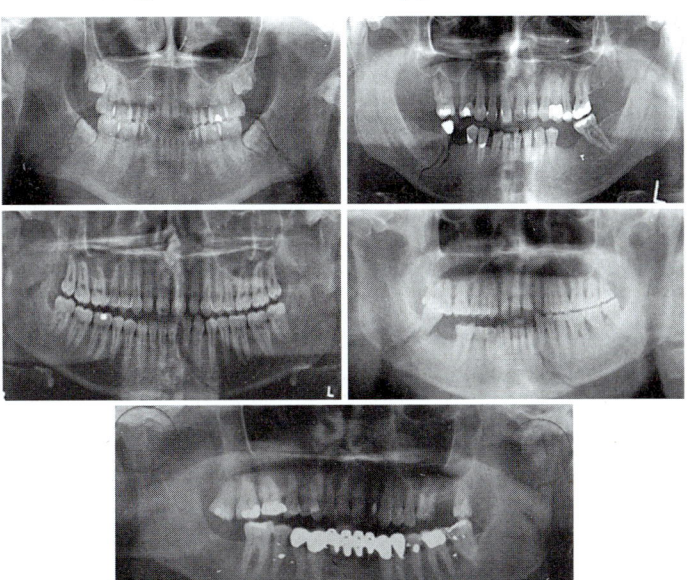

Orthopantamogram (OPG) is a panaromic X-ray of mandible; here there are OPG of various types of mandible fractures.

Treatment of mandibular fracture can be done by various techniques like simple interdental wiring, inter-maxillary fixation (IMF), open reduction and internal fixation with miniplates.

In cases of condylar fracture which are extra-articular and undisplaced, IMF is effective but when the fracture is intracapsular, miniplating or condylectomy is needed.

While doing plating in children, knowledge of ossification centre is necessary to avoid mandibular growth deformity.

ORBITAL BLOW OUT FRACTURE

It is fracture of orbital floor into maxillary antrum and does not involve orbital rim.

Mechanism of injury: Blunt trauma to eye globe by rounded object, this causes compression of orbital contents against thinnest orbital floor and contents herniate into antrum.

Clinical features are epistaxis, enophthalmos, diplopia in vertical plane due to entrapped inferior rectus and oblique, periorbital ecchymosis and anesthesia in distribution of infraorbital nerve.

X-ray occipitomental view shows a tear drop sign due to herniation. CT scan can be helpful.

Treatment is elevation of orbital floor by autogenous bone or septum or silicon or tantalum mesh.

CHAPTER 26

Miscellaneous Points in Nose

Length of adult nasal cavity: 7–8 cm.

Dome of nose: It is the highest point of lower lateral cartilage usually at the junction of medial and lateral crus. Height: 5 cm

Potato nose: Rhinophyma of nose.

Nasal cholesteatoma: It is the collection of granulation tissues and offensive cheesy material in nose in cases of rhinitis caseosa.

Woody nose: Rhinoscleroma.

Allergic nasal crease: It is a transverse crease on external nose, because of repeated rubbing of the nasal cavity in cases of allergic rhinitis.

Nasal valve: It is at the level of anterior end of inferior turbinate, lower end of upper lateral cartilage and corresponding septum.

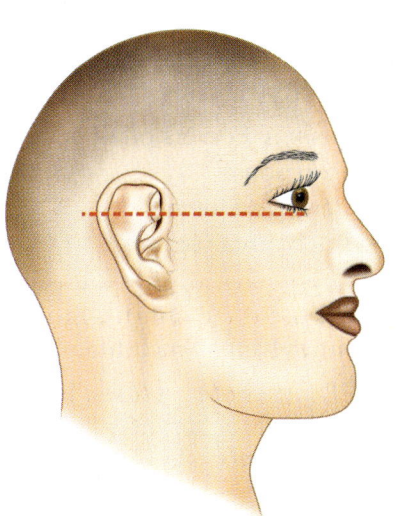

Frankfurt line: A line along the infraorbital border and superior margin of EAC.

Nasal cycle: Cyclical congestion and decongestion of nasal mucosa.

Every 4 to 12 hours. 80% subjects appreciate it. This is the reason for intermittent bilateral nasal obstruction in C-shaped DNS.

Total amount of mucous produced in nose and paranasal sinuses is approximately 1250 ml/day, i.e. 50 ml/hour and 25 ml/hour on one side of nose, total time taken by beating mucocilliary action to move mucous from anterior end of inferior turbinate to pharynx is about 30 minutes.

Things associated with the name of Killian: Killian's polyp (AC polyp), Killian's dehiscence, Killian's speculum, Killian's incision.

Things associated with the name of Cottle: Cottle's test is done to check obstruction caused at nasal valve area. The patient pulls the cheek outward and any obstruction at this site is relieved.

- Cottle's areas of septum
- Anterior caudal valve area
- Superior mid-portion
- Inferior mid-portion
- Posterior choanal area

Tests for mucociliary functions: Saccharin test, ciliary beat frequency, mucosal viscosity, electron microscopy. Usually it takes around 30 mins for nasal mucociliary clearance. If it takes more than one hour, this should raise the suspicion of ciliary dysfunction.

Anosmia

Loss of sense of smell.

Causes: DNS, nasal polyp, neoplasm of nasal cavity, enlarged turbinate, rhinitis, atrophic rhinitis, allergic or vasomotor rhinitis, neurological causes, fracture of base skull involving olfactory nerves, peripheral neuritis, diabetes, syphilis, intracranial tumors, meningitis, senile atrophy.

Hyposmia: Reduced sense of smell.

Cacosmia: Perception of foul smell because of intrinsic cause.

   Causes are: Dental infection, malignancy, foreign body in nose, lung abscess, maxillary sinusitis.

Parosmia: Perversion of smell and patient complaining of disgusting odors.
- Functional
- Peripheral neuritis
- Intracranial tumors
- Drugs, that is, streptomycin

   Olfactory examination is performed according to UPSIT (University of Pennysylvania Smell Identification Test) guidelines.

ENT causes of proptosis: Juvenile angiofibroma, carcinoma of ethmoid, carcinoma of maxilla, nasopharyngeal carcinoma, cavernous sinus thrombosis, fungal mass, orbital abscess, mucocele of frontoethmoid region, fibro-osseous dysplasia, faciomaxillary injuries.

Causes of unilateral pulsating proptosis: Arteriovenous fistula between ICA and cavernous sinus, carotico cavernous fistula
- Aneurysm of ophthalmic artery
- Cricoid aneurysm of orbit
- Rapidly expanding tumors, e.g. sarcoma

Telecanthus: Increase in intercanthal distance, increase >1/2 of interpupillary distance. ENT causes
- Fracture of ethmoid or midfacial region
- JNA (angiofibroma)
- Ethmoid malignancy
- Esthesioneuroblastoma

- Injuries
- Ethmoidal polyps

Cavernous sinus thrombosis: Any infection in dangerous area, orbit, sinuses and parapharyngeal space may be responsible for cavernous sinus thrombosis.

Infection reaches to cavernous sinus through,

Angular vein (face) → Ophthalmic (orbit) → Pterygoid plexuses (sinuses) → Lateral and medial petrosal sinus → Cavernous sinus

Myiasis of Nasal Cavity

- Maggots in nose
- Maggots are larvae of fly (genus *Chrysomyia*)
- Conditions in which maggots are found
  - Atrophic rhinitis
  - Poor personal hygiene
  - Leprosy
  - Syphilis
  - Sinonasal malignancy

Life cycle of maggots: Eggs hatch in 24 hours → larval stage for 2–7 days → pupae stage for 3–6 days → adult fly.

Common season for maggots in the year: August to October.

Removal of maggots: Should be picked up by forceps after instilling a few drops of chloroform, water, paraffin, oil or ether. Turpentine oil can be used but it is very irritating.

These larvae bury into the tissue once the light is shown, so repeated attempts should be made. Patient should be kept away from other patients in ward, preferably in mosquito net.

Trismus

- Inability to open mouth
- Causes
  - Quinsy
  - Parapharyngeal abscess
  - Alveolar infection
  - Submucous fibrosis
  - Acute parotitis
  - Tetanus
  - Ankylosis of TM joint

Malignancy of tonsil, maxilla, oral cavity, base tongue and JNA with infratemporal fossa extension, etc.

ENT diseases which are common in females:

- Atrophic rhinitis
- Otosclerosis
- Post-cricoid carcinoma

- Functional aphonia
- Glomus tumors

Differential diagnosis of nasal mass: Nasal polyp, inferior turbinate hypertrophy, foreign body, concha bullosa, inverted papilloma, angiofibroma, septal hematoma, septal abscess, rhinosporidiosis, sinonasal malignancy, etc.

Radiology in Rhinology

Occipitomental view (Water's): Maxillary, frontal and sphenoid sinus.

Occipitofrontal (Caldwell's): Ethmoid and frontal.

Lateral: Sphenoid.

Submentovertical (skull base): Ethmoid and sphenoid sinuses and zygomatic arches.

Oblique view: Ethmoid.

Differential diagnosis of maxillary sinus opacity: Maxillary sinusitis, AC polyp, mucocele, carcinoma, dental cyst, dentigerous cyst, fibrous dysplasia, benign tumors, blood following facial trauma.

CHAPTER 27

Nasopharyngeal Angiofibroma and Nasopharyngeal Carcinoma

Nasopharynx: Size 4 cm high, 4 cm wide and 2 cm deep.

Opening of eustachian tube in nasopharynx 1 cm behind and little lower to posterior end of inferior turbinate.

Fossa of Rosenmuller: Above and behind the eustachian tube opening.

Boundaries:
- *Anterior*: Eustachian tube and levator palatine.
- *Posterior*: Retropharyngeal space which contains node of Rouvière
- *Medial*: Nasopharyngeal cavity.
- *Lateral*: Tensor palatini, mandibular nerve and prestyloid compartment of parapharyngeal space.
- *Superior*: Foramen lacerum and floor of carotid canal.

Tumors of Nasopharynx

Benign: Papilloma, pleomorphic adenoma, angiofibroma, neurofibroma and neurilemmoma.

Malignant: SCC, lymphoma, sarcoma, adenocarcinoma, adenoid cystic carcinoma.

Miscellaneous: Chordoma, craniopharyngioma.

NASOPHARYNGEAL ANGIOFIBROMA

Histologically benign but locally invasive tumor of nasopharynx present exclusively in adolescent males.

Median age of presentation—15 years

Site of origin is found to be superior margin of sphenopalatine foramen.

Gross appearance is lobulated, pinkish mass.

Theories:
- Hormonal theory
- Embryonic remnant theory
- Enchondral bone theory

I. Ringertz theory: JNA arises from skull base periosteum; II. Som and Neffson theory: Hypertrophy of periosteum happens in response to hormonal influence; III. Bensch and Ewing theory: Tumor arises from embryonic fibrocartilage between basi sphenoid and basi occiput; IV. Brunner theory: Tumor originates from conjoined pharyngobasilar and buccopharyngeal fascia; V. Marten et al theory: Tumor arises due to deficiency of androgens or overactivity of oestrogen; VI. Sternberg theory: It could be a type of hemangioma like cutaneous hemangioma; VII Osborn theory: Could be due to either a hamartoma or residual fetal erectile tissues which are under the influence of hormones. The most commonly accepted theory is that JNA arises from sex steroid dependent hamartomatous tissue in the turbinate cartilage.

Why angiofibroma bleeds?
Vessels of angiofibroma are not lined by tunica media (smooth muscles) and hence they do not undergo vasoconstriction when bleeding starts. For this reason, biopsy of angiofibroma is contraindicated.

Differential diagnosis
- Antrochoanal polyp
- Adenoids

Tumors of nose and paranasal sinuses
- Granulomatous condition of nose and paranasal sinuses
- Rhinosporidiosis
- Hypertrophied inferior turbinate

Extensions of angiofibroma
- Anteriorly to nasal cavity
- Medially by destroying the nasal septum and entering into contralateral nasal cavity. Posteriorly through choanae → nasopharynx → foramen of Morgagni → neck Laterally through pterygomaxillary fissure → infratemporal fossa → cheek → oral cavity.
- Superiorly to ethmoidal sinuses
- Intracranial extension
  - Middle cranial fossa through infratemporal fossa and infraorbital fissure
  - Anterior cranial fossa through ethmoids

Feeders of angiofibroma

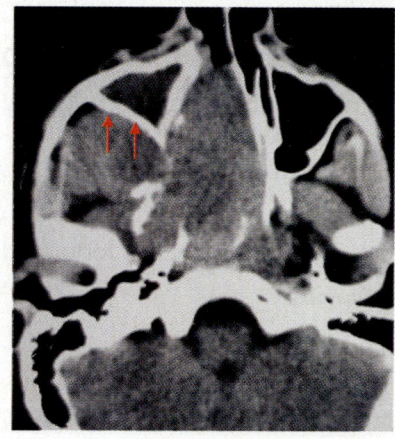

- Internal maxillary artery
- Ascending pharyngeal artery
- Sphenopalatine artery
- Contralateral maxillary artery
- Branches of internal carotid

Antral sign (Holmann-Miller sign): Radiological finding in nasopharyngeal angiofibroma; anterior bowing of posterior wall of maxillary sinus.

CT findings diagnostic of angiofibroma: Erosion of medial pterygoid plate on CT scan.

Staging of nasopharyngeal angiofibroma

	Fisch staging of juvenile nasopharyngeal angiofibroma
Stage I	The tumor is limited to the sphenopalatine foramen nasopharynx and nasal cavity without bone destruction
Stage II	The tumor invades the nasal sinuses or the pterygomaxillary fossa with bone destruction
Stage IIIa	The tumor invades the infratemporal fossa or orbit without intracranial involvement
Stage IIIb	The tumor invades the infratemporal fossa or orbit with intracranial and extradural involvement
Stage IVa	The tumor shows intracranial, extradrual and/or intradural invasion, without invasion of optic nerve, sella, or cavernous sinus
Stage IVb	The tumor in stage IVa with invasion of optic nerve, sella and/or cavernous sinus

How to reduce bleeding during surgery?

Hypotensive anesthesia: Drugs used are sevoflorane as inhalation agent with phentanyl, nitroprusside, nitroglycerin, labetalol, trimethaphan.

Preoperative embolization should be done one day prior to surgery.

The materials used are:
- Muscle pieces (finely sliced sternocleidomastoid)
- Gel foam
- Teflon powder
- Silicone sphere
- Liquid polymers
  Estrogen 5 mg twice daily two weeks prior to surgery
  Preoperative radiotherapy 3000 rad
  External carotid artery ligation

Approaches to remove angiofibroma
Inferior
  Transpalatal (Wilson)
  Transpalatal and transpterygoid
Anterior
  Transfacial (lateral rhinotomy)
Trans/endonasal and transmaxillary
  Facial degloving approach
Lateral
    Transzygomatic
    Frontotemporal craniotomy

Areas of recurrence in angiofibroma: Cheek, nasopharynx, orbit, infratemporal fossa, sphenoid.

Branches of external carotid artery
- Ascending pharyngeal artery
- Superior thyroid artery

- Lingual artery
- Facial artery
- Occipital artery
- Postauricular artery
- Internal maxillary artery (terminal)
- Superficial temporal artery (terminal)

Branches of thyrocervical trunk
- Inferior thyroid artery
- Transverse cervical artery
- Suprascapular artery

NASOPHARYNGEAL CARCINOMA

- 10–15 times more common in Chinese and South-East Asians.
- Factors associated with cancer of nasopharynx.
- Epstein-Barr virus (main), tobacco, diet—salted fish, nitrosamines

Occupation:
- Industrial fumes and chemicals
- Household smoke

Presentation:
- Lymphadenopathy 60%
- Epistaxis and nasorespiratory symptoms 40%
- Cranial nerve involvement, V, VI, IX, X 20%
- Aural symptoms

Serodiagnosis:
- IgA VCA (viral capsid antigen)
- IgA EA (early antigen)
  These serological titres can be used for follow-up of these cases.
  VCA can be used for screening of nasopharyngeal carcinoma.

Treatment: Radiotherapy.

Oral Cavity and Throat

CHAPTER 28

Sleep Apnea

Snoring: A noise generated from the upper airway due to partial obstruction either because of mass effect or collapse of walls.

Possible sites of obstruction for airway can be at:
• Nostrils, nasal cavity and nasopharynx
• Oropharynx
• Hypopharynx and larynx

Heroic snoring: Snoring is heard in adjacent room when the door is kept open.

Apnea: Cessation of airflow at nostril or mouth at least for 10 seconds.
Apnea index = Number of apnea attacks per hour.

Sleep apnea grading
• Mild 5–20 apnea/hour
• Moderate 20–40 apnea/hour
• Severe >40 apnea/hour

Sleep apnea syndrome can be diagnosed when there is
• > 30 episodes during 7 hours or
• > 7 episodes in one hour.

Examination: Modified Mallampati score is helpful in diagnosing the narrow airway at the level of oropharynx (explained in detail in the next chapter). Flexible nasopharyngolaryngoscopy is helpful.

Muller's maneuver: It is done by placing the tip of flexible nasopharyngolaryngoscope at the oropharynx and the tract below is visualized. When the patient inspires, if the walls collapse below the level of oropharynx and base of tongue collapses, it is called positive Muller's maneuver and in these cases UPPP will not give good results.

Investigations done X-ray PNS, nasopharynx
• X-ray chest
• Sleep pulse oximetry (screening test)
• Polysomnogram (gold standard)
  – EOG, ECG, EMG and ENG
  – Also look for nasal airflow and abdominal movements.

- Flexible sleep endoscopy
  Blood tests like thyroid function tests and lipid profile should also be done.

Management

- Weight reduction and lifestyle modifications like abstinence from alcohol
- Positional advice (lateral position while sleeping reduces apnea index)
- CPAP: Gold standard medical treatment
- Hypoglossal nerve stimulation

UPPP (Uvulopharyngopalatoplasty):

- Laser reduction of obstructive tissue
- Radiofrequency surgery
- Tracheostomy—Gold standard surgical treatment

Latest technique: Transoral robotic surgery has been started in treatment of obstructive sleep apnea. Disadvantage is the expensive nature of the surgery.

CHAPTER 29

Tonsils and Adenoid

Waldeyer's ring: Inner and outer rings.

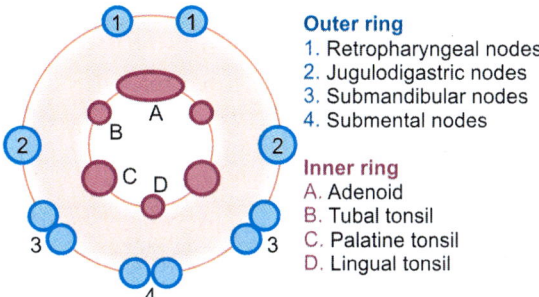

Outer ring
1. Retropharyngeal nodes
2. Jugulodigastric nodes
3. Submandibular nodes
4. Submental nodes

Inner ring
A. Adenoid
B. Tubal tonsil
C. Palatine tonsil
D. Lingual tonsil

Outer and inner Waldeyer rings

Inner ring is a group of lymphoid tissue around the pharynx. It helps in immunoglobulin production and maturation of B and T lymphocytes.

It consists of:
- Adenoid (also called Luschka's tonsil)
- Tubal tonsil (also called Gerlach's tonsil)
- Palatine tonsil
- Lingual tonsil
- Lymphoidal follicles on posterior pharyngeal wall
  Outer ring consists of:
- Retropharyngeal and parotid group of lymph nodes
- Jugulodigastric lymph nodes
- Submandibular lymph nodes
- Submental lymph nodes

PALATINE TONSIL

Pair of dense lymphoid tissue found on the lateral wall of oropharynx between the anterior (palatoglossus) and posterior (palatopharyngeus) muscles.

141

Two surfaces: Medial and lateral; medial is crypted. Two poles—upper and lower; upper is attached to soft palate and lower to the tongue.

Plica triangularis: It is a triangular fold of mucosal membrane which passes from anterior pillar to base of tongue. It can be easily appreciated while examining the oropharynx.

Plica semilunaris: It is a mucosal fold from the anterior pillar to posterior pillar on the superior pole of the tonsil.

Differences between adenoid and tonsil

Features	Palatine tonsil	Adenoid	Lingual tonsil
Location	Laterally in the oropharynx	Posterosuperior in the nasopharynx in midline between two torus tubarius	In the base of tongue in midline
Relation to age	Grows to maximum till 8 years and persists into adult life	Grows to maximum till 5 years and atrophy starts and completes at 12 years	Persists even after 8 years
Surface	Shows multiple crypts on medial surface	No crypts are present	Crypts present
Mucosal covering	Non-keratinized squamous	Ciliated columnar	Non-keratinized squamous
Capsule	Present which is condensed pharyngobasilar fascia	Absent	Absent
Blood supply	Named vessels as listed below	No named feeders; only adjacent plexus	No named feeders; only adjacent plexus
Pain on inflammation	Present	Absent	Present

Tonsillar bed
- *Pharyngobasilar fascia*: Paratonsillar vein
- *Superior constrictor*: Falciparum ligament and tonsillar artery
- Styloglossus
- Buccopharyngeal fascia
  Lymphoid cluster is present in upper pole and plica semilunaris.
  Lower pole has tonsillar branch of lingual artery and plica triangularis.

Blood supply of tonsil
- *Tonsillar artery*: Branch of facial artery
- *Ascending palatine*: Branch of facial artery
- *Descending palatine*: Branch of maxillary artery
- *Dorsal linguae*: Branch of lingual artery
- *Tonsillar branch*: Ascending pharyngeal artery

Venous drainage of tonsil: Paratonsillar vein and peritonsillar venous plexus that drain into pharyngeal venous plexus or facial vein.

Main source of bleeding during tonsillar surgery is venous. It should be kept in mind that an attack of hypoxia during anesthesia like subclinical asthma getting exaggerated with GA drugs is a common cause for bleeding during tonsillectomy.

Type of acute tonsillitis
- Acute catarrhal
- Acute follicular
- Acute parenchymatous
- Acute membranous

Bacteria etiology for acute tonsillitis
- Group A beta hemolytic streptococci
- *Haemophilus influenzae*
- *Staphylococcus aureus*
- *Streptococcus pneumoniae*

Causes of unilateral tonsillar swellings
1. Lymphomas (Hodgkin and NHL)
2. Carcinoma of tonsil (SCC)
3. Parapharyngeal swellings (lymph nodes, abscesses and schwannomas)
4. Peritonsillar and tonsillar abscesses

Indications of tonsillectomy
- Chronic tonsillitis
- Recurrent tonsillitis—at least 7 episodes in last year/5 episodes in each of last 2 years/3 episodes in each of last 3 years
  - What is one episode—sore throat with either one of the following features like fever, cervical lymphadenopathy, positive culture or tonsillar exudates.
- Sleep apnea syndrome
- Large size leading to dyspnea or dysphasia
- Unilateral enlarged tonsil for biopsy
- Attack of peritonsillitis—interval tonsillectomy is done
- As an approach to glossopharyngeal neurectomy and styloidectomy.

Signs of chronic tonsillitis
- Congestion of anterior pillar.
- Cheesy material comes out while pressing the tonsil (Irwin Moore's sign)
- Bilateral persistently enlarged jugulodigastric nodes.

Contraindications of tonsillectomy
- <4 years of age as even small bleeding can cause shock
- Cleft palate—overt or submucous cleft
- Bleeding diathesis
- Active URI

Hemorrhages involved in tonsillectomy
1. *Primary*: During the time of surgery or within 6 hours of postoperative period.
2. *Reactionary*: Can occur from 6 hours to 24 hours of operation.
3. *Secondary*: After 24 hours of operation. Can occur even up to 3 weeks after surgery.

Pathophysiology in relation to bleeding following tonsillectomy: Immediately cut blood vessel goes onto vasospasm following which there will be platelet aggregation and adhesion to the cut edges. Mature clot, i.e. web of fibrin forms around these aggregated platelets proximal to the cut end of the vessel by the time the spasm goes away. The vasospasm of the vessel remains for 4–6 hours and when the dilatation of the vessel starts, the hemostasis is maintained by the formation of clot. Only named arteries have enough pressure to displace the formed clots to continue to bleed, whereas unnamed smaller vessels cannot.

Bleeding can occur in tonsillectomy due to the following reasons:
1. Primary bleeding is due to either slippage of ligature or weak or failed vasospasm
    A. Nutritional deficiency mainly vitamin C (scurvy)
    B. von Willebrand's disease
2. Reactionary bleeding is due to failure of clot formation
    A. Sharply cut wound
    B. Deficient clotting factors or thrombocytopenia
    C. Vitamin K deficiency
    D. Diseases like von Willebrand's disease, hemophilia, etc.

Management of post-tonsillectomy bleeding: Identify the bleeder and ligate it if bleeding occurs in immediate postoperative period (primary or reactionary).

If bleeding is secondary, remove the clot, observe and start antibiotics.

If all the actions fail to control the bleeding keep a gauze pack or gel foam between the tonsillar pillars and suture them together. Even when this fails then give blood transfusion and bleeding will stop which justify that there was some clotting factor deficiency.

Pathophysiology of post-tonsillectomy hemorrhage is given in detail in the chapter of hemostatic drugs in pharmacology in ENT chapter.

What is intracapsular tonsillectomy?
Here 90% of the tonsillar tissue is removed by coblator. More useful in sleep apnea syndrome rather than tonsillitis. Widely done in western countries. Risk of bleeding is high.

Quinsy (peritonsillar abscess): Collection of pus between tonsillar capsule and superior constrictor. Usually occurs at the upper pole. Patient will have pain, excess salivation, characteristic hot potato voice, fever. Treated by incision and drainage and systemic antibiotics in acute phase followed by interval tonsillectomy.

Hot tonsillectomy: Tonsillectomy in acute stage. Bleeding is more and due to edema, the dissection and plane identification is difficult.

Differentials for membranes over the tonsil: Oral thrush (fungal infections seen in immunocompromised patients—*Candida albicans*).

Malignancy:
• SCC, adenoid cystic, adenocarcinoma and mucoepidermoid carcinoma.
• Lymphoma, melanoma

Infections:
• Streptococcal tonsillitis

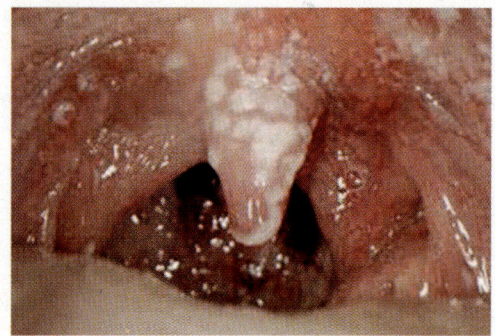

Oral thrush

- Diphtheria (greyish, bleeds on removal with associated bull's neck lymphadenopathy)
- Vincent angina
- IMN (infectious mononucleosis)
- Peritonsillar abscess

Blood diseases
- Leukemia, agranulocytosis
- Miscellaneous
- Aphthous ulcer, Beçhet's syndrome and traumatic ulcer

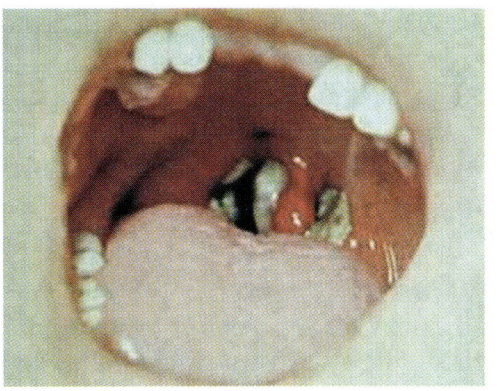

Causes of hard tonsil
- Malignancy
- SCC, lymphoma
- Calcification in tonsil
- Tonsillolith
- Enlarged styloid process (with lateral cervicofacial pain—Eagle syndrome)
- Foreign body in tonsil

ADENOID (LUSCHKA'S TONSIL)

Spontaneous regression—up to 12 years of age
Maximum size—at age of 5 years

Blood supply
- Plexus of vessels like ascending palatine branch of facial artery
- Ascending pharyngeal artery of external carotid artery
- Pharyngeal branch of maxillary artery

Lymphatic supply: Upper jugulodigastric, retropharyngeal and parapharyngeal lymph nodes.

Symptoms and sign of enlarged adenoid
- Nasal obstruction
- Nasal discharge
- Rhinolalia clausa
- Eustachian tube dysfunction leading to serous otitis media and conductive hearing loss
- Mouth breathing, snoring and sleep apnea syndrome
- Recurrent URI
- Characteristic adenoid facies.

Adenoid facies and other features
- Open mouth and mouth breathing
- Pinched nose
- Crowded incisors
- Gingival hyperplasia

- Hypoplastic upper lip and maxilla
- Loss of nasolabial fold
- Hanging mandible
- High-arched palate

Dull or duffer-like expression
- Pectus excavatum
- Harrison sulcus
- Pigeon chest

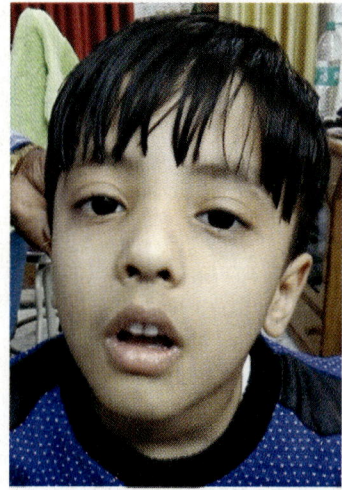

Adenoid facies

Differentials of adenoid hypertrophy: JNA, antrochoanal polyp, rhinosporidiosis, nasopharyngeal tumors.

Surgery for adenoid hypertrophy: Position is same as for tonsillectomy; most times it is done in combination with tonsillectomy. It can be shaved off with adenoid curette after palpating and estimating the size of the adenoid to avoid damage to the eustachian tube orifice. On palpation adenoid will feel like a bag of worms. Recent modalities like removal with endoscopic-guided microdebrider or suction coagulation. Bleeding after the adenoidectomy can be managed with posterior nasal packing.

Vincent's angina
- Also called trench mouth
- Diagnosed in trenches of World War II.
- Necrotizing gingivitis involving gums and oral cavity.

Organisms
- *Borrelia vincentii* (spirochete)
- Anaerobic bacteria like fusiform bacilli

Treatment
- Penicillin

Various Causes for Halitosis
1. Dental caries
2. Chronic tonsillitis
3. Chronic sinusitis
4. Atrophic rhinitis
5. Poor oral hygiene
6. Neglected vegetative foreign body in aero-digestive tract
7. Acid peptic disease and GERD

MODIFIED MALLAMPATTI'S CLASSIFICATION

This scoring is an assessment for easiness of direct laryngoscopy, intubation and predictor for sleep apnea. Higher the class, more difficult is the intubation, DL, esophagoscopy, bronchoscopy and even tonsillectomy. Large size tongue is usually associated with hypothyroidism, acromegaly, morbid obesity, amyloidosis and lymphangiomas.

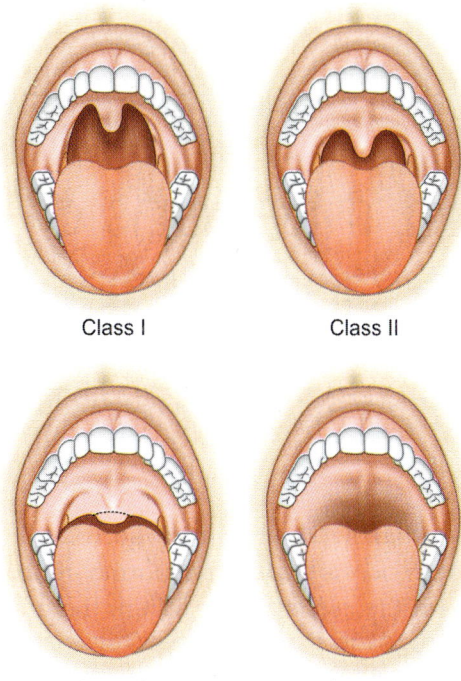

Class I   Class II

Class III   Class IV

Class	Description
I. On simple oral cavity exam.	Soft palate, uvula, anterior and posterior pillars of tonsil visible
II. On simple oral cavity exam.	Soft palate and uvula visible
III. On simple oral cavity exam.	Soft palate and base of uvula visible
IV. On simple oral cavity exam.	Soft palate not visible at all

CHAPTER 30

Premalignant Lesions of Oral Cavity and Oropharynx

1. *Leukoplakia*

a. Leukoplakia simplex—lesion is not raised from surrounding mucosa

b. Leukoplakia verrucosa—lesion is raised than normal mucosa

c. Leukoplakia ulcerosa—in the center of the lesion, there is an ulcer. This is often called erythroplakia. It has the maximum risk for conversion into malignancy. Ulceration is the result of microscopic fight between local body immune cells and cancer cells which are having non-self proteins, thus taken as foreign body by local immune cells and they tried to destroy cancer cells leaving ulcer behind. Local host immune cells are macrophages and killer T-lymphocytes.

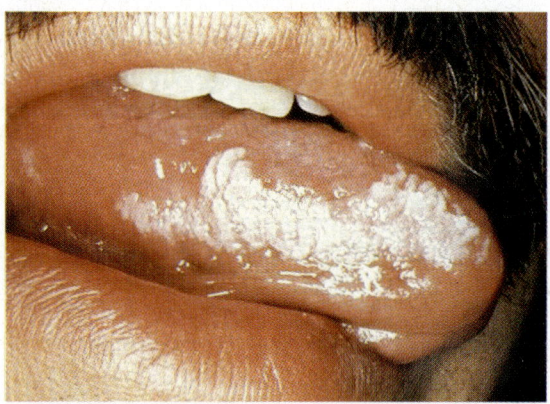

Verrucous leukoplakia without ulceration

Factors such as tobacco smoking, chewing, alcoholism, nutritional deficiencies (like B$_{12}$ or vitamin C and iron) and local irritation or trauma due to sharp tooth are responsible. Sharp tooth can be either sharp towards medial aspect, thus responsible for SCC of lateral border of tongue or sharp towards lateral aspect, thus responsible for SCC of buccal mucosa.

Tar of tobacco is also known as aryl hydrocarbon is a strong carcinogen. If it gains entry into traumatized mucosa of buccal or tongue lateral border can lead to very fast metamorphosis of normal cell into carcinomatous cells.

2. *Oral submucous fibrosis (OSMF):* Submucosa is replaced by fibrous tissue. The uvula is pulled anteriorly and palate will form a Gothic arch appearance. There can be formation of multiple fibrous strands within the oral cavity. Oral submucous fibrosis is common among betel-nut user in any form. Betel-nut contains arycholine—a compound similar to acetylcholine which can cause constant muscle spasm and gradually mouth opening will be restricted with fibrosis of lamina propria. This was for the first time diagnosed and named by Dr Pindborg, a British doctor Posted in South India during British rule. These patients later on develop severe oral ulceration on taking chillies. This condition can be treated with injection triamcinolone 40 mg in bilateral retromolar trigones and in the fibrous strands every 2 weeks for 6–8 times. Interval needs to be prolonged in females in reproductive age group. Tobacco usage should be stopped in any form.

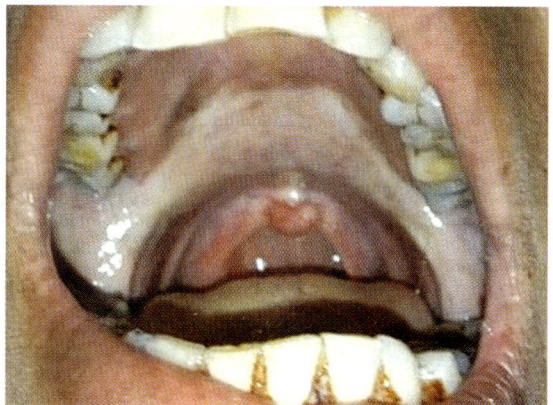

OSMF with Gothic arch palate with the uvula pulled anteriorly

3. *Bowen's disease*

4. *Oral lichen planus:* Chronic inflammatory autoimmune mucocutaneous disease; its oral lesions are pre-malignant in nature. It may be associated with hepatitis C infection.

Factors Inducing Malignancy

Remember EIGHT "S":

1. Smoking
2. Spirit (alcohol)
3. Sharp teeth
4. Spices
5. Submucous fibrosis
6. Syphilis
7. Sepsis
8. Sideropenic dysphagia

In patients undergoing surgery for either leukoplakia or oral carcinoma, it should always be associated with dental extraction or smoothening of the sharp edges of the teeth to prevent conversion into malignancy in earlier and recurrence in the later.

CHAPTER 31

Trachea and Bronchial Tree

TRACHEA

It is a musculocartilaginous tube extending down from the lower end of subglottis till carina where it divides into right and left bronchi (C6 to T5). Length of trachea in adult is 10–12 cm. Trachea has 16–20 incomplete, semicircular cartilaginous rings anteriorly whose ends are connected posteriorly by trachealis muscle. This maintains the lumen of the trachea intact at all the times.

Dimensions:
- Transverse diameter 20 mm
- Anteroposterior diameter 16–20 mm
- Tracheal bifurcation is located 25 cm from upper central incisors in adults.

Stridor: It occurs due to partial obstruction of larger airways—supraglottis, glottis, subglottis and/or trachea. It can be inspiratory (laryngeal), expiratory (tracheal) or biphasic.

Tracheostomy

It is the procedure of making an artificial fistula between the skin and trachea. The stoma is maintained with the help of a tracheostomy tube. This procedure can overcome proximal airway obstruction, decrease dead space volume, function as a new airway following laryngectomy, etc.

Normal anatomical dead space is 150 ml, which decreases by 30–50% following a tracheostomy.

Moser's dictum for tracheostomy: 'The time to do the tracheostomy is when you first think about its need'.

Signs of respiratory distress
- Tachypnea
- Suprastrenal, epigastric and intercostal retractions
- Using accessory muscles (sternomastoid, trapezius, scaleni)
- Nasal flaring
- Deranged blood gas analysis—pO_2 <50 %; pCO_2 > 50%.

Indications for tracheostomy
1. Congenital malformations like Pierre Robin sequence, subglottic stenosis, congenital laryngeal palsy, laryngeal webs, laryngomalacia, laryngeal clefts, etc.
2. Infections like epiglottitis, croupe, retropharyngeal abscess, laryngeal diphtheria, Ludwig's angina, peritonsillar abscess, laryngeal TB.
3. Tumors—laryngeal papillomatosis, hemangiomas, lymphangiomas, laryngeal carcinoma, oropharyngeal carcinoma, other benign tumors of oro/hypo pharynx and larynx.
4. Traumatic—maxillofacial fractures, penetrating or crush injuries to neck causing laryngeal fractures or dislocations, burns, instrumentations like esophagoscopy, laryngoscopy or bronchoscopy, flail chest, pneumothorax, etc.
5. Neurogenic—bilateral recurrent laryngeal palsy, coma, polio, etc.
6. Prolonged intubation
7. Proximal foreign body
8. ARDS
9. Pre-operative tracheostomy in cases of total laryngectomy
10. To maintain airway intra-operatively during oropharyngeal or laryngeal surgeries.

Size of tracheostomy tube
For <12 years of age
  Age/3 + 3.5 × 3 for FG (French gauge)

For >12 years of age
  Age/4 + 4.5 × 3 for FG

Simple formula for calculating tube size is: Age + 12 up to 18 years, e.g. a 4 years old child will need (4 + 12) = 16 number tracheostomy tube.

Above 18 years we have to choose according to the size of trachea which could range between 30 and 38 F or roughly size of his thumb diameter.

Difficulties during tracheostomy: Short neck, obesity, local inflammation, tracheal shift by large or malignant thyroid, cervical vertebral abnormalities like spondylosis, tracheal stenosis, laryngeal malignancies, subglottic hemangiomas, tracheal push/pull by lung pathology, aneurysm of brachiocephalic trunk.

During emergency tracheostomy it is advised not to sedate the patient.

Care of tracheostomy tube at home: Teach patient/relatives about the anatomy and physiology of the process, stoma and skin care. They should also be taught to identify stridor.

Cotton should be avoided as cotton fibers may be inhaled and cause granuloma formation.

Moist gauge piece should be kept over the tracheostomy tube for humidification. This prevents crust formation.

Better to use uncuffed tubes; if ELN palsy is there cuffed tube can be used but with regular uncuffing of the balloon to avoid tracheal stenosis.

Change tube regularly after washing the hands.

If double lumen tubes are used relatives should be taught how to remove inner tube and place it back.

Preferably two persons should be there while changing the tube

Suction should be ready all the time and to be done every 30 minutes.

Proper lighting should be maintained.

Extra tubes of varying sizes should be ready.

Check the tension of string around neck.

Suction at home: Mechanical suction or rubber bulb attached bottle. It is advised not to use excessive pressure and more than necessary introduction of catheter inside the trachea.

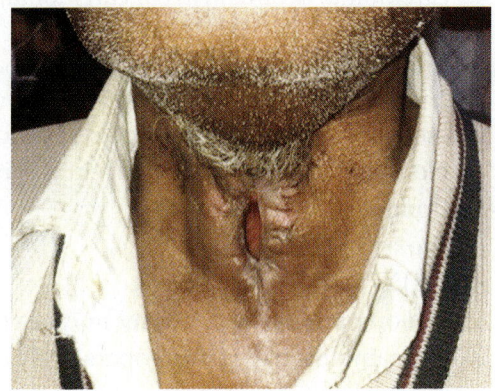

Catheters of different sizes should be kept ready.

Difficulties during the decannulation: Patient becomes habitual of tracheostomy. Immediately after decannulation the patient might have shortness of breath due to raised dead space and due to necrosis of sensory nerve fibers of trachea.

More chances of infection, granulation and fibrosis at tracheostome leading to difficult decannulation.

Tracheostome following a permanent tracheostomy

Immediate complications during tracheostomy:

1. Bleeding, injury to thyroid gland, carotid artery and jugular veins.
2. Apnea following tracheostomy due to CO_2 washout which ultimately causes respiratory depression. Treatment is by either closure of tracheostome temporarily or CO_2 can be given.
3. Cardiac arrest due to vagal stimulation or more commonly due to catecholamine release, hyperkalemia and rise in pH.
4. Injury to recurrent laryngeal nerve
5. Collapse of lung
6. Pneumothorax
7. Damage to cricoid cartilage and trachea

Intermediate complications

1. False passage created during tube changes
2. Crusting and blockage of tube
3. Surgical emphysema
4. Tracheoesophageal fistula
5. Dysphagia—common when large sized tubes are used and in children
6. Tracheobronchial cast of crust with respiratory distress
7. Secondary infection, lung abscess, atelectasis

Late complications of tracheostomy

1. Stricture in trachea
2. Subglottic stenosis when high tracheostomy is one damaging the cricoid
3. Tracheomalacia

4. Injury to brachiocephalic vein
5. Permanent tracheocutaneus fistula
6. Keloid occurs in prone patients
7. Difficult decannulation

Indication of lower tracheostomy: Respiratory papillomatosis.

Indication of higher tracheostomy: Carcinoma larynx—as tracheostome should be excised along with the larynx, otherwise there would be stomal recurrence.

Tracheostomy Tubes

Metallic

Advantages
- Bigger inner diameter allows the laminar flow of air
- Inner tube present, so tube can be cleaned at home
- Durable and hence one-time expense
- Fenestration present, so patient can vocalize

Disadvantages
- No cuff therefore, IPPV is not possible
- Cannot be used in comatose patients
- Erosion of anterior tracheal wall, perichondritis and granulation formation more common
- Radiotherapy cannot be given as scattering may occur
- Connection with anesthesia tube difficult

Examples of metallic tubes
- Silver Jackson tube: This has an outer tube, inner tube and obturator. Inner tube can be removed and cleaned leaving the outer tube in place.
- Alder Hey tube: Outer and inner tubes are fenestrated so patient can speak with tube in place.
- Durham tube: Adjustable flanges.
- Fuller's tube: Biflanged outer tube; best suited for short and thick necked patients. It keeps the trachea dilated.

Nonmetalic

Advantages:
- Cuffed type is present, so IPPV can be given and connection with anesthesia tube is easy
- Mechanical damage to trachea is minimal
- Cosmetically better
- Radiotherapy can be given

Disadvantages
- Thick walled so internal diameter is less, hence laminar flow is less
- Cuffs to be deflated at regular intervals

Examples of nonmetallic tube
- PVC: Cheap
- Portex: Less damage to trachea but very expensive
- Shiley: For children
- Salpeker: Has two cuffs, one can be deflated alternatively.

BRONCHIAL TREE

Bronchopulmonary Segments

- Right lung has 10 segments (mnemonic—**A PALM S**eed **M**akes **A**nother **L**ittle **P**alm)
- Left lung has 8 segments (mnemonic—**ASIA ALPS**).

Left side, in a few cases, has another segment called lingular segment and the total segments become 10.

Right main bronchus is shorter (5 cm) and wider, divided into 3 secondary bronchi—right upper lobe, right middle lobe and right lower lobe. Angle with trachea is 25°–30° and that is why foreign body is more common in right bronchus.

Left main bronchus is relatively longer (5.5 cm) and narrower. Angle with trachea is 45°. It divides into left upper and left lower secondary bronchi.

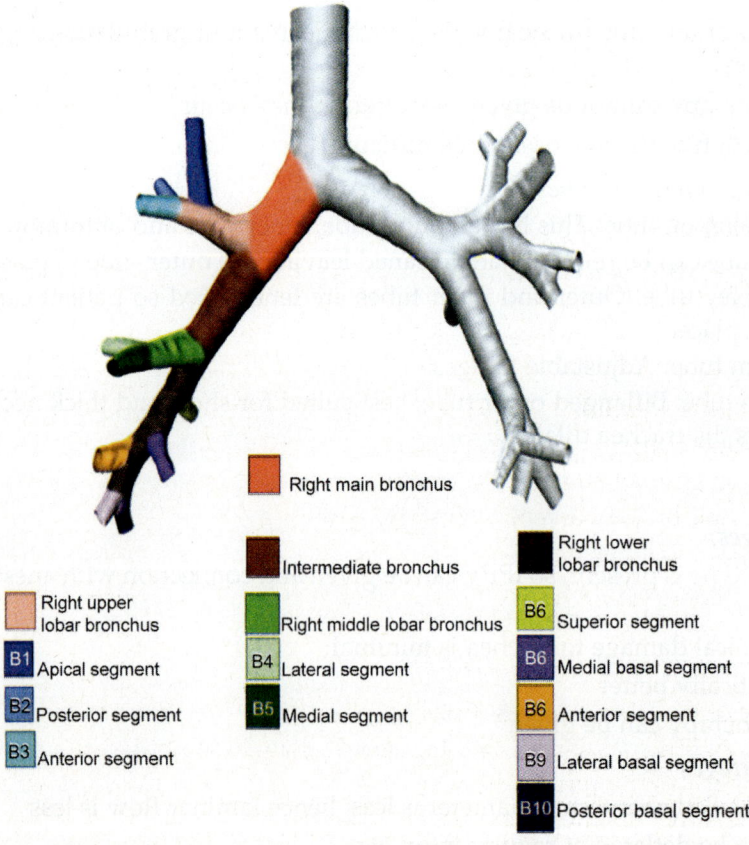

Right main bronchus

Intermediate bronchus

Right lower lobar bronchus

Right upper lobar bronchus

Right middle lobar bronchus

B6 Superior segment

B1 Apical segment

B4 Lateral segment

B6 Medial basal segment

B2 Posterior segment

B5 Medial segment

B6 Anterior segment

B3 Anterior segment

B9 Lateral basal segment

B10 Posterior basal segment

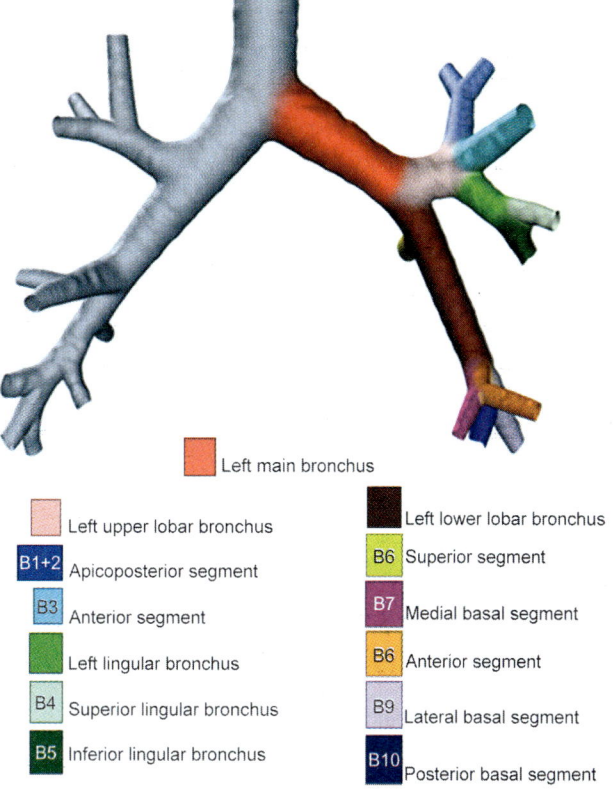

Left main bronchus

Left upper lobar bronchus

B1+2 Apicoposterior segment

B3 Anterior segment

Left lingular bronchus

B4 Superior lingular bronchus

B5 Inferior lingular bronchus

Left lower lobar bronchus

B6 Superior segment

B7 Medial basal segment

B6 Anterior segment

B9 Lateral basal segment

B10 Posterior basal segment

Indications for Bronchoscopy

Diagnostic
- Suspected foreign body
- Unexplained stridor, cough
- Vocal cord paralysis
- Primary unknown with secondary in neck
- Hemoptysis
- X-ray patches in lungs
- Collapse of lungs
- Localised emphysema
- Biopsy and bronchoalveolar lavage (BAL)

Therapeutic
- Removal of foreign body
- Removal of polyp
- Aspiration of pus/secretions

Signs of foreign body in trachea or bronchus are
1. Palpatory thud is a sign of blunt tracheal foreign body heard as a slap when the FB hits against the subglottis.
2. Ball and valve unilateral emphysema.
3. Unilateral collapse of lung.

4. Deteriorating O_2 saturation in a young child which is of sudden onset and which has no evidence of infective pathology.

5. Whistling sound in partial obstruction of trachea by foreign bodies like whistles.

Forceps space: The space formed around the periphery of foreign body during inspiration which can be used to negotiate and remove the foreign body is called forceps space. Hence it is advocated to use ventilating bronchoscope for foreign body removal as this will aid both easy removal of foreign body and also avoids apnea.

For the beginners there will be difficulty in negotiating the bronchoscope into the bronchus and for this the neck of the patient should be tilted so the trachea can come in line with the bronchus.

CHAPTER 32

Esophagus

It is a 25 cm long muscular tube from cricopharynx to stomach (C6–T11). It lies in the posterior mediastinum.

Its lumen is collapsed at rest and opens only during swallowing. Hence the level of esophagus can be identified with the help of a few constrictions during esophagoscopy. They are:

- Cricopharynx narrowest part—15 cm from upper central incisor
- Arch of aorta and left main bronchus at 23 and 25 cm from upper central incisor
- Diaphragm at 35 cm
- Gastroesophageal junction at 40 cm.

Position for rigid esophagoscopy: Barking dog position which is an extension at atlanto-occipital joint and flexion at neck on thorax.

Position for flexible esophagoscopy: Left lateral position.

Indication for rigid esophagoscopy

Diagnostic

- Dysphagia, aphasia
- Primary unknown
- Secondary neck
- Vocal cord paralysis
- Haemetmesis
- Suspected foreign body

Therapeutic

- Removal of foreign body
- Removal of benign lesion
- Diathermy
- Dilatation

Contraindications: Trismus, TB of spine, aneurysm of aorta, corrosive poisoning.

Signs to know that esophagoscope is in the stomach

Gastric secretion may appear, mucosal rougae appear

Killian's dehiscence: This is a potential gap between the two parts of inferior constrictor that is thyropharyngeus and cricopharyngeus. It is also called 'Gateway of tears' during rigid esophagoscopy.

Common site for foreign body lodgement: At the cricopharynx (cricoesophageal junction), as it is the narrowest constriction; peristaltic waves are weak, as they begin here.

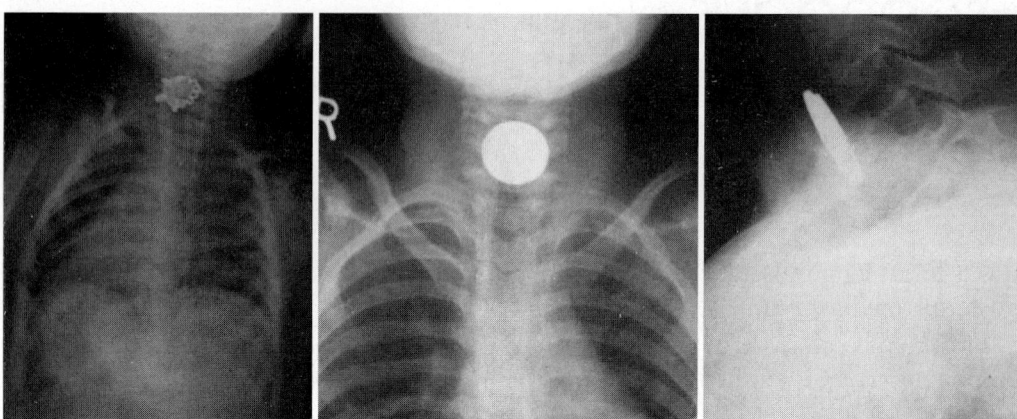

Various X-rays showing radio-opaque shadow in neck (soft tissue view). [FB found to be stuck at cricoesophageal junction]

Complications during the esophagoscopy

- Injury to teeth, lip, soft palate, tonsils and other parts in oropharynx
- Esophageal perforation

Signs of perforation

During operation

- Rise in pulse rate and fall in blood pressure—noted by anesthetists
- Sudden loss of resistance during introduction
- Dark bluish areas and bleeding are seen

After operation

- Fall in blood pressure
- Severe pain at interscapular region
- Subcutaneous emphysema
- Fever, if infection has set in after 48 hours

Management

- Keep the patient nil per oral strictly
- Pass Ryle's tube
- Bedrest and hydration
- Systemic antibiotics covering anaerobes

After 48 hours, if pulse rate and emphysema increases → refer to thoracic surgeon for surgical intervention.

Gastroesophageal Reflux Disease

It is the regurgitation of acidic gastric contents into the lower part of esophagus due to relaxed LES (lower esophageal sphincter). Patient will present with dyspepsia more in lying down, nighttime dry cough, laryngopharyngeal reflux, etc. Due to prolonged reflux, the patient might develop Barrett's esophagus which is a condition where there is metaplasia of esophageal epithelium of lower esophagus into gastric epithelium with Goblet cells. Barrett's esophagus is a premalignant condition for esophageal malignancy.

Factors which prevent the reflux
Esophageal sphincter (physiological)
- Mucosal folds
- Pinch-cock effect of diaphragm
- Gastroesophageal angle
- Negative pressure in chest
- Positive pressure in abdomen

Causes of esophageal stricture
- Reflux esophagitis
- Corrosive poisoning
- Malignancy
- Esophageal surgery
- Drugs (potassium therapy, aspirin)

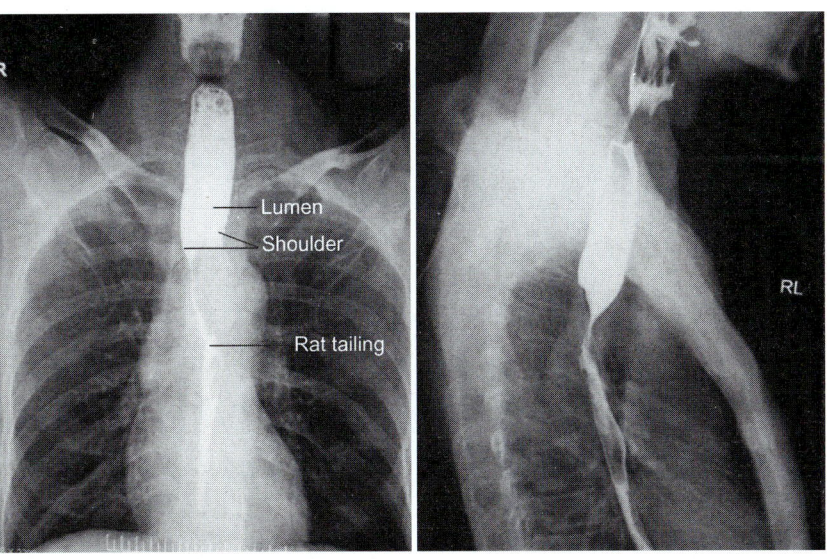

Barium swallow X-ray of esophageal malignancy showing stricture. Note the shoulders found in the lower end of lumen are unequal (As seen in malignancy, shoulders in achalasia cardia are equal and the narrowing occurs at the lower end of esophagus.)

Esophageal malignancy: Upper 1/3rd most common is squamous cell carcinoma; lower 1/3rd common is adeno-carcinoma; middle 1/3rd can develop any of the two variants.

Esophageal dilators: Gum elastic, Hurst (filled with mercury), Maloney, Chevalier Jackson.

Esophageal tubes: Southey, Atkinson, Maloney, Livingstone, Mosseou-Barbin, Celestin.

Schatzki ring: Lower esophageal ring seen in 15% of cases on barium swallow. This condition will present as dysphagia to solid food more than liquid.

Globus pharyngeus (functional dysphagia): Feeling of lump in the throat or something stuck in throat. On clinical examination no abnormality is detected.

Barium swallow of acquired tracheoesophageal fistula following an esophageal malignancy

Achalasia Cardia

It is a primary esophageal mobility disorder caused by impaired relaxation of lower esophageal sphincter and absent peristalsis. Dysphagia, regurgitation of food, heartburn and weight loss are the common presenting complaints.

Diagnosed by Barium swallow and esophageal manometry.

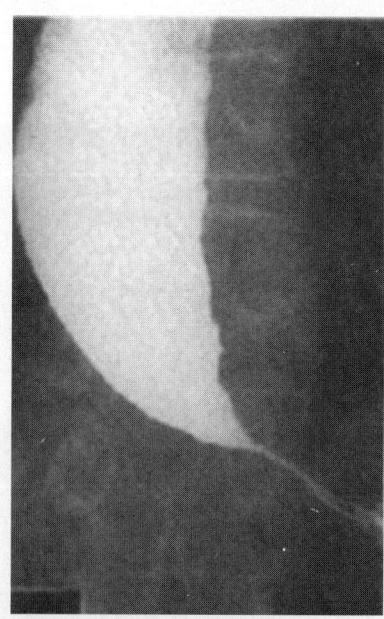

Barium swallow with classical bird's beak appearance in achalasia cardia. Note the shoulders are equal.

This condition can be treated by injection botulinum toxin, endoscopic dilatation and myotomy.

Laryngology, Head and Neck and Miscellaneous Topics

CHAPTER 33

Neck Swellings

MIDLINE NECK SWELLING

Solid	Cystic
Lingual thyroid	Ranula—plunging
Enlarged thyroid isthmus or pyramidal lobe	Dermoid cysts
Prelaryngeal lymphadenitis	Thyroglossal cysts
Pretracheal lymphadenitis	Thyroid cystic disease involving isthmus
Submental lymphadenitis	Innominate vein aneurysm
Thyroiditis	Subhyoid bursitis
Ectopic thyroid	
Neurofibroma	
Laryngeal tumors	

LATERAL SWELLING

Solid	Cystic
Lipomas	Cystic hygroma
Lateral cervical lymphadenopathy (inflammatory, metastatic)	Necrotic nodes
Carotid body tumor	Cold abscesses
Parapharyngeal tumor	Branchial cysts
Parotid tumors	Dermoids
Thyroid nodule in the lobes	Laryngocoele
Cervical rib	Parotid abscess
Schwannomas	Thyroid cysts

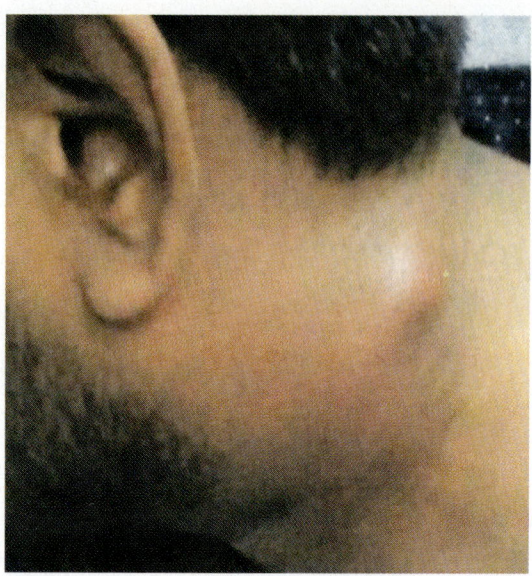

Cold abscess in the posterior triangle. Fluctuant, non-tender swelling

Thyroglossal cyst: Anywhere between thyroid and tongue.

Remnant of thyroglossal duct.

Midline 90% and lateral 10%. Can present as painless swelling in front of neck in adulthood. If infected, presents with pain and sinus formation.

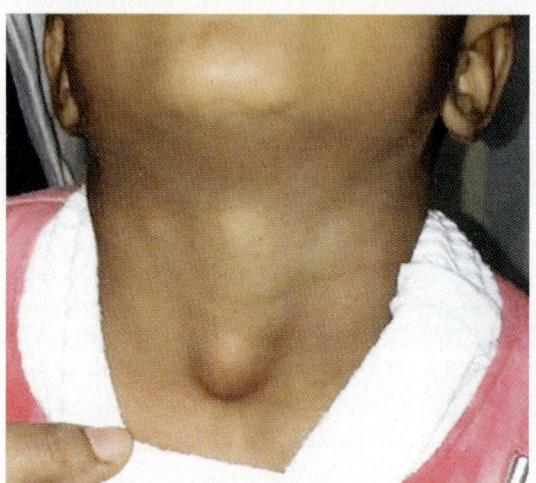

Thyroglossal cyst

Moves with protrusion of tongue. Diagnosis is clinical. Ultrasound is necessary to rule out ectopic thyroid and to confirm the presence of normal thyroid tissue. FNAC is needed only if there is any suspicion of malignant changes.

Treatment is surgical excision by Sistrunk's operation. Here the body of hyoid is also removed along with the cyst and thyroglossal duct. If left behind, the chance of recurrence is very high.

Branchial cyst: Congenital epithelial cyst in lateral neck due to failed obliteration of 2nd branchial cleft.

Cystic swelling at junction of upper 2/3rd and lower 1/3rd of anterior border sternomastoid.

60% left side

Lined by stratified squamous epithelium but mixed finding along with respiratory epithelium is also reported.

Might present as sinus or fistula also.

Operation: Excision.

Cystic hygroma: Cystic swelling seen in children may be present at birth.

Cystic lymphatic malformation believed to be a remnant of primitive jugular sac.

Lining—single layer flat epithelium.

Commonly seen as a transilluminant fluctuant swelling in posterior triangle of neck.

Treatment: Excision, hypertonic saline injection, busulfan injection.

Laryngocele: Air-filled cystic swelling because of dilatation of saccule of larynx; common in professionals like trumpet players, glass blowers due to consistent increased intralaryngeal pressure.

Swelling expands through thyrohyoid membrane.

External type—comes out through thyrohyoid membrane to present in lateral neck; 30% of cases.

Internal type—presents as a swelling of false vocal cord and aryepiglottic fold; 20% of cases.

Mixed type with swelling on both intralarygeal aspect and neck.

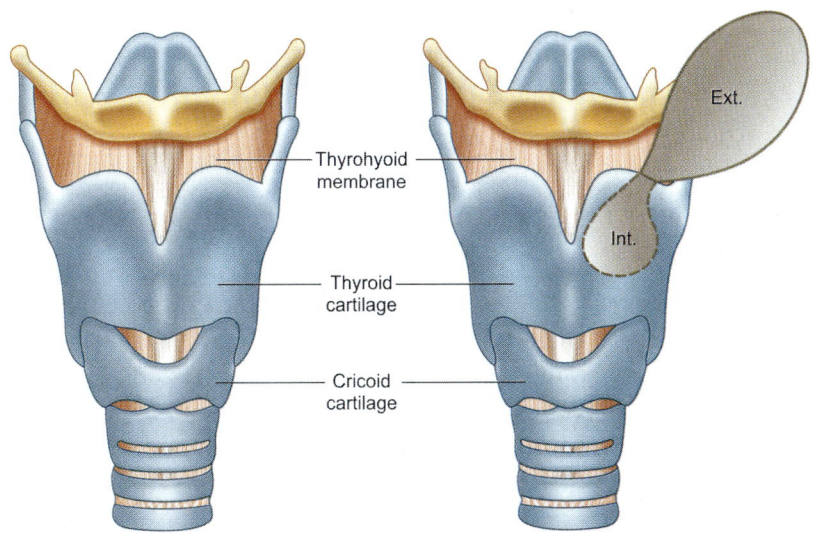

X-ray soft tissue neck (STN) with and without Valsalva maneuver.

Treatment: Excision for external type and ligating the laryngeal connection; large internal or mixed type might need laryngofissure to remove the dilated portion, whereas small internal laryngocoele needs micro laryngeal marsupialization.

CHAPTER 34

Cervical Lymph Nodes and Neck Dissection

Lymph nodes are secondary lymphoid system; they act as a filter for the antigens in the lymph and releasing Ig and immune competent cells. There are hundreds (800–1000) of lymph nodes in the body constituting to about 2–3% of body weight. Out of these, 300 are present in the cervical group. Grossly a lymph node has a capsule, external cortex and internal medulla.

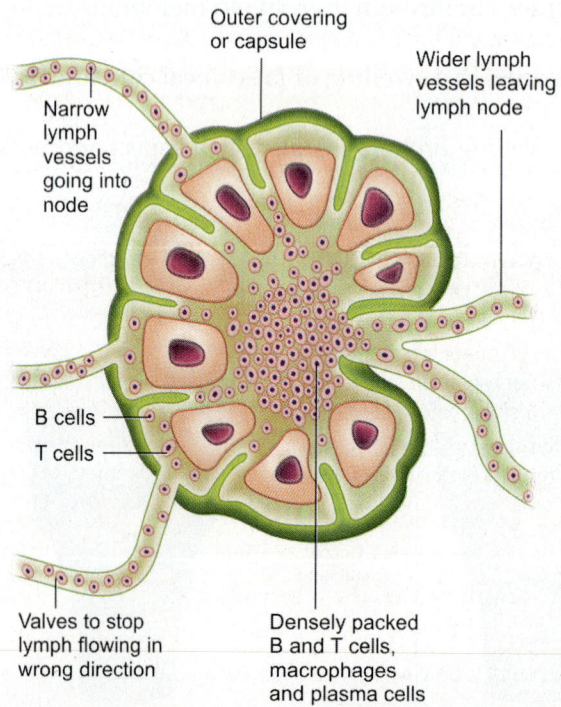

Size of lymph node should be more than 1 cm to become palpable. But the metastasis can be found in the lymph node which is not clinically palpable too.

Hence in any head and neck malignancy, it is advised to go for ultrasound of the neck to rule out the possible micro metastasis.

Structures in neck which can be confused with lymph nodes
- Transverse processes of C_1 and C_2 (bony hard and not mobile)
- Carotid bulb (transmitted pulsations)
- Superior horn of thyroid cartilage (mobile on deglutition and with movement of the thyroid cartilage)
- Tail of parotid gland
- Submandibular gland (palpable bimanually)
- Fibrosed jugular vein thrombosis
- Branchial and thyroglossal cysts
- Cervical rib
- Dermoid cysts

Level of neck nodes

Levels	Location	
Level I	I a—submental; They drain from floor of the mouth, anterior oral tongue, anterior mandibular alveolar ridge and lower lip	II b—submandibular; They drain from oral cavity, anterior nasal cavity, soft tissue structures of the midface and submandibular gland
Level II	Upper jugular nodes from the skull base to upper border of thyroid cartilage; they drain from oral cavity, nasal cavity, nasopharynx, oropharynx, hypopharynx, larynx, and parotid gland	
	II a—anterior to spinal accessory nerve	II b—posterior to spinal accessory nerve
Level III	Middle jugular nodes from the upper border of thyroid cartilage to cricoids cartilage. This group includes jugulo-omohyoid node. These nodes drain oral cavity, nasopharynx, oropharynx, hypopharynx and larynx	
Level IV	Lower jugular nodes from cricoids to clavicle. This level drains hypopharynx, cervical esophagus and larynx	
Level V	Posterior triangle nodes.	
	V a—spinal accessory nodes, draining the nasopharynx and oropharynx	V b—nodes along tranverse cervical vessels draining thyroid.
Level VI	Anterior compartment nodes include pre- and paratracheal nodes, precricoid (Delphian) node and the perithyroidal nodes, including the lymph nodes along the RL nerves. They drain thyroid gland, glottic and subglottic larynx, apex of the piriform sinus, and cervical esophagus	
Level VII	Anterosuperior mediastinal nodes between the common carotid arteries below suprasternal notch till brachiocephalic vein	

Retropharyngeal lymph nodes are not classified under any of the above groups.

Midline group of lymph nodes (Ia and VI) are involved, they are considered as ipsilateral lymph node and not as distant metastasis.

Malignancies of the following regions will cause bilateral node secondaries:
1. Nasopharynx
2. Base tongue
3. Pyriform sinus
4. Epiglottis
5. Thyroid

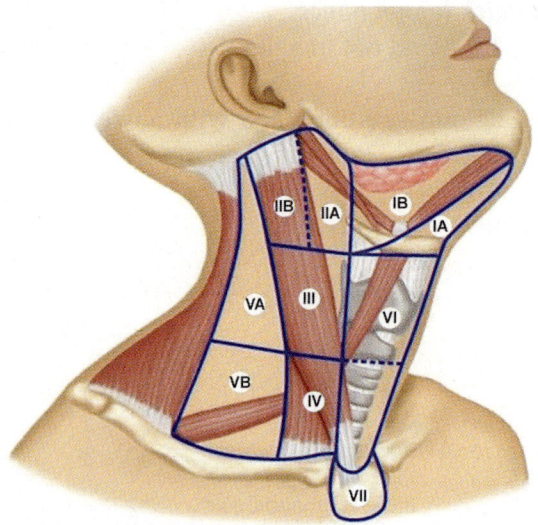

level IA is submental lymph nodes in triangle made by two anterior belly of digastric muscles and hyoid bone; IB is submandibular lymph nodes in triangle made by the anterior and posterior belly of digastric and lower border of mandible; IIA jugulodigastric lymph nodes present anterior to spinal accessory nerve; IIB jugulodigastric lymph nodes present posterior to spinal accessory nerve; VA posterior triangle lymph nodes present above the line drawn along inferior border of cricoid cartilage; VB posterior triangle lymph nodes present below the cricoid line

Technique to palpate cervical lymph nodes: Patient is kept seated and the examiner stands behind the patient. Neck of the patient is slightly flexed to relax the neck muscles. The pads of index and middle fingers are rolled over the skin of the neck. When the swelling is palpated, the size, consistency, mobility and surface are noted down.

Proper preoperative evaluation of the lymph nodes will give an idea about the etiology of the disease (inflammatory or neoplastic) and if malignant, it helps in TNM staging of the disease.

Neck dissection (ND): Kocher proposed removal of metastatic lymph nodes in malignancies (1880).

First radical neck dissection was performed by George Crile (1906).

Selective neck dissection was suggested and popularized by Ballantyne in 1980.

Radical neck dissection (ND) : It includes the removal of all ipsilateral lymph from level I–V and spinal accessory nerve, internal jugular vein, and sternocleidomastoid muscle.

Modified radical neck dissection: It refers to the excision of all lymph nodes routinely removed by the radical neck dissection, with preservation of one or more out of spinal accessory nerve, internal jugular vein and sternocleidomastoid muscle.

Selective neck dissection: It refers to preservation of one or more of the lymph node groups that are routinely removed in the radical neck dissection. Types are:

• Anterior ND—level VI
• Supraomohyoid ND—levels IA and IB, level IIA or levels IIA and IIB, level III
• Lateral ND—level IIA or levels IIA and IIB, level III, and level IV
• Posterolateral ND—levels II, III, IV and V, the post-auricular nodes, suboccipital nodes and the external jugular nodes

Various incisions for neck dissection:

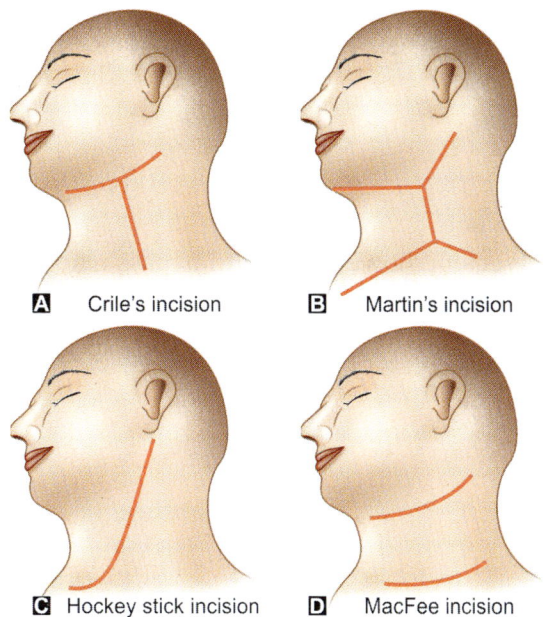

A Crile's incision   B Martin's incision

C Hockey stick incision   D MacFee incision

A—Crile (Y-shaped, not radiated)

B—Martin (double Y)

C—Hockey stick

D—MacFee (parallel double neck incision, postirradiation)

Other incisions are inverted hockey stick, horizontal T and Conley.

When the IJV/IJVs is/are tied in neck dissection, it will lead to increased intracranial tension—on unilateral removal it is increased by 3 times and on bilateral removal 5 times. But the cerebral venous flow takes alternate routes like posterior jugular vein, occipital vein, deep cervical veins, vertebral plexus, etc. so that the ICT is maintained.

When the IJV ligature slips and bleeding occurs postoperatively in RND, cortical mastoidectomy to expose sigmoid sinus, it should be cut and packed so that there will be no distal bleeding.

If bilateral neck dissection is to be done, uninvolved side/less involved side or modified neck side should be done first so that malignant seeding will not happening in the normal side.

Nerves encountered during (radical neck dissection) (RND):

- Greater auricular nerve
- Mandibular branch of facial nerve
- Vagus
- Brachial plexus
- Accessory spinal nerve which has to be removed
- Hypoglossal

- Lingual
- Others

Contraindications for RND

- Primary untreatable
- Medically unfit patient
- Distant metastasis
- Vertebral involvement
- Base of skull involvement
- Carotid artery involvement, however, carotid bypass may be done first
- Brachial plexus involvement.

CHAPTER 35

TNM Staging of Head and Neck Cancers

AJCC TNM staging of head and neck malignancy.

A. Oral Cavity

T_X—primary tumor cannot be assessed

T_0—there is no evidence of primary tumor

T_{is}—carcinoma is in situ

T_1—tumor is 2 cm or less in greatest dimension

T_2—tumor is 2–4 cm in greatest dimension

T_3—tumor is >4 cm in greatest dimension

T_4 (lip)—tumor invades through cortical bone, inferior alveolar nerve, floor of mouth, or skin of face, i.e. chin or nose

T4a—tumor invades adjacent structures like cortical bone into deep extrinsic muscle of tongue, maxillary sinus, skin of face

T4b—tumor invades masticator space, pterygoid plates or skull base and/or encases the internal carotid artery.

B. Oropharynx

T_X—primary tumor cannot be assessed

T_0—there is no evidence of primary tumor

T_{is}—carcinoma is *in situ*

T1—tumor is 2 cm or less in greatest dimension

T2—tumor is 2–4 cm in greatest dimension

T3—tumor is >4 cm in greatest dimension

T4a—tumor invades the larynx, deep/extrinsic muscle of the tongue, medial pterygoid, hard palate, or mandible

T4b—tumor invades the lateral pterygoid muscle, pterygoid plates, lateral nasopharynx, or skull base or encases the carotid artery.

C. Larynx

Subsites: Supraglottis, glottis and subglottis

T_X—primary tumor cannot be assessed

T_0—there is no evidence of primary tumor

T_{is}—carcinoma is *in situ*

Supraglottis

T_1—tumor is limited to one subsite of the supraglottis with normal vocal cord mobility

T2—tumor invades mucosa of more than one adjacent subsite of the supraglottis or glottis or region outside the supraglottis, without fixation of the larynx

T_3—tumor is limited to the larynx with vocal cord fixation and/or invades any of the following: Postcricoid area, pre-epiglottic tissues, paraglottic space, and/or minor thyroid cartilage erosion

T_{4a}—tumor invades through the thyroid cartilage and/or invades tissues beyond the larynx

T_{4b}—tumor invades prevertebral space, encases the carotid artery, or invades mediastinal structures.

Glottis

T_1—tumor is limited to the vocal cords(s) (may involve anterior or posterior commissure), with normal mobility

T_{1a}—tumor is limited to one vocal cord

T_{1b}—tumor involves both vocal cords

T_2—tumor extends to the supraglottis and/or subglottis, and/or with impaired vocal cord mobility

T_3—tumor is limited to the larynx with vocal cord fixation and/or invades paraglottic space, and/or minor thyroid cartilage erosion

T_{4a}—tumor invades through the thyroid cartilage and/or invades tissues beyond the larynx

T_{4b}—tumor invades prevertebral space, encases the carotid artery, or invades mediastinal structures.

Subglottis

T_1—tumor is limited to the subglottis

T_2—tumor extends to the vocal cord(s), with normal or impaired mobility

T_3—tumor is limited to the larynx, with vocal cord fixation

T_{4a}—tumor invades cricoid or thyroid cartilage and/or invades tissues beyond the larynx

T_{4b}—tumor invades prevertebral space, encases the carotid artery, or invades mediastinal structures.

D. Hypopharynx

T_1—tumor is limited to one subsite of the hypopharynx and 2 cm or less in greatest dimension

T_2—tumor invades more than one subsite of the hypopharynx or an adjacent site, or measures more than 2 cm but not more than 4 cm in greatest dimension without fixation of the hemilarynx

T_3—tumor is more than 4 cm in greatest dimension or with fixation of the hemilarynx

T_{4a}—tumor invades thyroid/cricoid cartilage, hyoid bone, thyroid gland, esophagus, or central compartment soft tissue

T_{4b}—tumor invades prevertebral fascia, encases the carotid artery, or involves mediastinal structures.

E. Nasal Cavity and Paranasal Sinuses

T_X—primary tumor cannot be assessed

T_0—no evidence of primary tumor

T_{is}—carcinoma is *in situ*

Maxillary sinus

T_1—tumor is limited to the maxillary sinus mucosa, with no erosion or destruction of bone

T_2—tumor is causing bone erosion or destruction, including extension into the hard palate and/or middle nasal meatus, except extension to the posterior wall of the maxillary sinus and pterygoid plates

T_3—tumor invades any of the following: Bone of the posterior wall of the maxillary sinus, subcutaneous tissues, floor, or medial wall of the orbit, pterygoid fossa, or ethmoid sinuses

T_{4a}—tumor invades anterior orbital contents, skin of cheek, pterygoid plates, infratemporal fossa, cribriform plate, sphenoid or frontal sinuses

T_{4b}—tumor invades any of the following: Orbital apex, dura, brain, middle cranial fossa, cranial nerves other than maxillary division of trigeminal nerve, nasopharynx or clivus

Nasal cavity and ethmoid sinus

T_1—tumor is confined to the ethmoid sinus with or without bone erosion

T_2—tumor invades two subsites in a single region or extends to involve an adjacent region within the nasoethmoidal complex, with or without bony invasion

T_3—tumor extends to invade the medial wall or floor of the orbit, maxillary sinus, palate, or cribriform plate

T_{4a}—tumor invades any of the following: Anterior orbital contents, skin of nose or cheek, minimal extension to anterior cranial fossa, pterygoid plates, sphenoid or frontal sinuses

T_{4b}—tumor invades any of the following: Orbital apex, dura, brain, middle cranial fossa, cranial nerves other than V2, nasopharynx, or clivus.

F. Salivary Glands

T_1—tumor is 2 cm or less without extraparenchymal extension

T_2—tumor is greater than 2 cm but not more than 4 cm without extraparenchymal extension

T_3—tumor is more than 4 cm and/or extraparenchymal extension

T_{4a}—tumor invades the skin, mandible, ear canal, and/or facial nerve

T_{4b}—tumor invades the skull base and/or pterygoid plates and/or encases the carotid artery.

Node staging (N) under the TNM staging system for head and neck tumors (excluding nasopharynx and thyroid)

N_X—regional lymph nodes cannot be assessed

N_0—there is no regional nodes metastasis

N_1—metastasis is in a single ipsilateral lymph node, 3 cm or less in greatest dimension

N_{2a}—metastasis is in a single ipsilateral lymph node, more than 3 cm but not more than 6 cm in greatest dimension

N_{2b}—metastasis is in multiple ipsilateral lymph nodes, not more than 6 cm in greatest dimension

N_{2c}—metastasis is in bilateral or contralateral lymph nodes, not more than 6 cm in greatest dimension

N_3—metastasis is in a lymph node more than 6 cm in greatest dimension.

Distant metastasis (M):

M_X—distant metastasis cannot be assessed

M_0—there is no distant metastasis

M_1—there is distant metastasis

Stage grouping

Stage 0 Tis N0 M0

Stage I T1 N0 M0

Stage II T2 N0 M0

Stage III T3 N0 M0

    T1 N1 M0

    T2 N1 M0

    T3 N1 M0

Stage IVA T4a N0 M0

    T4a N1 M0

    T1 N2 M0

    T2 N2 M0

    T3 N2 M0

    T4a N2 M0

Stage IVB T4b any N M0

    Any T N3 M0

Stage IVC any T any N M1

Clinical stage grouping by T and N status

	T1	T2	T3	T4a	T4b
N0	I	II	III	IVa	IVb
N1	III	III	III	IVa	IVb
N2	IVa	IVa	IVa	IVa	IVb
N3	IVb	IVb	IVb	IVb	IVb

G. Nasopharynx

T_1—tumor is confined to the nasopharynx

T_{2a}—tumor extends to the oropharynx and/or nasal cavity, without parapharyngeal extension

T_{2b}—tumor extends into the parapharyngeal space

T_3—tumor involves bony structures and/or paranasal sinuses

T_4—tumor has intracranial extension and/or involves cranial nerves, infratemporal fossa, hypopharynx, orbit, or masticator space.

Regional lymph nodes

N_0—there is no regional lymph node metastasis

N_1—unilateral metastasis in lymph node(s) is 6 cm or less in greatest dimension, above the supraclavicular fossa

N_2—bilateral metastasis in lymph nodes is 6 cm or less in greatest dimension, above the supraclavicular fossa

N_{3a}—tumor is greater than 6 cm in dimension

N_{3b}—tumor extends to the supraclavicular fossa

Stage grouping

Stage 0 Tis N0 M0

Stage I T1 N0 M0

Stage IIA T2a N0 M0

Stage IIB T1 N1 M0

   T2 N1 M0

   T2a N1 M0

   T2b N0 M0

   T2b N1 M0

Stage III T1 N2 M0

   T2a N2 M0

   T2b N2 M0

   T3 N0 M0

   T3 N1 M0

   T3 N2 M0

Stage IVA T4 N0 M0

   T4 N1 M0

   T4 N2 M0

Stage IVB any T N3 M0

Stage IVC any T any N M1

H. Thyroid

Primary tumor (T)

T_X—primary tumor cannot be assessed

T_0—there is no evidence of primary tumor

T_1—tumor is 2 cm or less in greatest dimension and is limited to the thyroid

T_2—tumor is more than 2 cm but not more than 4 cm in greatest dimension and is limited to the thyroid

T_3—tumor is more than 4 cm in greatest dimension and is limited to the thyroid or any tumor with minimal extrathyroid extension

T_{4a}—tumor of any size extends beyond the thyroid capsule to invade subcutaneous soft tissues, larynx, trachea, esophagus, or recurrent laryngeal nerve

T_{4b}—tumor invades prevertebral fascia or encases the carotid artery or mediastinal vessels

All anaplastic carcinomas are considered T4 tumors

T_{4a}—intrathyroidal anaplastic carcinoma—surgically resectable

T_{4b}—extrathyroidal anaplastic carcinoma—surgically unresectable

Regional lymph nodes (N)

N_X—regional lymph nodes cannot be assessed

N_0—there is no regional lymph node metastasis

N_{1a}—there is metastasis to level VI (pretracheal, paratracheal and prelaryngeal/ Delphian lymph nodes)

N_{1b}—there is metastasis to unilateral, bilateral or contralateral cervical or superior mediastinal lymph nodes.

Distant metastasis (M)

M_X—distant metastasis cannot be assessed

M_0—there is no distant metastasis

M_1—there is distant metastasis

Uses of TNM staging: It is a method of conveying clinical experiences to other without ambiguity.

- Epidemiology
- Planning the therapy
- Explaining the prognosis
- Comparing the result of different centres
- Exchange of information and research

If there is any doubt about the correct TNM staging, it is advised to go for less advanced (lower) stage.

If there are multiple simultaneous primary, then go for the highest T category of tumor.

CHAPTER 36

Anatomy of Larynx

It is the organ of phonation.

It extends from the base of tongue to subglottis.

It is located in the anterior neck in the midline from C3 to C6. It is located higher in females and children.

Larynx consists of cartilages (paired—arytenoid, corniculate and cuneiform and unpaired—thyroid, cricoid and epiglottis), muscles (intrinsic and extrinsic), membranes and mucosa.

Manual Garcia, a music professor, is considered as the father of laryngology. He is the first to see his own vocal cords with the help of two mirrors in 1855.

Embryology

It develops from the cranial end of laryngotracheobronchial groove in 3rd week of IUL.

4th arch derivatives	6th arch derivatives	Hypobranchial eminence
Thyroid cartilage	Cricoid cartilage	Epiglottis
Cuneiform cartilages	Arytenoids cartilages	
	Corniculate cartilages	

Corniculates are also called 'cartilage of Santorini'.

Cuneiforms are called 'cartilage of Wrisberg'.

Differences between adult's and child's larynx—7S:

1. Size
2. Shape—funnel shaped and omega-shaped epiglottis in children
3. Soft cartilages in children and hard and even ossified cartilages in adult
4. Superiorly placed in children (C2–C3)
5. Lot straighter in children
6. More sensitive in children, hence more the chances of spasm
7. Subglottis is the narrowest portion in children, whereas glottis is the narrowest part in adult larynx.

Thyroid lamellae angle is wide in females (120°), whereas it is narrow in males (90°) thus the A-P length of larynx is more in males.

Length of vocal cord:

Male 18–23 mm

Female 16–17 mm

Petiole is the stalk-like process through which epiglottis is attached to thyroid cartilage.

Oblique line in thyroid cartilage gives attachment to inferior constrictor, sternothyroid and thyrohyoid.

Arytenoid cartilage: Paired; pyramidal. It has the following parts, namely:

- *Base*: It articulates with cricoid cartilage.
- *Muscular process*: Directed laterally. All intrinsic muscles are attached to it.
- *Vocal process*: Directed anteriorly giving attachment to vocal cords

Intrinsic muscles of larynx

- *Abductor*: Posterior cricoarytenoid
- *Adductors*: Lateral cricoarytenoid, interarytenoid, cricothyroid, thyroarytenoid
- *Tensors*: Cricothyroid, vocalis, thyroarytenoid

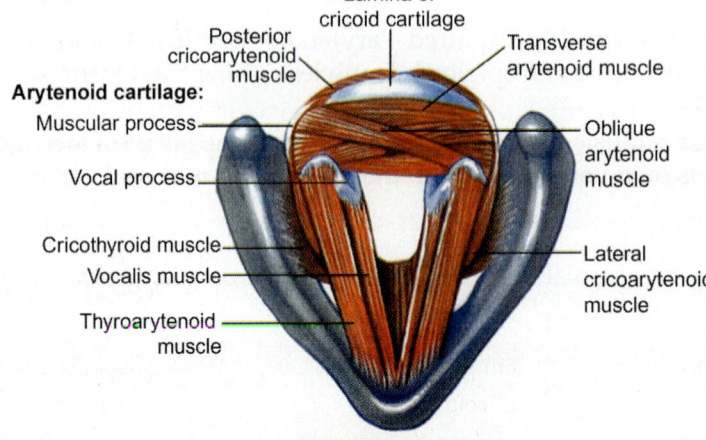

Intrinsic muscles of larynx

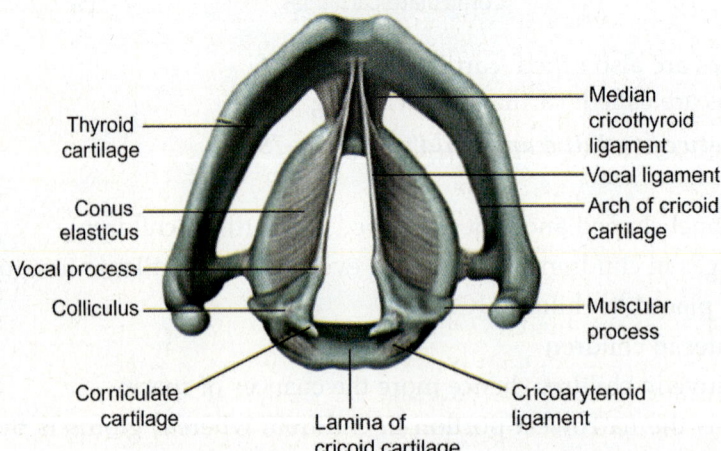

Conus elasticus and ligaments of larynx

Extrinsic muscles of larynx
- *Strap muscles:* Sternothyroid, thyrohyoid, stylopharyngeous and palatopharyngeous
- *Pharyngeal muscles:* Inferior constrictor.

Laryngeal ligaments and membranes
1. Extrinsic
   a. Thyrohyoid membrane
   b. Hyoepiglottic ligament
   c. Cricotracheal ligament
   d. Median and lateral thyrohyoid ligaments
2. Intrinsic
   a. Cricothyroid membrane with central thick Conus elasticus
   b. Quadrilateral membrane—upper border is aryepiglottic fold, lower border is false vocal cord.

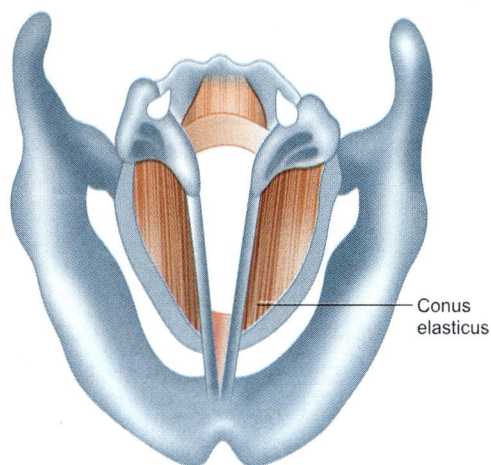

Conus elasticus (cricovocal membrane): Extends from superior border of cricoid to vocal ligament.

Thickened upper portion of this extends from anterior commissure to vocal process. This delays tumor spread.

Quadrangular membrane: It is attached anteriorly to lateral border of epiglottis and extends to either sides posteriorly to medial surface of arytenoids.

Broyle's ligament (yellow spot): At anterior commissure there is no inner perichondrium over the thyroid cartilage; intracartilaginous continuation of anterior commissure ligament, which gets attached to the outer perichondrium is known as Broyle's ligament. Malignant involvement at this site is likely to involve the laryngeal cartilage early. In that case surgery is required.

Paraglottic and pre-epiglottic space: Paraglottic space has vocalis muscles, thyroarytenoid muscles and ventricles. This space is a common site for lateral spread of carcinoma from the surface of larynx and it can involve the intrinsic muscles of vocal cord, thus it impairs the mobility of VC. It communicates with pre-epiglottic space anteriorly and superiorly. From pre-epiglottic space it can spread to opposite paraglottic space taking a full circle.

Pre-epiglottic space is commonly filled by fat. It is bounded anteriorly by thyroid cartilage, thyrohyoid membrane and hyoid bone; superiorly by hyoepiglottic ligament and posteriorly by epiglottis.

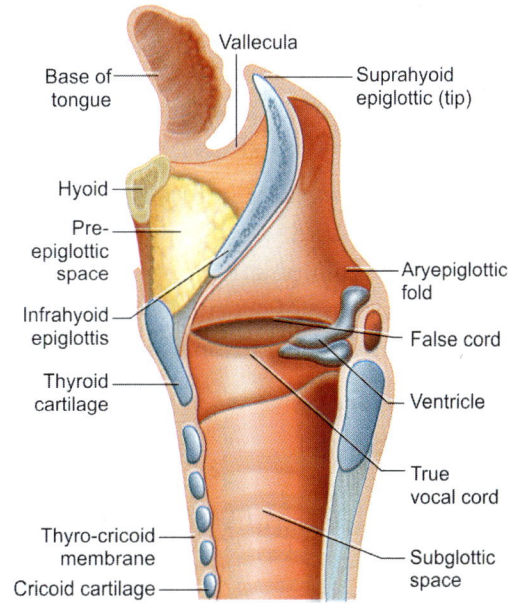

Sagittal section of larynx

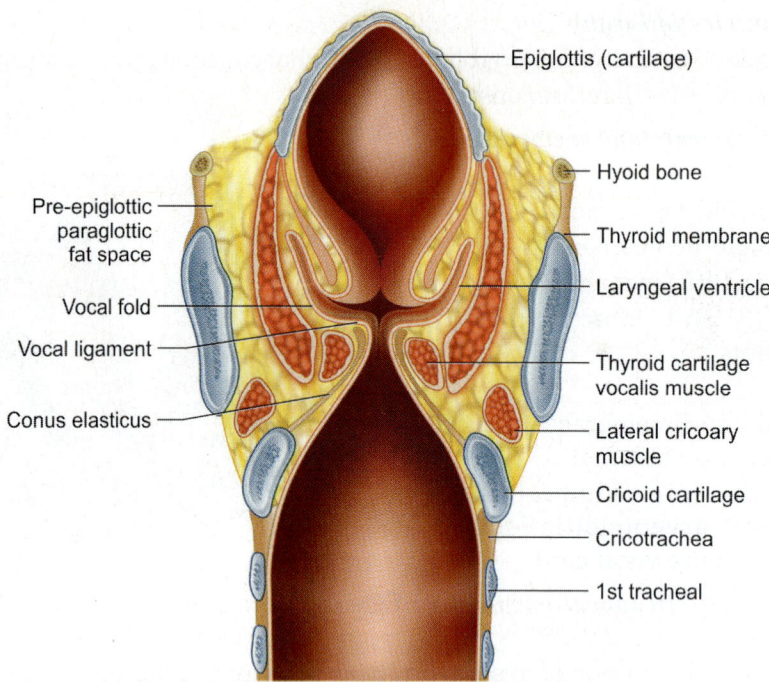

Laryngeal joints: There are 2 joints, namely
1. Cricothyroid joint
2. Cricoarytenoid joint; both of these are synovial joints

Hidden areas of larynx: These are the areas that are difficult to visualize during indirect laryngoscopy. They include:
- Anterior commissure
- Ventricles
- Subglottic area
- Laryngeal surface of epiglottis
- Apex of pyriform sinus

Squamous epithelium in larynx
- True vocal cord
- Posterior commissure
- Upper margin of aryepiglottic folds
- Posterior upper portion of epiglottis

Cavities of larynx
1. Laryngeal inlet
2. Vestibule
3. Ventricle (oil can of larynx)
4. Rima glottis
5. Subglottic space

Anatomy of vocal cords: VC has the following layers in it
1. Stratified squamous epithelium
2. Lamina propria—superficial layer
3. Lamina propria—intermediate layer
4. Lamina propria—deep layer
5. Vocalis muscle

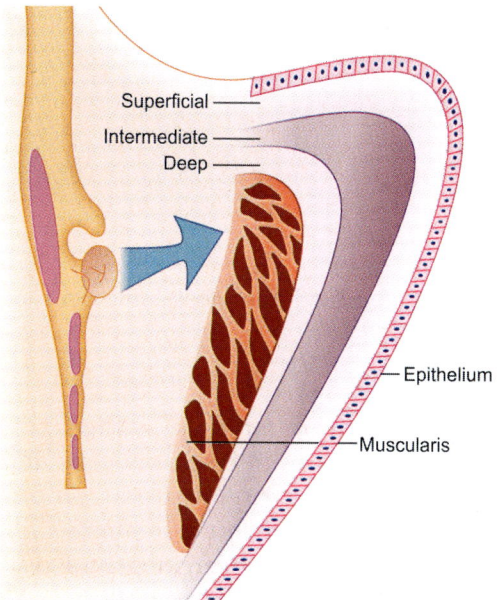

Lymphatic drainage: Vocal cord is devoid of lymphatics. They are present only in subepithelial layer (Reinke's space). Hence it is called lymphatic watershed.

Functions of larynx: Primary function is protection of airway
- Phonation
- Fixation of chest
- Respiration
- Cough reflex

CHAPTER 37

Carcinoma of Larynx

Carcinoma of larynx, histologically:
- Squamous cell carcinoma constitutes the most common type (up to 85–90%)
- Verrucous carcinoma—1 to 4%
- Rest are adenocarcinoma, adenoid cystic carcinoma and chondrosarcoma.

Tobacco smoking is the main factor in laryngeal malignancies: Tobacco smoke has more than 300 compounds in it. It has 16 co-carcinogens and 9 carcinogens. It has gases like SO_2, CO_2, CO, ammonia, etc. Aryl hydrocarbon of smoke is converted by aryl hydrocarbon hydroxylase, an enzyme found in pulmonary macrophage or type 2 alveolar cell into epoxide, the most potent carcinogen of respiratory tract. Epoxide then brings changes in normal cells of larynx or respiratory tract and converts to cancer cells.

It is to be noted that cancer of larynx almost always starts from anterior parts of larynx and never originates from posterior parts of larynx, although posterior parts can be involved when cancer spreads posteriorly. Reason behind is that pulmonary macrophages also known as policeman of larynx take round only along the posterior parts of larynx and can detect cancer and kill it immediately. But this is not the case in anterior parts of glottis where it does not come in contact with pulmonary macrophage.

Reasons of early invasion and spread of cancer at anterior commissure:
- No intervening perichondrium, so cord blends with cartilage.
- Mucosa and cartilage are found close.
- Inferiorly cricothyroid membrane is placed, so early spread to extralaryngeal tissues.
- Abundance of mucous glands.
- Mucociliary flow (inhaled carcinogen) from trachea also converges here.

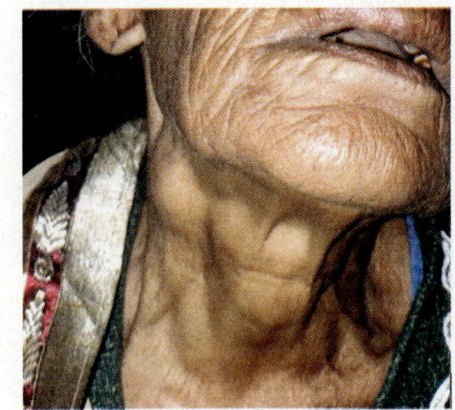

This patient presented with a triad of otalgia, odynophagia and neck swelling seen in pyriform sinus malignancy.

Indications of direct laryngoscopic (DL) examination
Diagnostic
- Hoarseness
- Stridor
- For talking biopsy of lesion and assessment of extent of tumor
- Vocal cord paralysis
- Primary unknown

Therapeutic
- Vocal polyp
- Papillomatosis
- Foreign body removal

Investigations for carcinoma of larynx: Routine baseline investigations like complete blood count, urine routine and microscopy, blood urea, creatinine, serum electrolytes, blood sugar, coagulation profile, ECG, X-ray chest
- X-ray of soft tissue of neck
- To see the airway.
- Involvement of cartilages.
- Barium swallow and meal

Contrast enhanced CT neck: Local extension and lymph nodes in neck.

Direct laryngoscopy: To know the extent of tumor and to take biopsy.

Biopsy: To know the histological type and grade of tumor, so prognosis can be predicted.

Differential diagnosis carcinoma of larynx
- Chronic laryngitis
- Tuberculosis
- Syphilis
- Fungal granuloma
- Benign tumors

Causes of fixed vocal cord in carcinoma of larynx

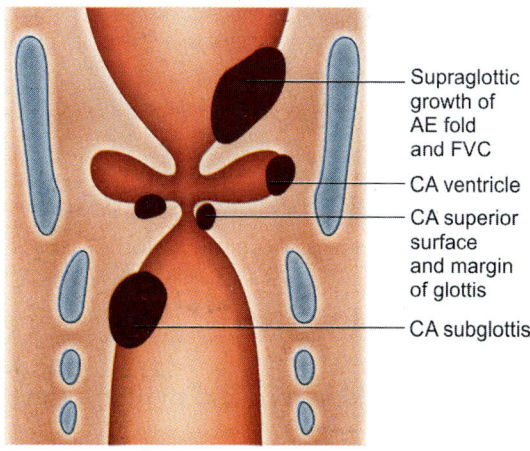

Classification of carcinoma of larynx

Deep invasion of thyroarytenoid (vocalis) muscle
- Involvement of cricoarytenoid joint
- Involvement of arytenoid or cricoid cartilage
- Perineural invasion
- Bulk of tumor (mechanical)

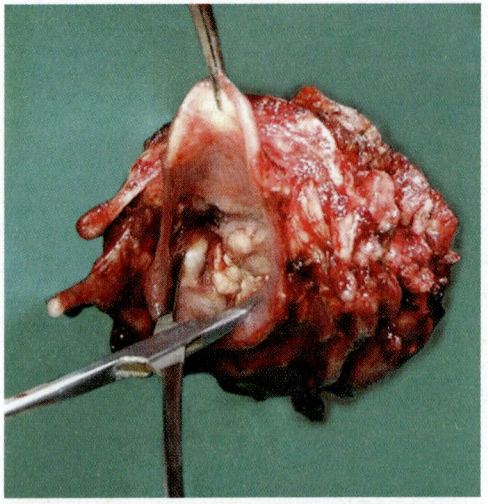

Glottic carcinoma invading the thyroid cartilage and strap muscles anteriorly through Broyle's ligament

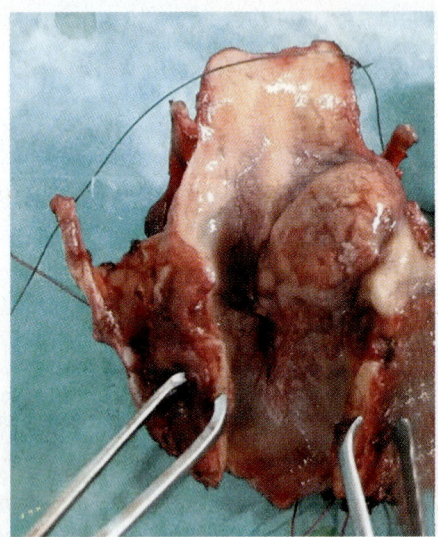

Another operative specimen of total laryngectomy showing glottis cancer with supra, subglottis and extralaryngeal spread

How to judge the paraglottic involvement?
Fixed hemilarynx:
- Distance increases between the false cord and pyriform sinus because of presence of edema/swelling.
- CT scan.

Transglottic tumors: Those tumors of larynx which cross the ventricle, thus involving more than two regions of larynx are called transglottic tumors. These tumors involve the paraglottic space extensively and need extensive surgery. These are not the ideal cases for conservative surgeries.

First laryngectomy was performed by Billroth in 1873 on New Year Eve.

MANAGEMENT OF CARCINOMA OF LARYNX

Glottic T1a—chordectomy (endoscopically laser assisted or coblation).

Supraglottic T1a—horizontal partial laryngectomy.

Glottic T1b or T2—vertical lateral or frontolateral partial laryngectomy (removal of cord or with anterior commissure)—vertical hemilaryngectomy (removal of arytenoid along with vocal cord).

Supraglottic T1b or T2—horizontal partial or horizontal hemilaryngectomy (removal of arytenoid).

T3 carcinoma of larynx—total laryngectomy

T4 carcinoma of larynx can spread anteriorly into: (a) Thyroid cartilage or strap muscles (usually through calcified thyroid cartilage common above 45 years of age or through broyales ligaments).

b. Lateraly into thyroid gland and pretrachial lymph node.

c. Superiorly base of tongue.

d. Posteriorly pharynx and esophagus.

These all T4 lesions need extended total laryngectomy.

Lymph node can be addressed by

1. prophylactic neck dissection,
2. elective neck dissection.

Postoperative radiotherapy should be given after one and a half month of surgery. Radiotherapy could be sole treatment for T1 and T2 lesions in indicated patient but not in young patient.

Rehabilitation of laryngectomized patient

Preoperative:

- Should stop smoking.
- Patient should be introduced with other laryngectomized patients.
- Anatomical and physiological changes should be explained preferably in a group.
- Speech therapist should see the patient.
- Family should be fully explained regarding potential problems.
- Different options for voice should be discussed with patient.
- Training for esophageal speech should be started.

Postoperative precaution: As soon as the patient becomes ambulatory, deep breathing exercise should be encouraged.

Voice rehabilitation options available after surgery are:

- Esophageal voice
- Artificial larynx

- Neoglottis operation
- Neoglottis operation with valves (TEP)

Esophageal voice: 50–60% can develop this type of voice depending on the motivation and speech therapist's treatment.

Advantages
- No expenses
- No instrument required
- No battery required
- No aspiration problems

Disadvantages
- Difficult in adults
- A few can learn this technique
- Monotonous speechless word
- Patient has to belch continuously

Electrolarynx: It is an electromechanical device that picks up vibration from pharynx, base of tongue, oral cavity and converts it into speech.

Disadvantages
- Metallic voice
- Expensive
- Battery is required
- Draws public attention
- One hand is always busy

Indications for using LASER in carcinoma of larynx
- Verrucous carcinoma
- Recurrence after RT (radiotherapy)
- Reduction of respiratory obstruction
- Palliation
- Laser cordectomy

Contraindications of laser in carcinoma of larynx
- Subglottic or supraglottic extension
- Anterior commissure involvement
- Vocal process involvement

Causes of laryngeal stenosis
- Surgeries like partial laryngectomy
- High tracheostomy cutting through the cricoid ring
- Trauma—acute > chronic; causes are RTA, burns, intubation, etc.
- Chondroma
- Squamous cell carcinoma
- Infections like scleroma, tuberculosis, leprosy, etc.
- Wegener's granulomatosis
- Relapsing polychondritis

CHAPTER 38

Papillomatosis of Larynx

Multiple, nonkeratinizing squamous epithelium.

Cause: Human papillomavirus 6, 11 strains

Tracheostomy: Should be avoided as far as possible because of explosive growth afterwards.

Other sites: Tracheobronchial tree, chest, lips, soft palate, tonsil and tracheostomy site.

Treatment
- MLS (microlaryngeal surgery)
- 4 weeks apart, otherwise adhesions may form.
- Laser can cause less bleeding and less charring; coablation can also be handy.
- Topical 5-flourouracil
- Systemic cis-retinoic acid
- Interferons
- Cryotherapy
  Radiotherapy is contraindicated as malignant transformation may occur.

CHAPTER 39

Vocal Cord and its Benign Diseases

Rima glottis: It is the space between the true vocal cords.

0 mm	Phonation
3 mm	Paramedian
6–7 mm	Cadaveric
12–14 mm	Inspiration
19–20 mm	Deep inspiration

Rima vestibuli: Space between the false vocal cords.

Glottis
- True vocal cords, anterior commissure and posterior commissure
- Normal glottic space is 8 mm in adults
- If it is <3 mm, then the patient develops SOB and stridor.

Vocal nodules: Also called Singer's nodule, screamer's nodule, teacher's nodule. Bilateral localized thickening in vocal cords at the junction of anterior 1/3rd and posterior 2/3rd.

Treatment
- Early cases are reversible with speech therapy
- Microlaryngeal surgery (MLS) if it is organized

Vocal polyp: Ballooning of epithelium usually following sudden voice abuse leading to hematoma, later ingrowth of connective tissue.

Commonest site is anterior commissure.

Unilateral and pedunculated, sometimes moves with respiration.

Bleeding diathesis like thrombocytopenia should be kept in mind as a cause of hematoma.

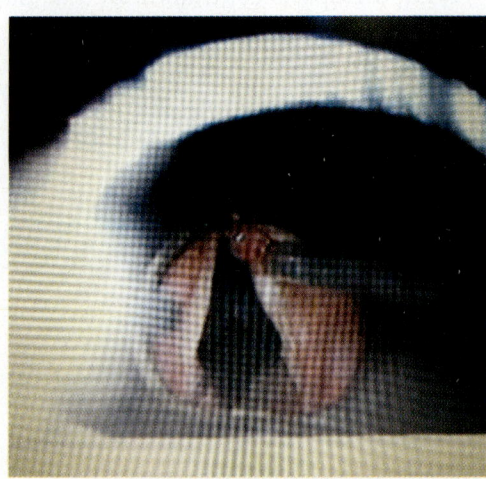

Microlaryngoscopic picture of right VC polyp

Treatment: MLS followed by speech therapy.

- **Vocal cord paralysis.**
- Vocal cord positions.

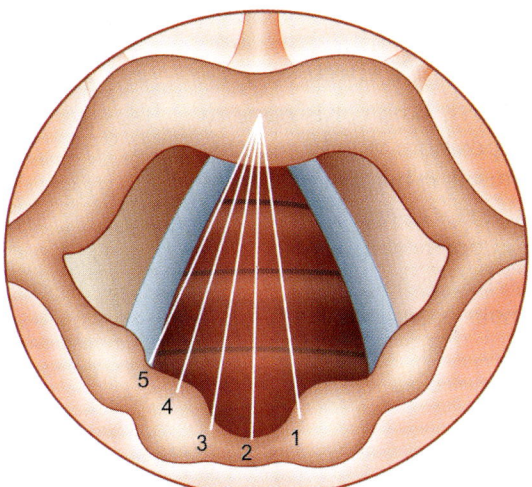

1. Median vocal cord in midline
2. Paramedian vocal cord 1.5 mm from midline
3. Intermediate vocal cord 3.5 mm from midline
4. Partial abduction vocal cord 7 mm from midline
5. Full abduction vocal cord 9.5 mm from midline
   or a gap of 19 mm between two vocal cords

Causes

- *Malignancy 25%*: Bronchus, lung, esophagus, thyroid and nasopharynx
- *Surgical trauma 20%*: During thyroid, lung, esophageal and cardiac surgery
- Idiopathic 15%
- Nonsurgical trauma 15% road traffic accidents
- Neurological causes 15%
- Miscellaneous 5%
- Viral infection, GB syndrome, diabetes, collagen disorders
- Left vocal cord paralysis > right, ratio is 4:1
- Because of longer course of recurrent laryngeal nerve

Important relation of right recurrent laryngeal nerve

- Right subclavian artery
- Apex of right upper lobe of lung
- Supraclavicular laryngeal nerve

Important relations of left recurrent laryngeal nerve

- Aortic arch
- Left atrium
- Esophagus
- Mediastinal lymph node

Ortner's syndrome: Cardiomegaly of left atrium causes paralysis of left recurrent laryngeal nerve.

Semon's theory: In advancing organic lesion of recurrent laryngeal nerve, the abductor fibers are affected first.

Wagner and Grossman theory: It states that superior laryngeal nerve supplying the cricothyroid muscle has additive effect.

Bilateral abductor paralysis: Both cords come to median or paramedian positions due to additive action of cricothyroid muscle in bilateral recurrent laryngeal nerve paralysis as seen in diagram position of vocal cord in position B.

    Voice may be good

    Stridor may be the main presenting complaint; it can be present at rest, if not appears during exertion or after an attack of URI.

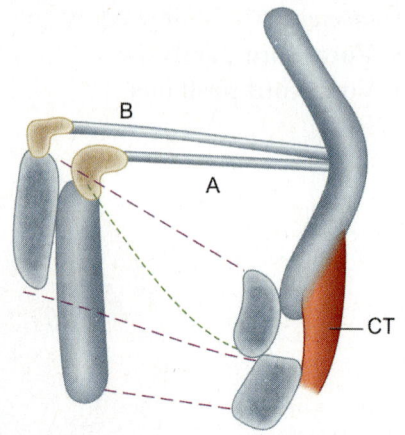

A: The position of vocal cord in A is when there is no paralysis.

B: When vocal cord is stretched and in paramedian plane due to recurrent laryngeal nerve paralysis and unopposed action of cricothyroid muscle which pulls cricoid cartilage backward under thyroid cartilage.

Wagner and Grossman theory

Treatment

- Tracheostomy
- Must wait for 6 months for any surgical procedure

Other surgical options are

- Partial or complete arytenoidectomy (cold/LASER)
- Laryngofissure/direct
- Laryngoscopy/LASER
- Lateralisation by slings

Cordectomy (partial or complete)—LASER is used more nowadays due to clean dissection and less bleeding.

Re-innervation procedures with ansa hypoglossi or phrenic nerve.

Bilateral adductor paralysis: Position of cords—cadaveric.

Clinical features: Voice aphonia, aspiration, and pneumonia.

Treatment: Tracheostomy, epiglottopexy, vocal cord plication, and fat laryngoplasty.

Isshiki's thyroplasty: Phonosurgery to improve the mechanics and functions of vocal cord.

- Type I. Medialization of cord
- Type II. Lateralization of cord
- Type III. Shortening of cord (lowers the pitch of voice)
- Type IV. Lengthening of cord (increases the pitch of voice)

Voice quality in normal male and female

Male

- Bass (very low-pitched voice) like good actor and show anchor.
- Baritone (most of male have this voice) they are good singer like a few famous singers.
- Tenor (males who have female-like voice).

Female

- Contralto (females who have male-like voice—low pitched)
- Mezzo-contralto—(most of female voice—mid-frequency)
- Soprano (best female voice—like famous female singers).

CHAPTER 40

Voice Disorders

Phonation is initiated by area 4 in the Sylvian fissure of cerebral cortex.

Hoarseness is rough, harsh, low-pitched and breathy voice.

Vocal abuse: Overuse of laryngeal and pharyngeal musculature by shouting, yelling, continuously singing at a high pitch and excessive talking. It is common in vendors, teachers, singers, etc.

Vocal misuse: Incorrect use of voice which includes pitch, quality and intensity, e.g. mimickers.

Stammering (stuttering): Involuntary prolongation and cessation of sounds.

That is b-b-b-ball (ball), that is part of word is repeated.

Compare with nonfluency where complete word is repeated, e.g. it is, it is then sentence is completed, e.g. it is a beautiful day.

Mogiphonia

Person voice is normal otherwise, but when he addresses a gathering of crowd he cannot start the sentence and stammering appears.

Dysphonia plica ventricularis: Voice is produced by false voice vocal cords.

Causes
- Chronic laryngitis
- Functional (psychological)
- Voice is low pitched and rough

Treatment: Voice therapy and counselling.

Functional aphonia (hysterical aphonia)
- Seen in emotionally labile females.
- If asked, patient will cough normally.

Puberphonia
- Persistence of childhood voice after puberty.
- Emotionally immature boys.
- By performing Gutzman test, voice improves.

Treatment: Counselling, type IV thyroplasty.

Spasmodic Dysphonia

Can be seen in Parkinsonism or even without it and treatment is tab pacitane or inj botulinum A toxin into adductor or abductor of vocal cord.

Phonaesthenia: Weak voice because of fatigue in phonatory muscles, i.e. thyroarytenoid and interarytenoid.

I/L findings: Elliptical space triangular space key hole.

Treatment: Voice therapy.

Rhinolalia: It is change in tone of voice due to nasal or nasopharyngeal problems.

Rhinolalia aperta: Nasal twang is present because of continuous escape of air through the nose.
- Cleft palate, palatal perforation, palatal paralysis
- Postoperative, e.g. adenoidectomy, UPPP (uvulopalato pharyngoplasty)

Rhinolalia clausa: This is due to lack of air escape through the nose and voice is flat.
    Bilateral nasal obstruction or nasopharyngeal obstruction, e.g. bilateral polyp, nasal mass.

Rhinolalia mixta: When both the conditions co-exist, e.g. cleft palate with polyp.

CHAPTER 41

Chronic and Tubercular Laryngitis

Primary tuberculosis of larynx is very rare.

Predilection to posterior commissure.

Associated with pulmonary tuberculosis.

Presents with hoarseness, productive cough and referred otalgia.

Laryngoscopic findings are
- Waxy pale larynx
- Turban epiglottis
- Mouse-nibbled appearance of vocal cord
- Club-shaped arytenoids and
- Interarytenoid mammillations.

Treatment: ATT (antitubercular treatment).

Chronic Laryngitis

Etiological factors
- Smoking
- Alcohol
- Voice abuse
- Chronic infection of upper respiratory tract, that is, sinusitis
- Male: Female ratio 8:1
- Hoarseness, worst in morning

Types:
- Simple diffuse chronic laryngitis
- Chronic diffuse hyperplastic

May present as vocal nodule, vocal polyp, contact ulcer, Reinke's edema or dysphonia plicae ventricularis.

Causes of laryngeal perichondritis: Radiotherapy, tuberculosis, trauma, malignancy.

CHAPTER 42

Lymphoma in Head and Neck

WHO classification of lymphoid malignancies		
B cell	*T cell*	*Hodgkin's lymphoma*
Precursor B-cell neoplasm Precursor B lymphoblastic leukemia/lymphoma (precursor B-cell acute lymphoblastic leukemia) includes subtypes with recurrent genetic abnormalities	Precursor T-cell neoplasm **Precursor T lymphoblastic lymphoma/leukemia (precursor T cell acute lymphoblastic leukemia)**	Nodular lymphocyte-predominant Hodgkin's lymphoma
Mature (peripheral) B-cell neoplasm **B-cell chronic lympho-cytic leukemia/small lymphocytic lymphoma**	Mature (peripheral) T-cell neoplasm T-cell prolymphocytic leukemia	Classical Hodgkin's lymphoma Nodular sclerosis classical Hodgkin's lymphoma
B-cell prolymphocytic leukemia	T-cell granular lymphocytic leukemia	Lymphocyte-rich classical Hodgkin's lymphoma
Lymphoplasmacytic lymphoma (Waldenström's macroglobulinemia)	Aggressive NK cell leukemia	Mixed-cellularity classical Hodgkin's lymphoma
Splenic marginal zone B-cell lymphoma (± villous lymphocytes)	Adult T-cell lymphoma/leukemia (HTLV-1+)	Lymphocyte-depletion classical Hodgkin's lymphoma
Hairy cell leukemia	Extranodal NK/T-cell lymphoma (HTLV-1+)	Lymphocyte-depletion classical Hodgkin's lymphoma
Plasma cell myeloma/plasmacytoma	Enteropathy-type T-cell lymphoma	
Extranodal marginal zone B-cell lymphoma of MALT type	Hepatosplenic γδ T-cell lymphoma	
Mantle cell lymphoma	Subcutaneous panniculitis-like T-cell lymphoma	
Follicular lymphoma	Mycosis fungoides/Sézary's syndrome	
Nodal marginal zone B-cell lymphoma (± monocytoid B cells)	Anaplastic large cell lymphoma, primary cutaneous type	

Contd.

Contd.

WHO classification of lymphoid malignancies (Contd.)		
B cell	T cell	Hodgkin's lymphoma
Diffuse large B-cell lymphoma (including subtypes)	**Peripheral T-cell lymphoma, not otherwise specific (NOS)**	
Burkitt's lymphoma/ Burkitt's cell leukemia	Angioimmunoblastic T-cell lymphoma	
Primary mediastinal large B-cell lymphoma	**Anaplastic large cell lymphoma, ALK+**	
Plasmablastic lymphoma	Primary cutaneous γδ T-cell lymphoma	
Primary effusion lymphoma		
Large B-cell lymphoma arising in HHV-8+ multicentric Castleman's disease		
Intravascular large B-cell lymphoma		
ALK+ large B-cell lymphoma		

Note: Malignancies in bold occur in at least 1% of patients.

Abbreviations: HHV, human herpesvirus; HTLV, human T-cell lymphotropic virus; MALT, mucosa-associated lymphoid tissue; NK, natural killer; WHO, World Health Organization.

Source: Adapted from SH Swerdlow et al: *WHO Classification of Tumours of Haematropoietic and Lymphoid Tissues,* 4th ed. World Health Organization, 2008.

Hodgkin Lymphoma

Clinical-palpable nontender lymphadenopathy. >50% will have mediastinal lymphadenopathy at the time of diagnosis. One-third of patients present with fever, night sweats and weight loss, fever is Pel-Ebstein type, some unusual manifestation could be unexplained itching, erythema nodosum, cerebellar degeneration, nephrotic syndrome, immune hemolytic anemia, thrombocytopenia, hypercalcemia and pain in lymph nodes on alcohol ingestion.

Hodgkin lymphoma is divided into

1. Nodular lymphocyte—predominant
2. Nodular sclerosis
3. Mixed-cellularity common with HIV infection
4. Lymphocyte depletion common with HIV infection

Differential diagnosis

1. Tub
2. Mononucleosis
3. Non-Hodgkin lymphoma
4. Phenytoin-induced adenopathy
5. Non-lymphoid malignancies.

Investigation: FNAC but biopsy of whole lymph node is better. CBC, ESR, LDH, chest X-ray, CT scan of chest, abdomen and pelvis, USG of neck and abdomen and most useful is PET scan.

Treatment: Localised disease brief course of chemotherapy followed by radiotherapy have high cure rate, i.e. >90%.

Other stages of Hodgkin need chemotherapy

Common chemotherapy is:

1. ABVD: Doxorubicin 25 mg/m^2 IV bolus, day 1 and 15 (adriamycin or k/a—hydroxydaunorubicin H of CHOP) + bleomycin 10 mg/m^2 IV bolus, days 1 and 15 + vinblastine 6 mg/m^2 IV bolus days 1 and 15 + dacarbazine 375 mg/m^2 IV infusion days 1 and 15 (similar to procarbazine). No of cycles given depend on PET CT and neuro-thrombocytopenia.

2. Stanford V regime-doxorubicin 25 mg/m^2 IV day 1 and 15, vinblastine 6 mg/m^2 IV days 1 and 15, mechlorethamine 6 mg/m^2 IV day 1, vincristine 1.4 mg/m^2 IV days 8 and 22, bleomycin 5 mg/m^2 IV days 8 and 22, etoposide 60 mg/m^2 IV days 15 and 16, prednisone 40 mg/m^2 orally for 22 days 2 in Europe BEACOPP regime in high doses are better and good. It is developed by German oncology group and includes—bleomycin, etoposide, doxorubicin, cyclophosphamide, vincristine, procarbazine and prednisone in IIB, IIIB, and stage IV. Total 4 cycles are given often involved radiotherapy is mixed with chemotherapy. No drug is given on days 15–21 days.

   Dosing regime: Bleomycin—10 mg/m^2 IV push days 8

   Etoposide: 100 mg/m^2 IV infusion day 1–3

   Adriamycin: 25 mg/m^2 day 1

   Cyclophosphamide: 650 mg/m^2 IV infusion day 1

   Oncovin/vincristine: 1.4 mg/m^2 IV infusion day 8

   Procarbazine: 100 mg/m^2 orally days 1–7

   Prednisone: 40 mg/m^2 days 1–14

3. Patient who get relapse of disease after effective chemotherapy are not curable and need autologus bone marrow transplantation.

4. In relapse cases immunotoxin, brentuximab, vedontin + ABVD will give better response.

5. Predecessors of BEACOPP were COPP and MOPP.

Treatment of non-Hodgkin lymphoma

1. Small lymphocytic lymphoma CVP/CHOP regime plus Rituximab. Young patient can be considered for bone marrow transplantation.

2. Mucosa associated lymphoid tissue lymphoma. Treatment with chlorambucil plus rituximab + *H. pylori* eradication.

3. Mantle cell lymphoma. Cyclophosphamide + vincristine + doxorubicin + dexamethasone + cytarabine + methotrexate + rituximab.

4. Follicular lymphoma. CVP/CHOP or rituximab + CHOP.

5. Diffuse large B-cell lymphoma. Rituximab + CHOP (America).

6. Burkitt's lymphoma cyclophosphamide in high doses + management of HIV.

7. Mature T-cell/mycosis fungoides lymphoma. Treatment includes—radiotherapy + topical nitrogen mustard + phototherapy + electron beam radiation + interferon.

8. Adult T-cell lymphoma median survival 7 months. Treatment—interferon + zidovudine + arsenic trioxide.

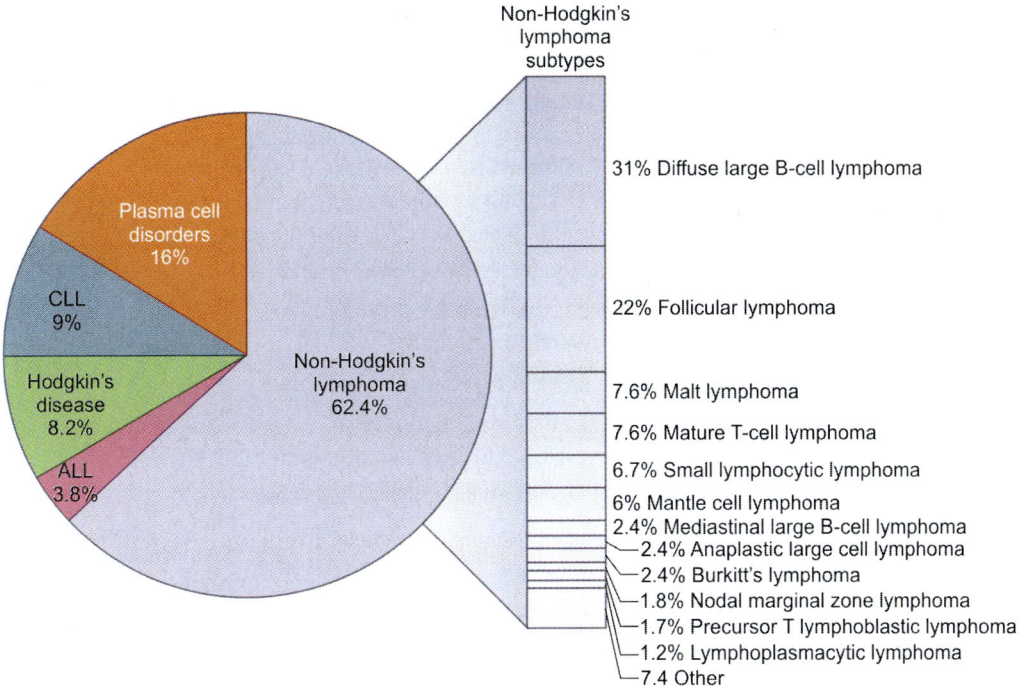

9. Anaplastic large T/null cell lymphoma. Rituximab which is b-cell specific and should not be used.

   Treatment is like large b-cell lymphoma like crizotinib + cd 30 immunotoxin + brentuximab.

10. Peripheral T-cell lymphoma has a fatal outcome, it has heterogenous morphological group like: (a) Nasal type previously termed lethal midline granuloma nose, often converts into leukemia, (b) enteropathy type T-cell lymphoma which occurs in untreated gluten-sensitive enteropathy.

Staging evaluation for non-Hodgkin's lymphoma
Physical examination
Documentation of B symptoms
Laboratory evaluation
Complete blood counts
Liver function tests
Uric acid
Calcium
Serum protein electrophoresis
Serum β_2-microglobulin
Chest radiograph
CT scan of abdomen, pelvis, and usually chest
Bone marrow biopsy
Lumbar puncture lymphoblastic, Burkitt's, and diffuse large B-cell lymphoma with positive marrow biopsy
Gallium scan (SPECT) or PET scan in large cell lymphoma

Abbreviations: CT, computed tomography; PET, positron emission tomography; SPECT, single photon emission computed tomography.

Infectious agents associated with the development of lymphoid malignancies	
Infectious agent	*Lymphoid malignancy*
Epstein-Barr virus	Burkitt's lymphoma
	Post-organ transplant lymphoma
	Primary CNS diffuse large B-cell lymphoma
	Hodgkin's lymphoma
	Extranodal NK/T-cell lymphoma, nasal type
HTLV-1	Adult T-cell leukemia/lymphoma
HIV	Diffuse large B-cell lymphoma
	Burkitt's lymphoma
Hepatitis C virus	Lymphoplasmacytic lymphoma
Helicobacter pylori	Gastric MALT lymphoma
Human herpesvirus 8	Primary effusion lymphoma
	Multicentric Castleman's disease

Abbreviations: CNS, central nervous system; HIV, human immunodeficiency virus; HTLV, human T-cell lymphotropic virus; MALT, mucosa associated lymphoid tissue; NK, natural killer

CHAPTER 43

Cancer Chemotherapy and an Introduction to Radiotherapy

CHEMOTHERAPY FOR HEAD AND NECK TUMORS
Classification of Chemotherapeutic Agents

Category	Examples
Alkylating agents	Cisplatin Carboplatin Cyclophoshamide Busulphan chlorambucil
Antibiotics	Doxorubicin Mitomycin C Bleomycin Actinomycin D Daunorubicin
Antimetabolites	Methotrexate 5-flurouracil 6-mercaptopurine Cytosine arabinoside Thioguanine
Enzymes	L-asparaginase
Hormones	Adrenocorticoids Androgens Estrogens Anti-estrogens Progestogens
Nitrosoureas	Carmustine Lomustine Streptozotocin
Plant alkaloids	Vincristine Vinblastine
Random synthesis	Dacarbazine Hydroxyurea procarbazine

Traditional approach for solid head and neck tumors is given below

Early stage local and regional disease → Surgery/radiotherapy

Recurrent disease and/or metastasis → Radio/chemotherapy

Advanced late stage disease → Chemotherapy.

Tumors are clinically detectable when they attain the weight of 1 gram (10^9 cells). When the tumor cells are between 10^{12} and 10^{13} (1000 gr–10000 gr), mortality due to cancer becomes almost certain. The growth of cancer cells is exponential but the rate of growth decreases with increasing size of the tumor.

Tumor killing by chemotherapy drugs follow first order kinetics, i.e. the number of tumor cells killed by chemotherapy drug remains fairly constant in one exposure. Hence chemotherapy is of good role when the tumor is in initial stage or can be used for palliative care to decrease the tumor mass.

Pharmacological classification of chemotherapeutic drugs

I. *Directly acting cytotoxic drugs*:

1. Alkylating agents

2. Anti-metabolites

3. Natural products: Antibiotics, vinca alkaloids, taxanes, epipodophyllotoxins, camptothecin analogues, enzymes, biological response modifying drugs.

4. Miscellaneous: Cisplatin and carboplatin.

II. *Indirectly acting by altering the hormonal mileau*: Corticosteroids, estrogen and ERM, 5α-reductase inhibitors, GnRH agonists, progestins.

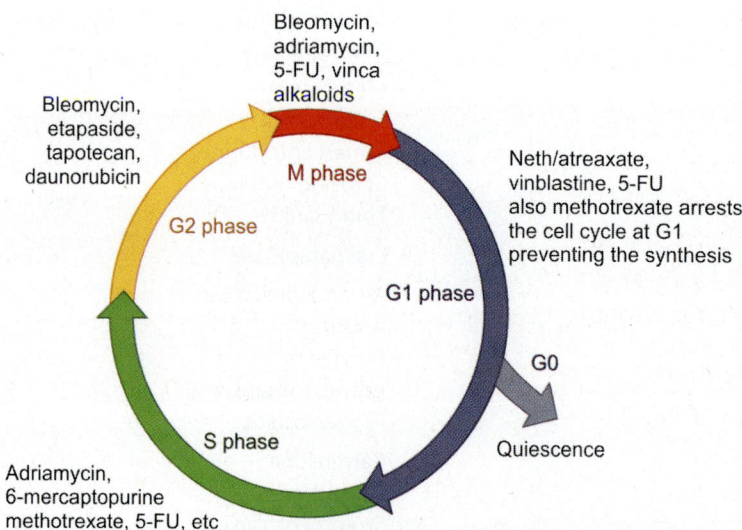

Drugs that do not depend upon the phase of cell cycle are cyclophosphamide, cisplatin, chlorambucil, actinomycin-D, L-asparginase, etc.

Kinetic classification of antitumor drugs

Class II	Class III
Bone marrow cell kill does not increase with increase in dose	Bone marrow cell kill increases with increase in dose
Methotrexate	Adriamycin
Hydroxyurea	Chlorambucil
6-Mercaptopurine	Cyclophosphamide
Vinblastine	5-Fluorouracil
Vincristine	Cisplatin
	Carboplatin
	Methyl-gag
	Mitomycin C

Precautions to be observed in cases receiving chemotherapy

1. Never give another cycle of chemo before the cell counts are confirmed to be normal following the previous cycle.
2. Methotrexate to be given after extended leucovorin (folinic acid) rescue in patients with renal compromise.
3. Doses of cyclophosphamide, adriamycin and 5-FU should be halved in patients who have received thoracic, abdominal and pelvic irradiation.
4. Doses of class III should be halved if the regimen contains more than one of them.
5. Bleomycin should not be given in patients with respiratory disease.
6. Adriamycin should not be given in cardiac illness.
7. Drugs which are excreted in urine, e.g. methotrexate should be given with proper hydration of the patient.

RADIOTHERAPY

Treatment modality based on using high energy rays from radioactive substances. Radiotherapy can be used alone or in combination with other treatment modalities.

Two landmarks in history regarding radiation in medicine are the discovery of X-ray in 1895 by Roentgen and Radium in 1898 by Marie Curie.

Henry Becquerel found the biological effects of radium in living cells.

Units of Radiation

1 Gray (Gy) = 100 rad = 100 cGy

- Curative 6500–7000 rad
- Palliative 4000 rad
- Preoperative 4500 rad

Types of radiation: Electromagnetic (X-ray and Gamma ray) and particulate (proton, electron, neutron, etc.).

Radiation delivery: External beam and internal delivery by placing the radioactive material in the tissue (brachytherapy).

Mechanism of tumor lysis: By directly damaging the DNA or by production of free radicals.

Types of RT: First line RT, adjuvant RT, palliative RT.

Most radiosensitive tumors
- Lymphoma
- Embryonal tumors
- Anaplastic tumors
- All HPV positive head and neck cancers are radiosensitive.

Radioresistant tumors
- Sarcoma
- Melanoma
- Bone and soft tissue tumors

Toxic effects of RT: Acute toxicity—mucositis, erythema, dermatitis, odynophagia.

Contraindications of radiotherapy
- Previous radiotherapy given
- Verrucous carcinoma
- Fibrous dysplasia
- Juvenile papilloma
- Patient refusal
- Cachexic patient (not an absolute contraindication)

Brachytherapy (interstitial): Radiation given at the site of disease.

Advantages
- Higher does can be given without damage to surrounding tissues.
- Duration of radiotherapy can be reduced.
- Dose distribution is superior as it is concentrated.

Sites for brachytherapy
- Tongue
- Maxilla
- Lip
- Nasopharynx

Sources of brachytherapy
- Radium
- Gold 198 seeds
- Tantaleum 182 wires
- Radium 192 seeds
- Caesium 137 needles

Intensity modulated radiotherapy: This has become the standard protocol for patients receiving RT for head and neck tumors in the last 5–10 years in the Western countries. For this, the disease is outlined into **gross tumor, areas at high risk for microscopic spread and areas at low risk for microscopic spread** by extensive pre-treatment evaluation of the disease. Gross tumor receives 70 Gy, high risk areas receive 65 Gy and low risk areas receive 50 Gy. The dose is fractioned into 2 Gy/day. This technique reduces the toxicity significantly.

Palliative treatment: It is the treatment given to alleviate the symptoms without any intent to cure the disease.

It can be in the form of RT or CT (chemotherapy).

Adjuvant chemotherapy: Cytotoxic drugs given to improve survival before, during and after standard treatment.

Induction chemotherapy: Drugs given to improve the survival prior to the standard treatment.

Care during the radiotherapy
- Soft diet—to avoid pain because of mucositis
- Care of teeth—remove unhealthy teeth
- Avoid alcohol
- Avoid smoking
- Avoid spicy food
- Avoid shaving—electric shaver can be used
- Avoid soap—at affected area
- Avoid plaster
- Avoid sunlight

After how many days post-RT surgery should be done?
Minimum 6 weeks, by that time edema subsides.

Advantages of preoperative radiotherapy
- Tissues are well oxygenated, so better results
- Tumor size may decrease

Disadvantages of preoperative radiotherapy
- More bleeding
- Tissues planes are difficult to find
- Poor oxygenation at diseased areas
- Chances of flap necrosis are more.

CHAPTER 44

Occult Primary

Neck swelling which in turn found to be malignant metastasis from an unknown primary malignancy is called nodal metastasis from an occult primary malignancy. Its prevalence is 5% among all head and neck malignancies. In more than 90% cases of neck secondary from an occult primary, the primary is a squamous cell carcinoma from Waldeyer's ring, with one out of 4 cases arising from tonsils. The remaining may be adenocarcinoma, melanoma or other rare malignancies.

The symptoms are painless neck swelling growing in size over months. The swelling can be painful if there is suppuration of the involved node. Prevalence is more among males than in females. Just like other head and neck malignancies, tobacco and/or alcohol addiction is a major risk factor in these cases.

Evaluation

This evaluation includes:

1. *History:* To get information like loss of weight and appetite, skin lesions like mole and their removal, ear ache, nasal obstruction, throat pain, shortness of breath, voice change, dysphagia, cough with expectoration, etc.

2. *Clinical examination:* Palpation of the swelling to look for the consistency, number, fixity, etc. Posterior rhinoscopy to examine nasopharynx, oral cavity, bimanual palpation of base of tongue and tonsils, indirect laryngoscopy to view hypopharynx, larynx, thorough skin examination to look for moles and other suspicious lesions, palpation of thyroid, etc.

3. *Fine needle aspirate of the lymph node:* To confirm the malignant nature of the disease and to obtain idea about the primary. This is the most beneficial test as it gives the histological clue regarding the occult which in turn helps to identify the site of primary.

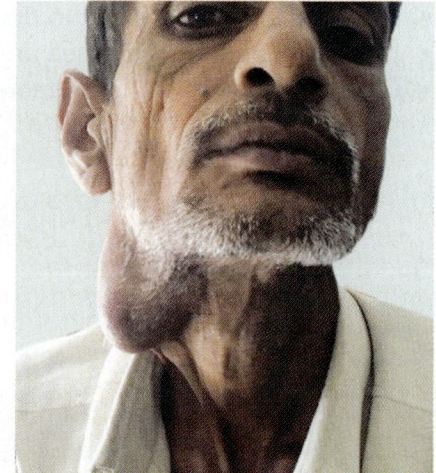

Picture of a patient with occult right neck fixed node. Pan-endoscopy did not reveal any primary

4. *Examination under anesthesia* like direct laryngoscopy, rigid esophagoscopy, naso-pharyngoscopy, etc. along **with directed biopsy** and bilateral tonsillectomy.
5. *Radiological investigation* includes chest X-ray, CECT of head and neck, gadolinium enhanced MRI of head and neck (from skull base to thoracic inlet), PET-CT scan (last option when the primary is still unknown). In 26% of cases where the primary was still unknown, PET CT identified the primary malignancy.

NECK DISSECTION IN OCCULT PRIMARY

When the primary is found out and if its operable surgical excision should be done along with radical neck dissection (gold standard management). If no primary is found till end and node are mobile, radical neck dissection is to be done. In these patients, in case if primary appears later, then surgical excision should be done. If lymph nodes are fixed to carotid and/or inoperable, then palliative radiotherapy and/or chemotherapy should be given.

Second primary: It is also called synchronous tumor. It is the presence of two different primary malignant tumors in the same region, prevalence is 10% among head and neck tumors.

Residual cancer: It appears within 6 months after treatment.

Recurrence is when cancer appears after 6 months of treatment.

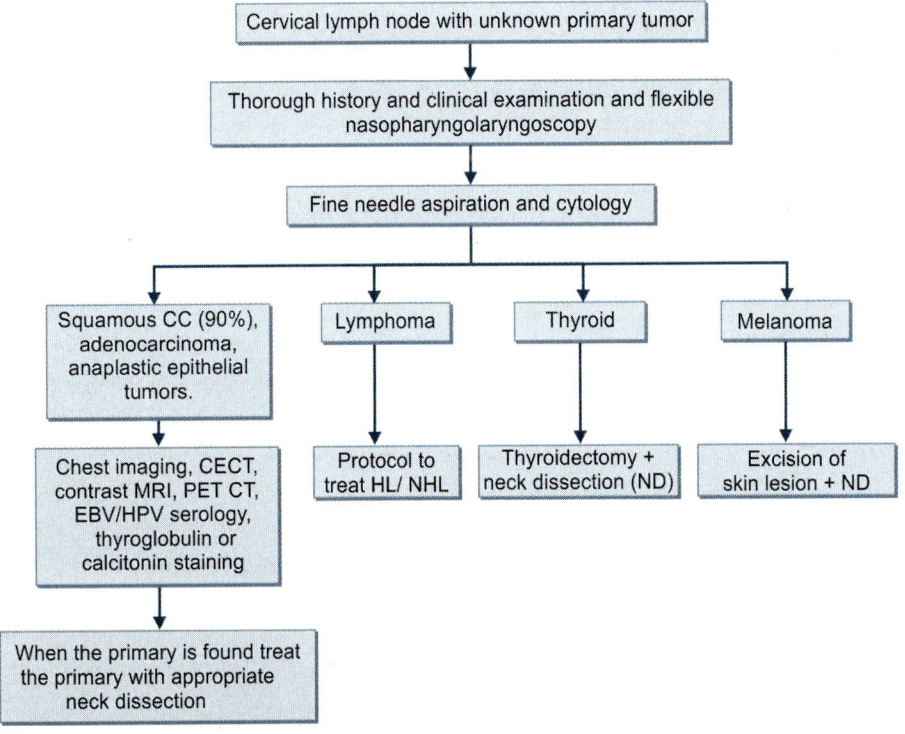

CHAPTER 45

Salivary Glands

Saliva secretion per day
- 500–700 ml
- 3/4th from submandibular gland
- pH is around 6.5

Functions of saliva
- Lubrication of food
- Bacteriostatic: Lysozyme
- Helps in digestion: Amylase
- Excretory function: Urea
- Solvent
- Taste

Factors which affect the quantity and quality of saliva: Drugs, taste, smell, radiotherapy, tactile stimulation, psychic.

Xerostomia: Sjögren's syndrome, uraemia, diabetes, Plummer-Vinson syndrome.

Minor salivary glands
600–1000 in numbers, present at following places: Oral cavity, nose, sinus, postnasal space, oropharynx, larynx and trachea.

Sialolithiasis: Two types
1. Calcium (opaque)—can be seen in X-ray
2. Magnesium (non-opaque)—cannot be seen in X-ray.

Most commonly occurring in submandibular gland. The reasons are
- Secretions are rich in calcium salts than parotid gland stones.
- Wharton's duct drainage is antigravity.
- Parotid duct is intermittently squeezed by buccinator muscle

Treatment is by removal of stone by an intraoral incision. After removal of the stone, the wound is not sutured and left open to heal forming a new opening for the duct. Recently sialolithiasis are removed by sialendoscopy. Advantage is it is a scarless, daycare procedure and its advent has decreased the need for removal of the gland.

Tumors of Salivary Glands

Benign: Pleomorphic adenoma
- Warthin's tumor
- Oncocytoma
- Hemangioma

Malignant: Mucoepidermoid carcinoma—most common in children

Acinic cell carcinoma: Best prognosis
- Adenoid cystic carcinoma perineural spread
- Squamous cell carcinoma
- Undifferentiated carcinoma

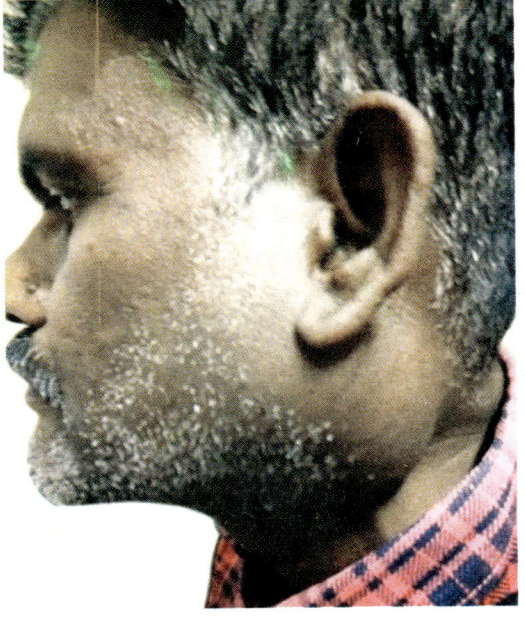

Hard swelling in left parotid later on found to be carcinoma of parotid by FNAC examination. The swelling was fixed to skin as well as underlying tissues.

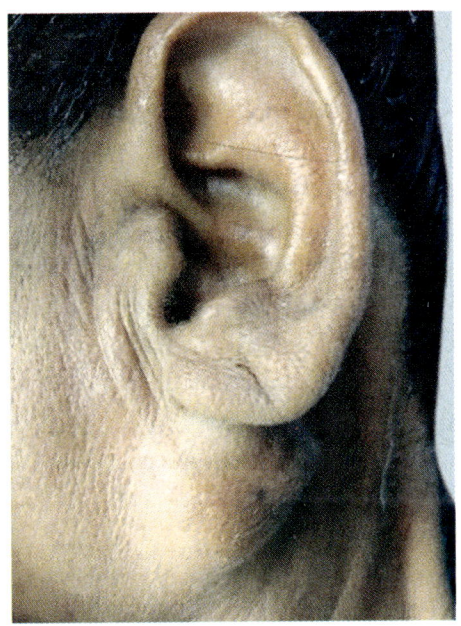

Clinical picture of a patient with pleomorphic adenoma; the swelling was mobile and free from skin.

Tumors of salivary glands: 80% are located in parotid, of which 80% are benign and pleomorphic adenoma in nature.
- 10% are located in submandibular gland.
- Rest in minor salivary glands, majority of which are malignant.

CHAPTER 46

Thyroid Glands

Malignancies of Thyroid

Papillary: Microcarcinoma, follicular variant and diffuse sclerosing variants.

   Most common at early age, best prognosis, lymph node involvement is common.

Follicular: Minimally invasive, widely invasive and poorly differentiated subtypes.

   Associated with past history of radiation, seen in older age group and lymph node involvement is rare.

Medullary: Variants including mixed medullary follicular carcinoma.

   Arises from parafollicular 'C' cells which secrete calcitonin. Associated with MEN II.

Anaplastic: Worst prognosis.

   Hurthle cell carcinoma.

Others: Lymphoma, sarcoma.

   Secondaries.

Low risks for malignancy and high risk for malignancy

Female	Male
Young adult	Older age or children
Subcentimeter nodules	Large solitary solid mass
Stable size	Rapid increase in size
Multinodular gland or cyst	Palpable lateral lymph nodes
No local symptoms	Evidence of local invasion
Suppressed TSH	Radiation exposure
Benign FNAC	Malignant in FNAC

Risk group categories in thyroid nodules

Low	High
Age <45	> 45
Size <4 cm	> 4 cm
Extent—intraglandular	Extraglandular
FNA grades—low	High
Distant metastasis—absent	Present
Transverse diameter > AP	AP > TRANS

Use of thyroid scan
- Hot/cold nodule
- Solitary or multinodular swelling
- Functional pulmonary metastasis can be detected
- Ectopic thyroid tissue can be detected

Incidentalloma

It is a thyroid nodule accidentally found during neck ultrasound. They are dangerous if detected after 45 years of age.

Assessing a thyroid swelling: Structural assessment—physical examination, ultrasound, CT scans, MRI functional assessment—thyroid function test, anti-Tg, anti-TPO, radio iodine scans, FDG-PET.

Dangerous thyroid swellings will show the following features:
- Age > 45
- Size > 4.5 cm
- AP diameter more than transverse
- Microcalcifications in USG
- Irregular margins
- Neck metastatic nodes
- Hypoechoic
- Solid within cystic swelling
- Increased vascularity

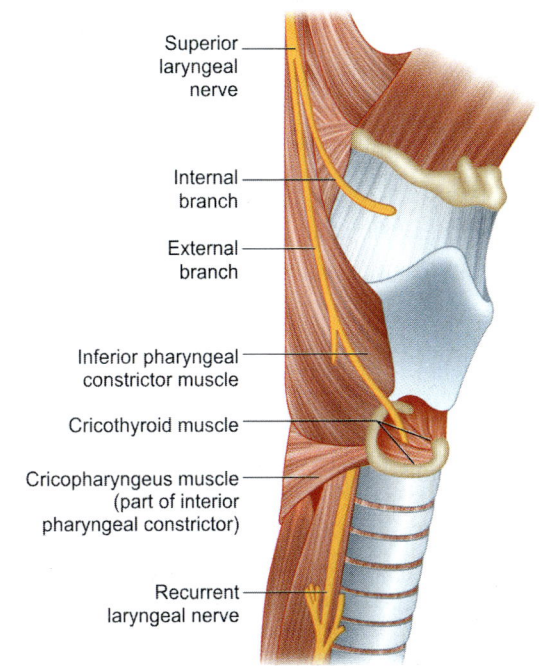

Superior laryngeal and recurrent laryngeal nerve distribution

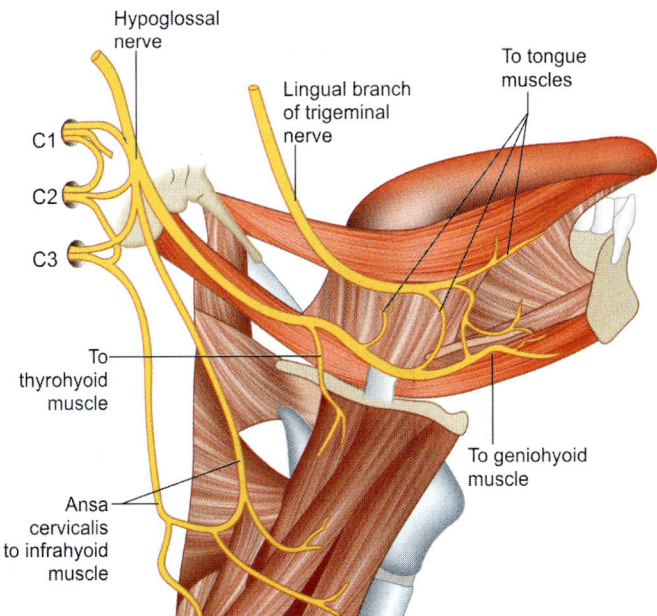

Relationship of ansa hypoglossi terminal branches to the strap muscles of neck directs the surgeon to cut the upper fibres of sternothyroid muscle to expose thyroid during thyroid surgeries

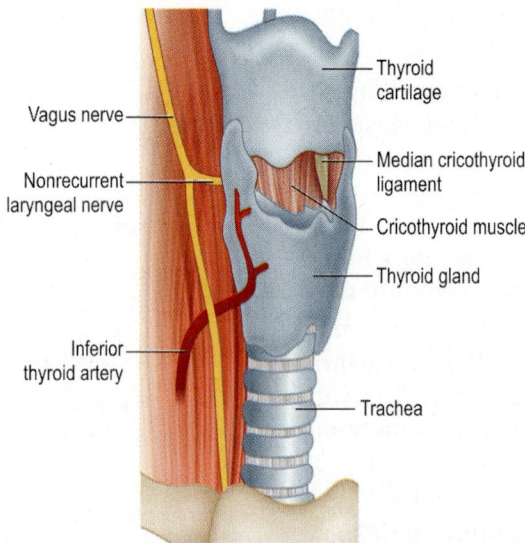

Non-recurrent laryngeal nerve in the right side (MC) due to retroesophageal right subclavian artery

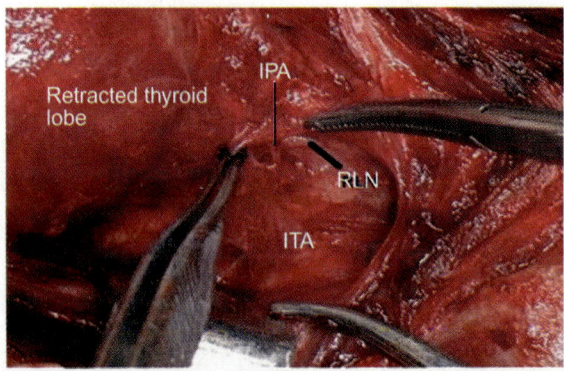

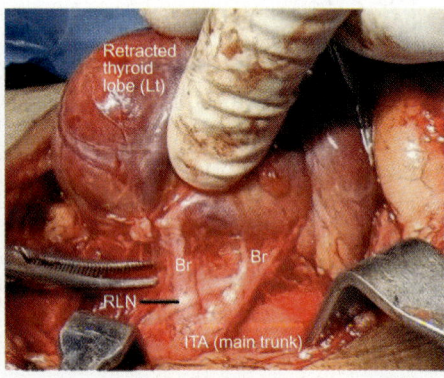

Right RLN passing posterior to inferior thyroid artery and artery to inferior parathyroid (IPA)

Left RLN passing in-between the branches of inferior thyroid artery

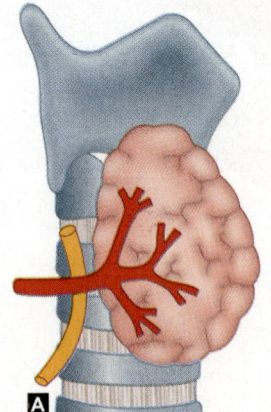

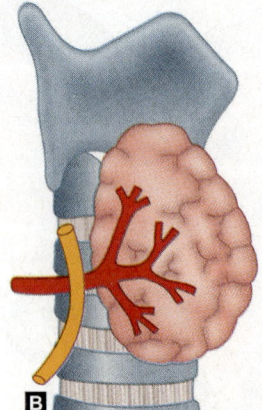

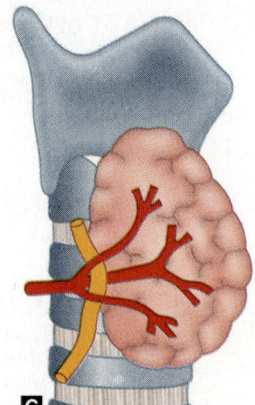

Anatomical variations in the course of RLN in relation to the branches of inferior thyroid artery; (A) Posterior to ITA; (B) Anterior to ITA; (C) In-between the branches of ITA

Approach to Solitary Thyroid Nodule

Differential diagnosis for a solitary thyroid nodule can be of either benign diseases of thyroid or malignant diseases.

Benign: Thyroid adenoma (toxic and non-toxic), hyperplastic nodules, thyroid cysts, thyroiditis, thyroid lymphoma

Malignant: All as mentioned previously.

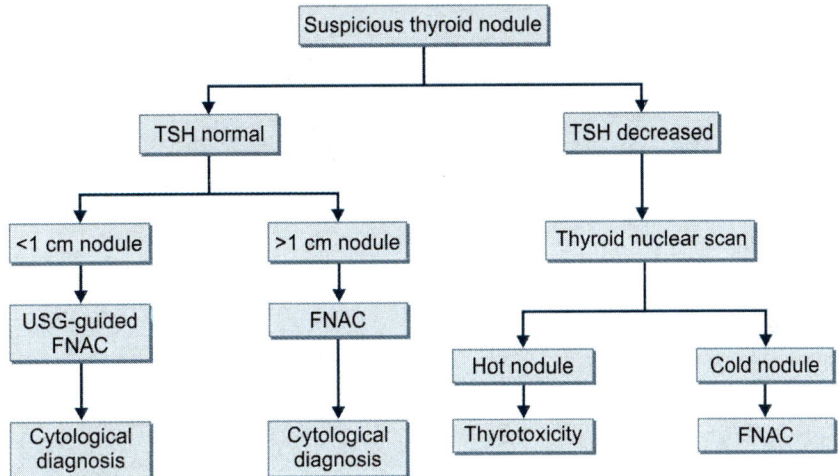

Fine needle aspirate cytology of thyroid

Category	Description	Management
Thy-1	Non-diagnostic, insufficient sample.	Repeat FNAC
Thy-2	Benign	Clinical follow up
Thy-3	Atypia of undetermined significance or follicular lesion	Repeat FNAC
Thy-4	Follicular neoplasm	Lobectomy
Thy-5	Malignant	Total thyroidectomy or lobectomy

CHAPTER 47

Skull Foramina

Foramen magnum
- Lower part of medulla
- Tonsil of cerebellum may project
- Meninges
- Spinal accessory nerve
- Vertebral artery
- Sympathetic plexuses
- Posterior spinal artery
- Anterior spinal artery
- Apical ligament
- Membrana tectoria

Foramen jugular
- Inferior petrosal sinus
- Meningeal branch of ascending pharyngeal artery
- Internal jugular vein
- 9th, 10th and 11th cranial nerve
- Meningeal branch of occipital artery

Foramen rotundum
- Maxillary nerve

Foramen ovale
- Mandibular nerve
- Lesser petrosal nerve
- Accessory meningeal artery
- Emissary vein

Foramen spinosum
- Middle meningeal artery
- Meningeal branch of mandibular nerve
- Emissary vein

Foramen lacerum
- Nothing significant

Superior orbital fissure
a. Lateral portion
    - Lacrimal nerve
    - Frontal nerve
    - Trochlear nerve
    - Superior ophthalmic vein
b. Middle portion
    - Abducent nerve
    - Nasociliary nerve
    - Upper and lower division of oculomotor nerve
c. Medial portion
    - Inferior ophthalmic vein
    - Sympathetic plexus around ICA

Inferior orbital fissure
- V2 (maxillary division of trigeminal nerve)
- Infraorbital artery and vein

Structure passing between base of skull and superior constrictor (sinus of Morgagni)
- Eustachian tube
- Tensor palatine
- Levator palate
- Branch of ascending pharyngeal artery

Anterior condyloid foramen (hypoglossal canal): XIIth nerve.

Structure passing through the cavernous sinus
- IIIrd, IVth and Vth
- VIth
- ICA

Structure between superior constrictor and middle constrictor
- Stylopharyngeous
- Glossopharyngeal nerve

Structure between middle constrictor and inferior constrictor
- Internal laryngeal nerve
- Superior laryngeal artery

Structure below inferior constrictor
- Recurrent laryngeal nerve
- Inferior laryngeal artery.

CHAPTER 48

Spaces in Head and Neck

Pharynx

Parapharyngeal space: Shape is like inverted pyramid having base towards sphenoid and apex towards lesser horn of hyoid bone.

Boundaries
- *Medial:* Inferior tonsil
- *Superiorly:* Eustachian tube
- *Lateral:* Ramus of mandible and deep lobe of parotid
- *Posterior:* Cervical spine covered with prevertebral fascia and muscles
- *Anterior:* Pterygoid muscles

Contents

Contents	Prestyloid	Poststyloid
Arteries	Nil	ICA
Veins	Nil	Internal jugular
Nerves	Inf alveolar, lingual	IX, X, XI, XII
Glomus bodies	Nil	+
Lymph nodes	Nil	++

Tumors
- Neurogenic
- Schwannoma
- Neurofibroma
- Paraganglioma
- Glomus vagale
- Lipoma
- Dermoid
- Hemangioma
- Carotid body tumors
- Mixed salivary gland tumors
- Aneurysm of ICA
- Lymphoma

Parapharyngeal Space Infection

Common causes are tonsillar infection, dental infection, CSOM, lateral sinus thrombophlebitis and lymph node suppuration.

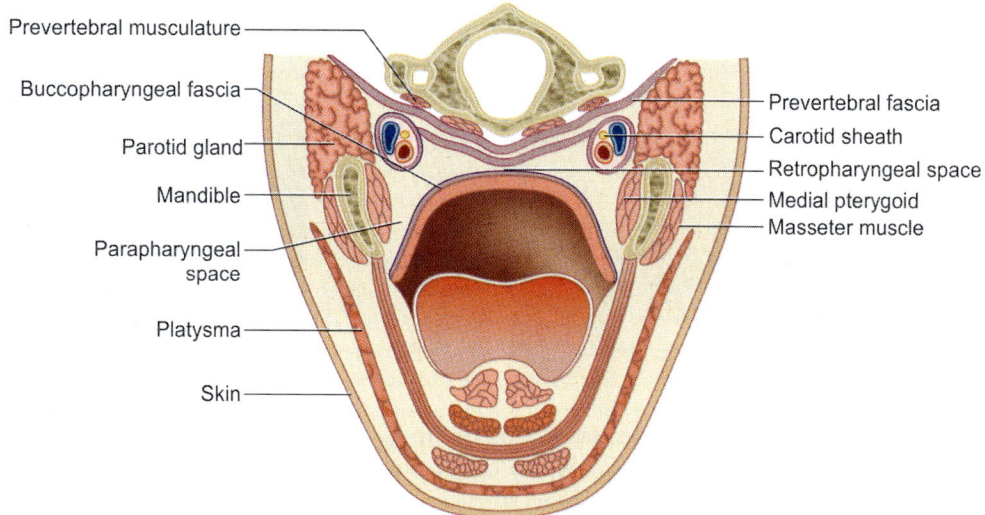

Parapharyngeal space: (1) Buccopharyngeal fascia, (2) mandible, (3) parapharyngeal space, (4) parotid gland, (5) carotid sheath, (6) mastoid process, (7) prevertebral musculature, (8) prevertebral fascia, (9) retropharyngeal space, (10) lateral pharyngeal wall, (11) tonsil.

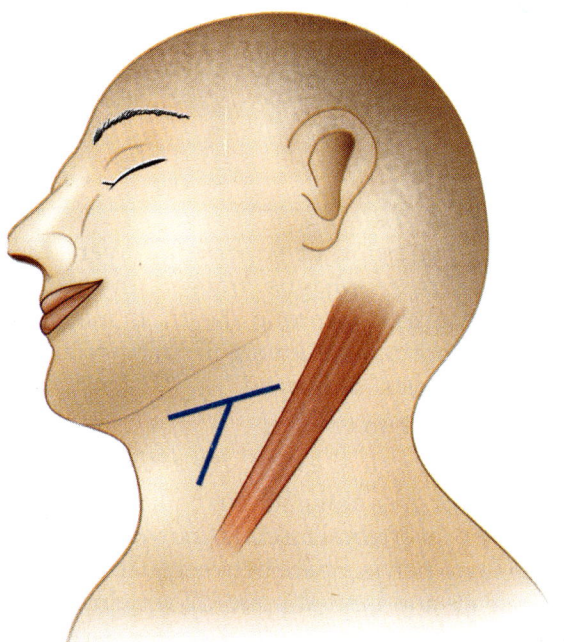

Incision for parapharyngeal abscess

Retropharyngeal Space (Gillette Space)

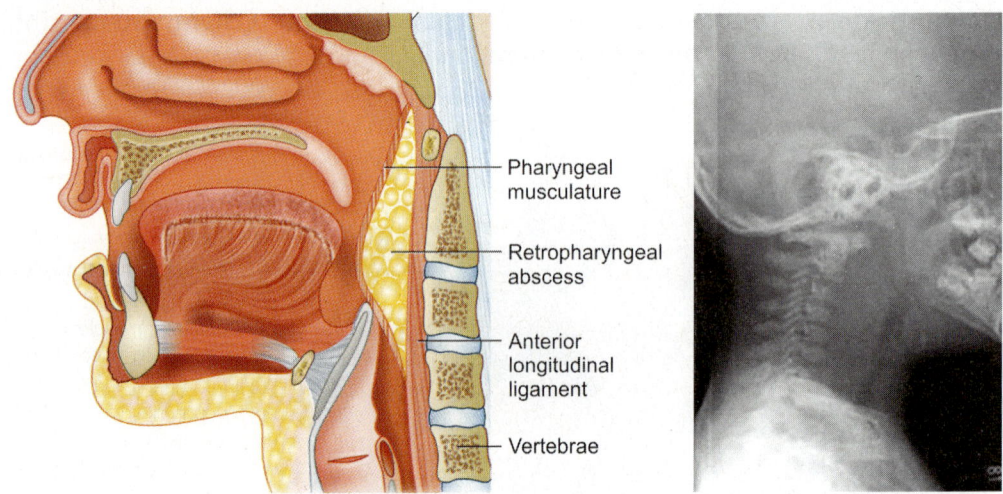

Pharyngeal musculature

Retropharyngeal abscess

Anterior longitudinal ligament

Vertebrae

Retropharyngeal abscess (3), anterior long ligament (2), vertebrae (1) and pharyngeal musculature (4); next image shows X-ray of a patient with retropharyngeal abscess. Note the increased soft tissue density in front of cervical vertebrae.

A good knowledge of neck spaces needs knowledge of cervical fascia (Colle's fascia). Cervical fascia compartments are:

1. Superficial fascia
2. Deep cervical fascia

Superficial cervical fascia encircles head and neck; thin anteriorly and thick posteriorly. Structures seen within it is platysma.

Deep cervical fascia has 3 layers

A. Superficial investing layer
   1. Posterior triangle
   2. Suprasternal space of burn
   3. Supraclavicular space.
B. Middle visceral layer is extension of superficial layer and encircle following structures—pharynx, larynx, esophagus, trachea, thyroid gland, strap muscle, carotid and jugular with vagus k/a carotid sheath. In mediastinum carotid sheath blends with adventitia of aorta, hence a significant portal of spread of infection called "Lincoln highway of neck" is formed.
C. Prevertebral fascia. It divides into two:
   1. Alar layer gets attached to wall of esophagus at C7 level.
   2. Prevertebral fascia proper goes along longus colli muscle up to pelvis. This space between alar facia and prevertebral fascia is known as danger space and infection in this space can go up to pelvis. Space between alar and buccopharyngeal fascia known as Rouviér space and limited up to C7 vertebra.

Prevertebral space: This space lies between vertebral bodies and prevertebral fascia. It extends from base of skull to coccyx.

Submandibular space: This space lies between the mucous membrane of floor of mouth, tongue and superficial fascia extending between the hyoid bone and mandible. It is further divided into:

1. *Sublingual:* Above mylohyoid
2. *Submaxillary:* Below mylohyoid

Infection of this space is known as **Ludwig's angina.** Causes are dental infections, fracture of mandible, injuries to oral mucosa and submandibular sialadenitis. (Wilheim Friedrich von Ludwig in 1836).

Criteria of Ludwig's Angina

1. Cellulitis and not an abscess.
2. Does not involve submandibular gland.
3. Floor of mouth is swollen and tongue pushed up and anteriorly.
4. Involves both sublingual and submaxillary space.

Paratonsillar space: Between the wall of pharynx and mucous membrane of the fauces.

Parotid space: Bounded by posterior part of ramus, styloid process and its muscles, sterno-mastoid and posterior belly of digastric. It contains parotid gland and lymph nodes.

Others

- Carotid space
- Masticator space
- Pterygoid space

Larynx

Pre-epiglottic space (Space of Boyer)

- Boundaries
- *Superior:* Hyoepiglottic ligament
- *Anterior:* Thyroid cartilage and thyrohyoid membrane
- *Posterior:* Epiglottis

Laterally it is continuous with paraglottic space. It contains fat, loose areolar tissues and a few glands.

Paraglottic space

- *Lateral:* Thyroid ala
- *Superomedial:* Quadrangular membrane
- *Inferomedial:* Conus elasticus
- *Posterior:* Pyriform fossa

It is continuous with pre-epiglottic space.

The immediate relation of this space with pyriform sinus highlights the spread of tumors from both sides and early fixation of hemilarynx in cases of pyriform cancer. Similarly endolaryngeal malignancy with paraglottic involvement may show the involvement of pyriform sinus.

The involvement of this space by malignancy of larynx may be palpated in neck.

Reinke's space: Subepithelial space of vocal cord. It contains loose areolar tissue.

Bounded superiorly and inferiorly by arcuate lines. Anteriorly by the anterior commissure and posteriorly by vocal process.

Ear

Prussak's space
- *Floor:* Lateral process of malleus
- *Lateral:* Pars flaccida
- *Superior:* Superior malleolar fold which is attached with notch of Rivinus

Anterior pouch of von Troltsch: Space between tympanic membrane and anterior malleolar fold.

Posterior pouch of von Troltsch: Space between tympanic membrane and posterior malleolar fold.

Miscellaneous

Space of burns: Space within suprasternal notch, sometimes lymph nodes can be found here in cases of cancer of thyroid and larynx.

Pterygopalatine Fossa

A pyramidal shaped space between posterior part of maxilla anteriorly and pterygoid process of sphenoid bone posteriorly.

Other boundaries
- *Medial:* Perpendicular plate of palatine bone
- *Lateral:* Pterygomaxillary fissure, infratemporal fossa
- *Superior:* Undersurface of sphenoid bone
- *Inferior:* Pyramidal process of palatine bone, i.e. angle between maxilla and pterygoid process

Communications
- *Medial:* Sphenopalatine foramen, nose.
- *Lateral:* Infratemporal fossa through pterygomaxillary fissure.
- *Posterior:* Foramen rotundum, middle cranial fossa, Vidian nerve.
- *Inferior:* Lesser and greater palatine canals.
- *Anterior:* Medial end of inferior orbital fissure.

Infratemporal Fossa

It lies below the middle cranial fossa between ramus of mandible and lateral wall of pharynx.
- *Medial:* Medial pterygoid and interpterygoid fascia
- *Lateral:* Mandible
- *Superior:* Greater wing of sphenoid and small portion of squamous temporal bone
- *Anterior:* Posterior wall of maxilla with pterygomaxillary fissure and inferior orbital fissure
- *Posterior:* Carotid sheath and styloid apparatus.

Contents: Medial and lateral pterygoid muscles, maxillary artery with its branches, veins, pterygoid plexus and branches of mandibular nerve.

Tumors of infratemporal fossa: Angiofibroma, meningioma, fibrosarcoma and chondrosarcoma, tumors of parotid and maxilla.

Approaches
- Conservative lateral
- Radical lateral
- Anterior transantral
- Extended anterolateral
- Superior
- Inferior

CHAPTER 49

Recent Advances in ENT

LASER

Light amplification by stimulated emission of radiation. They are used in surgeries to incise, excise or vaporise the tissue. Laser (CO_2) was first used in ENT by Strong and Jako in the year 1972.

Various lasers available in use are CO_2, Nd:YAG (neodymium: Yttrium-aluminium-garnet), KTP (potassium titanyl phosphate) and argon. Each of them has different wavelengths, tissue interactions and are used in different conditions. If an ENT surgeon is supposed to possess only one laser, it is CO_2 laser which is very precise and helps in atraumatic surgeries. Whereas Nd: YAG, the second commonly used laser in ENT, is used in deeper tissue planes (as it is not absorbed by water).

Laser–tissue bio-interactions

- *Photo-stimulation*: Low level, improved wound healing and pain relief
- Photo-coagulation of protein
- *Vapourisation*: Immediate cell death (tissue destruction)
- Photo-mechanical
- Photo-chemical

Characteristics of Laser beam

1. Monochromatic light with same wavelength
2. Unidirectional and focused

Advantages of laser

1. Immediate tissue destruction reducing the duration of procedures.
2. Bloodless dissection leading to clean operating fields.
3. Precision and minimal injury to adjacent tissues, thus significantly less postoperative pain.

Types of laser

Laser	Wavelength (nm)	Color	Remark
Argon	488–514	Blue visible	Absorbed by pigmented tissues, so used in photocoagulation of hemangioma, retina, stapes surgery and tympanoplasty
KTP-532	532	Blue green visible	Absorbed by pigments. Used in micro-ear surgery
Nd: YAG	1060	Invisible	Transmittable in flexible endoscopes. Used in tracheal and bronchial surgeries
CO_2	1060	Invisible	As CO_2 Laser beam is invisible, helium/neon aiming beam is required to focus, cannot be transmitted through flexible fibres. Very effective for vaporization

Precautions during LASER surgery
- Designate the area for laser with emission warning.
- Only authorised persons are allowed inside the room.
- Eye protection is not only for staff but for patient also. Plain glasses are good enough.
- Non-inflammable gases should be used for anesthesia.
- Endotracheal tubes should be wrapped with aluminium foil or should be laser proof.
- All the exposed area of patient should be made wet with moist towel.

Uses in laryngology: Vocal nodules, polyps, webs, stenosis, papillomas, malignancy.

Uses in otology: Stapes surgery—primary and revision, acoustic neuroma, breaking of adhesions within middle ear, etc.

Uses in rhinology: Rhinophyma, hemangioma, papilloma, etc.

Others: UPP (uvulopharyngopalatoplasty), pharyngeal pouch, tumors of tongue, tumors of oral cavity, leukoplakia, etc.

CRYOSURGERY

It is the technique of applying temperatures below freezing point to kill the tissues. First used in 1851 by Arnott. Liquid nitrogen was first used for this purpose in 1961 by Cooper and Lee.

The physiological changes caused by cryosurgery probe to living tissues are rupture of cell membrane, intracellular dehydration due to freezing of water, protein denaturing, disruption of cell metabolism due to ischemia and local intravascular thrombosis.

Temperature as low as –20°C is reached and then tissue is thawed. The procedure is repeated multiple times. Time duration for a single cycle is 5–6 minutes.

Cryosurgery is based on Joule Thompson principle, i.e. cooling is produced when expanding gas passes through the narrow passage.

Common gases used are nitrous oxide producing –70°C and liquid nitrogen producing –196°C.

Four methods
1. Rapid freeze and rapid thaw
2. Rapid freeze and slow thaw
3. Slow freeze slow thaw (most effective)
4. Slow freeze rapid thaw

Uses
1. *Oral cavity*: Tonsillectomy, granular pharyngitis, non-malignant ulcers, etc.
2. *Nose*: Epistaxis, vasomotor rhinitis, benign tumors like papilloma, hemangioma, JNA, inferior turbinoplasty, etc.
3. Palliative procedures in malignant oral ulcers.
4. Others: Meniere's disease, hypophysectomy.

COBLATOR

Coblation is also called "controlled ablation". Initially it was used in arthroscopic surgeries, later ENT surgeons started using it.

Principle: Radiofrequency ablation of tissue without involving heat production. When these waves are passed through saline, it produces plasma field by breaking water into sodium and chloride ions. This plasma field breaks the organic bonds in the tissue leading to its disintegration; thus the action is purely chemical and non-thermal.

Stages of plasma generation are
1. Vapour gas piston formation
2. Vapour film pulsation (tissue dissolution occurs)
3. Reduction of amplitude of current across the electrodes
4. Dissipation of electron energy at the metal electrode surface.

Differences between coblator and electrocautery

	Coblator	Electrocautery
Temperature	40–70°C	400–600°C
Thermal penetration	Minimum	Deep
Effects on target tissue	Gentle dissolution	Rapid burning, charring and cutting
Effects on surrounding tissue	Minimum	Unavoidable charring and permanent damage

ENT surgeries commonly performed with coblator are: (1) Adenotonsillectomy; (2) Tongue base reduction; (3) Tongue channeling; (4) Uvulo palato pharyngoplasty; (5) Cordectomy; (6) Removal of benign lesions of larynx like papilloma; (7) Kashima's procedure for bilateral abductor paralysis; (8) Turbinate reduction; (9) Nasal polypectomy; and (10) JNA.

CT NAVIGATION AND IMAGE GUIDED SURGERY IN ENDOSCOPIC ENDONASAL SURGERIES

Nasal and paranasal sinus endoscopic anatomy is very complicated and thus the risk of causing any grievous injury during surgery is always there. This is where the image guided systems, also known as navigation systems, is fast becoming an important and useful tool. Navigation guides the surgeon to confirm the location of anatomical

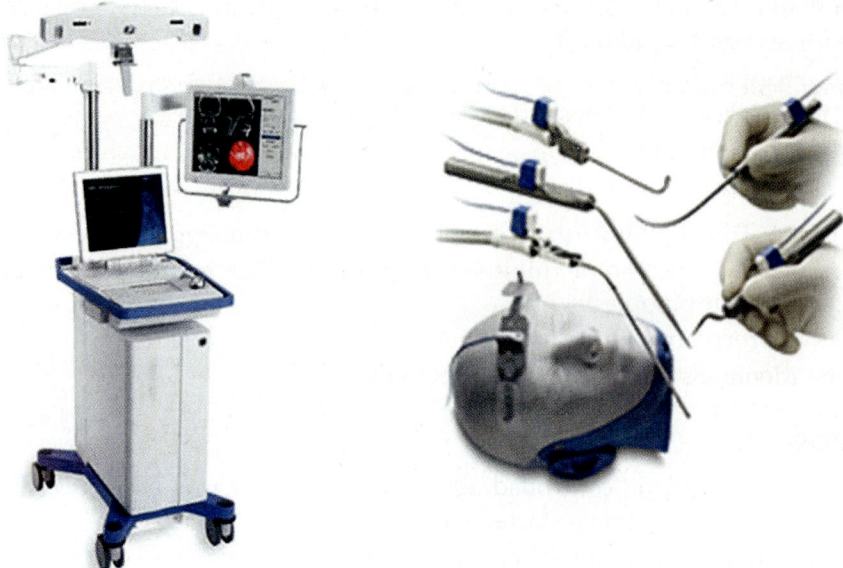

structures intraoperatively. It is like a GPS for surgical field. The surgical precision is up to 2 mm.

Preoperative CT scan of the patient (at least 0.5 mm cut) is loaded into the navigation system. Marker leads are placed on patient's face in specific reference points. The specially designed instruments are to be used. The position of the instrument can be monitored in the loaded CT scan image continuously during the surgery.

Limiting factor for the technique is the expenditure. But considering the facts of increased endonasal skull base surgeries and increased medicolegal cases, it is going to be a necessity of the future.

Appropriate indications for image guided FESS by AAO-HNS are
1. Revision sinus surgery
2. Distorted sinus anatomy of development, postoperative or traumatic origin
3. Extensive sinonasal polyposis: Pathology involving the frontal, posterior ethmoid and sphenoid sinuses
4. Disease abutting the skull base, orbit, optic nerve or carotid artery
5. CSF rhinorrhea or conditions where there is a confirmed or suspected skull base defect
6. Benign and malignant sinonasal neoplasms.

CONTACT ENDOSCOPY

Gold standard investigation to diagnose head and neck malignancies is "Histopathological biopsy". But in cancer of larynx, biopsy can cause troubles like bleeding, voice change, painful swallowing and infections other than those caused by the disease per se. There can also be necessary for multiple biopsies in some patients.

Contact endoscopy is a non-traumatic, easily repeatable *in vivo* technique to show the histopathological picture of the disease. Invented in the year 1979 and used to diagnose cancer larynx from 1995.

Other than laryngeal cancer it can also be used to diagnose oral, hypopharynx, nasal and nasopharyngeal lesions, etc. Also can be used to identify recurring cholesteatoma.

Technique: Real time and *in vivo* examination of the pattern of vascularisation as well as cellular architecture of the superficial layers of the mucosa with the help of endoscope. Commonly used endoscopes are 0 and 30° rigid endoscopes with camera having magnification up to 60X to 150X. Cellular architecture can be studied after staining the tissue with methylene blue.

Advantages
1. Non-invasive and fast
2. Can be used to examine wide area
3. Avoids risks of bleeding and cancer spread
4. Mapping of tumor margins
5. OPD procedure

BAROTRAUMA (DYSBARISM) IN ENT
1. Otic barotrauma
2. Sinus barotrauma
3. Dental barotrauma

Otic Barotrauma/Aviation Pressure Deafness/Aero Otitis Media
Middle ear disease following sudden change and difference in the air pressure between outside atmosphere and middle ear cavity. Commonly it occurs during landing of commercial airplanes, fighter jets, descent from hilly terrains and deep sea diving.

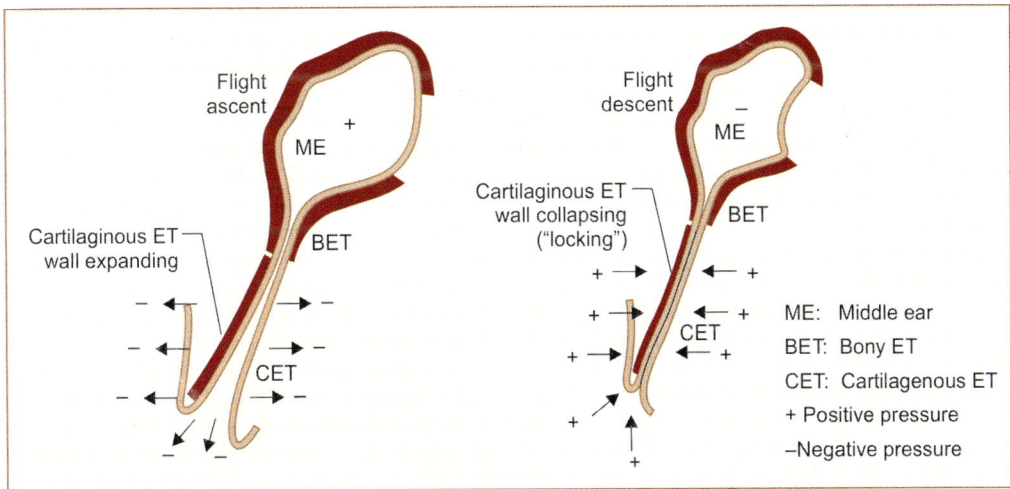

Barotrauma becomes more common in upper respiratory tract inflammations. Commercial passenger airplanes usually fly at the height of 36,000 ft (atm. pressure at 18,000 ft is half of pressure at ground level and at 34,000 ft it is 1/4th of pressure at ground level) above the ground level and air pressure within it is maintained for that height which is negative than ground level. Now during landing, air is pumped into the cabin to equalize to the ground level pressure but because of inflammation around eustachian tube the air pressure remains negative inside the middle ear but it becomes equal to outside atmospheric pressure in EAC. This negative pressure in middle ear leads extravasation of fluid from the middle ear mucosa and sometimes even bleeding. And there is ear pain, hearing loss and blocked feeling of ears for the patient. If this pressure gradient is more than 90 mm of Hg, then eustachian tube gets locked and is very difficult to manage. These patients can be managed by keeping them inside hypobaric chamber to gradually equalize the pressure inside middle ear and EAC/ nasopharynx. If the pressure gradient is 100–500 mm of Hg, the tympanic membrane can rupture, inner ear membranes can also rupture and cause fistula. Inner ear barotrauma can be diagnosed by presence of vestibular and cochlear symptoms.

Causes of failure of pressure equilibration in flight descents are: Sleeping during descent, eustachian tube dysfunction due to anatomical abnormality, edema due to rhinitis, URTIs, chronic middle ear diseases and pregnancy.

Teed's grading of middle ear barotrauma
- *Grade 0*: Normal
- *Grade 1*: Retraction with redness in Shrapnell's membrane and handle of malleus.
- *Grade 2*: Retraction with redness of entire ear drum.
- *Grade 3*: Same as grade 2 plus evidence in the tympanum or hemotympanum.
- *Grade 4*: Perforation of eardrum.

Sinus Barotrauma

This condition is similar to otitic barotrauma but due to pressure gradient between the nasal cavity and the sinus cavities. Causes are the same as of otitic barotrauma. But sinus barotrauma is 3 times less common than otitic barotrauma.

Frontal sinus is the commonest sinus to get involved in sinus barotrauma (68%) followed by ethmoid sinus (16%) and maxillary sinus (8%). Sphenoid sinus is rarely

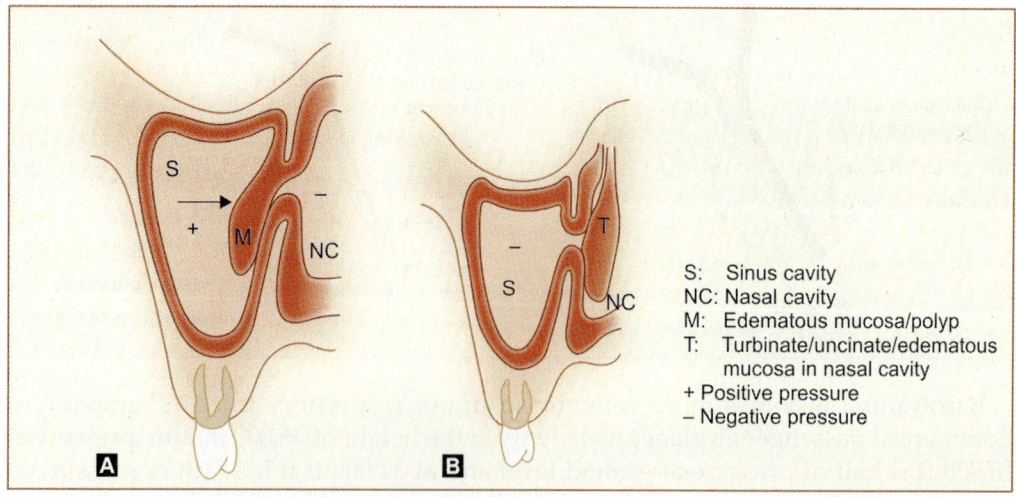

(A) Series of events happening during ascent when pressure in sinus is more than surrounding causing closure of ostium from within; (B) Descent where ostium is blocked from outside due to pushing of mucosa/polyp from nasal cavity to ostium due to higher pressure in nasal cavity

involved. The incidence of sinus barotrauma is directly proportional to the length of the sinus ostia (frontal 15–20 mm, maxillary 5–8 mm and sphenoid 2–4 mm). Occurrence increases with presence of local sinonasal diseases.

Gradient: 100–150 mm Hg → Edema and mucosal hyperemia

150–300 mm Hg → Seromucous/serohemorrhagic

Effusion: >300 mm Hg → Interstitial or intracavity bleeding.

The sinus barotrauma presents with headache (commonest), epistaxis, hypoaesthesia of infraorbital region and sinus dehiscence presenting as subcutaneous emphysema, pneumocephalus, etc.

Treatment of sinus barotrauma is mostly similar to otitic barotrauma. Other than this, nasal decongestants and treatment of underlying nasal pathology plays a role too.

Dental Barotrauma (Barodontalgia)

When a patient faces sudden change and difference in atmospheric pressure, there will be flaring up of pre-existing dental diseases. The pre-existing dental diseases include faulty dental restoration, dental caries without pulp involvement, peri-apicitis, recent dental treatment, etc.

Dental barotrauma is classified into 4 classes as follows.

Class	Pathology	Features	Treatment
I	Reversible (acute) pulpitis	Sharp transient pain on ascent	Zn oxide eugenol
II	Irreversible (chronic) pulpitis	Dull throbbing pain on ascent	Root canal therapy or extraction
III	Necrotic pulp	Dull throbbing pain on descent	Root canal therapy or extraction
IV	Periapical pathology (abscess/cyst)	Severe persistent pain	Root canal therapy or extraction

Delayed dysbarism: This is a side effect of 100% oxygen therapy. This can cause all three types of barotrauma. When the patient is under 100% O_2, all the cavities will get filled with oxygen. After the therapy is over, the O_2 get used up leading to negative pressure development in middle ear (due to absent inflation of middle ear in sleep), sinus cavity (edema around ostia) and dental caries cavity. This creates a pressure gradient between the cavity and ambience leading to delayed symptoms of barotrauma.

CHAPTER 50

High Yielders Topics

COMPARISON OF CT AND MRI

Characteristics of CT and MRI

	CT	MRI
Basic principle	X-rays	Radio waves
Radiation risk	High	Nil
Bony structures	+++	–
Soft tissues	+	+++
Blood vessels	+	+++
Metal implants	Can be done	Not safe
Position change	+	–

Differences between SMR and septoplasty

SMR	Septoplasty
Radical operation	Conservative operation
Flap elevated on both sides	Flap elevated on one side
Most of cartilage removed	Most of cartilage preserved
Revision difficult	Easier
Perforation incidence high	Low
Not done in children	Can be done

Differences between otitis externa and mastoiditis

Otitis externa	Mastoiditis
Displacement of pinna front	Downward and outward
Tenderness anterior to pinna	Mastoid antrum
Tragal tenderness present	Absent
Retroauricular sulcus obliterated	Not obliterated
Eardrum normal	Congested or perforated
X-ray mastoid normal	Cloudiness of air cells

Differences between safe and unsafe CSOM

	Safe	Unsafe
Perforation	Central	Marginal or total
Discharge	Continuous	Intermittent
	Profuse	Scanty
	Mucopurulent	Purulent
	Non-foul smelling	Foul smelling
	Non-blood stained	Blood stained
Cholesteatoma	Rare	Seen
Polyp	Rare	Common
Complications	Less	Common
Hearing loss	High	Less

Differences between BPPV (benign paroxysmal positional vertigo) and Meniere's disease

	BPPV	Meniere's
Nausea and vomiting	–	+
Recruitment	–	+
Tinnitus	–	+
Sensorineural loss	–	+

Differences between allergic and vasomotor rhinitis

	Allergic	Vasomotor
Sneezing	More	Less or absent
Rhinorrhea	More	More and first symptom
Lacrimation	More	Less
Skin test	+ve	–ve
Eosinophil counts	High	Normal
Vidian neurectomy	Not helpful	Helpful
Cause	Allergy	Vasomotor imbalance

Differences between ethmoidal and antrochoanal polyp

Antrochoanal polyp	Ethmoidal polyp
Single	Multiple
Maxillary sinusitis	Ethmoidal sinusitis
Infective	Allergic
At childhood	At puberty
Backward	Forward
Dumb-bell or trilobed	Grape like clustered

Differences between Eustachian tube of adult and child

Child	Adult
Narrow	Wide
Horizontal 10°	45°
Short	Long

Differences between acute epiglottis and acute laryngotracheobronchitis (LTB)

	Acute epiglottis	Acute LTB
Age	2–4 years	3 years
Onset	Rapid	Slow
Past history	—	Often
Cough	—	Barking
Dyspnea	Severe	—
Stridor	Inspiratory	Biphasic
Posture	Sitting and learning forward (Tripod)	Lying
Drooling	Marked	—
Neck node	Large	Small
X-ray	Thumb sign	Steeple sign

TESTS IN OTOLARYNGOLOGY

Fistula test: To detect the erosion on bony labyrinth. Tragus is pressed, patient feels vertigo and clinically nystagmus is noted.

- *False negative fistula test:*
  - Dead labyrinth
  - Cholesteatoma or granulation cover the fistula
  - External auditory canal not sealed properly
- *False positive fistula test:* Meniere's disease (Hennebert's sign), syphilis congenital, lax footplate.

Patch test: This is done to find out how much hearing improvement can be provided to the patient following myringoplasty. The perforation is closed with a patch of paper and audiometry is done. This is compared with the previous audiogram to find out the gain.

Dix Hallpike test (1952): Done in patients with vestibular symptoms. Before performing history of cervical spine or back diseases should be ruled out. While performing the test start with the normal or near normal ear. Keep the patient seated in the couch with legs extended. Head is turned 45 degrees to the test side and fixed by examiner. Patient eyes are fixed in front of him. In a quick movement the patient should lie on his/her back so that his/her head will be hanging at 20 degrees beyond the end of the couch and eyes' movement is noted. Observe for nystagmus (presence, direction, latency, magnitude, frequency, duration) for 30–60s, the same is observed in the other side also. Posterior canal, lateral canal and superior canal BPPV can be diagnosed with this test.

Cold caloric test (Kobrak test): This should be the last vestibular test in vertigo battery to be performed. Patient should be advised not to drive immediately after the test. Contraindications are uncontrolled hypertension, cardiac diseases, epilepsy, psychosis, eye surgery, ear surgery, TM perforation or atrophic TM. Positioning of the patient should be to bring the lateral canal to vertical plane—supine with head inclining forward by 30 degrees. Temperature of the fluid for irrigation should be 4 degrees.

Tobey-Ayre test: Done to detect lateral sinus thrombosis. Normally compression of each IJV raises CSF (cerebrospinal fluid) pressure by 50–100 mmHg, however, in thrombosis there is no rise or very slow rise of 10–20 mmHg.

- *False positive:* Collateral channels.
- *False negative:* Normal sinus is very small or absent.

Lille crow test: Compression of IJV leads to engorgement of retinal veins. Its absence means sigmoid sinus is thrombosed.

Romberg's test: Patient stands with feet together and arms by his side and is asked to close his eyes, if he sways, test is positive.

Gutzmann's test: Backward and downward pressure on the thyroid cartilage produces low pitch voice due to relaxation of stretched cords in case of puberphoina (mutational falsetto voice).

Schirmer's test: Topo-diagnostic test for facial nerve

- 5 cm long bloating paper
- 5 mm bend to be put in lower fornix
- 5 minutes
- Results significant, if difference is >50%

Allen's test: Before taking free vascularised flap based on radial artery; compression of radial artery is done to see whether after clamping it maintains sufficient blood circulation in the hand.

ABLB (Fowler) test: For recruitment of sound.

Stair test (Ogura): For assessment of pulmonary functions for conservative surgery of larynx.

Match blowing test: A bedside test for pulmonary function. If the patient can blow off a burning matchstick at a distance more than 30 cm, then his or her FEV_1 is supposedly normal and good which indirectly indicates there is no hidden asthma which may get precipitated by anesthetic drug during anesthesia of ENT surgery.

Breath holding time test: The duration the patient can hold his breath after maximal inspiration. This is a marker of lung compliance. Normal should be more than 30 seconds in healthy young individuals.

SIGNS IN OTOLARYNGOLOGY

Aquino's sign: Blanching of mass behind the tympanic membrane on carotid compression; seen in glomus tumors.

Battle's sign: Bluish discoloration of skin over the mastoid region due to fracture of lateral skull base/petrous temporal bone.

Bocca's sign: Absence of post-cricoid crepitus; seen in post-cricoid mass or edema.

Mouvre's sign: Cartilaginous crepitations seen normally when moved against the cervical vertebral column.

Boyce's sign: Zenker's diverticulum; soft swelling in the neck, which gurgles on palpation.

Browne's sign: Blanching of tympanic mass on siegelization; seen in glomus tympanicus.

Bryce's sign: Hissing sound on compression or reduction of lateral neck swelling; seen in External laryngocoele or combined laryngocoele.

Delta sign: Delta-shaped opacity in CECT or MRI within the sinus cavity; seen in lateral sinus thrombophlebitis.

Dodd's sign: Also called crescent sign—seen in X-ray as an air shadow between the nasal mass and posterior pharyngeal wall. This is found in antrochoanal polyp and absent in nasopharyngeal angiofibromas.

Furstenberg's sign: In encephalocoeles with patent intracranial communications, there is expansile pulsations during straining or coughing or compression of IJV due to increased ICT.

Guerin's sign: Hematoma over hard palate in rupture of greater palatine artery in Le Fort 1 fracture.

Griesinger's sign: Pitting edema over occipital region behind the mastoid process because of thrombophlebitis of mastoid emissary veins. Seen in lateral sinus thrombophlebitis.

Halo/Ring sign: Seen in traumatic CSF rhinorrhea in initial days following trauma. When CSF is collected in a handkerchief the CSF will spread out more than the blood content; hence the RBCs will stay in the centre surrounded by CSF outside.

Hennebert's sign: False positive fistula test; seen in Meniere's disease (25%) and tertiary syphilis (25%). This is due to hypermobility of footplate or fibrous strands between the footplate and saccule.

Hitselberger's sign: Anesthesia in EAC areas supplied by Arnold's nerve (X); seen in acoustic neuroma.

Holman-Miller antral sign: Anterior bowing of posterior maxillary sinus wall seen in the lateral view X-ray of PNS; seen in juvenile nasopharyngeal angiofibroma.

Hondousa sign: Widening of the space between ramus and body of maxilla; seen in cases of JNA with infratemporal fossa involvement.

Irwin Moore's sign: Cheesy purulent material comes out of the tonsils on squeezing with tongue depressor. Seen in chronic tonsillitis.

Laugier's sign: Blood behind the tympanic membrane; seen in lateral skull base fractures.

Lighthouse sign: Pulsatile discharge coming out of a small perforation; seen in ASOM after perforation or CSOM with acute episode having a small perforation.

Lyre's sign: Seen in angiograms of carotid body tumors; splaying of internal and external carotid arteries.

Omega sign: Omega-shaped epiglottis in congenital laryngomalacia seen during laryngoscopy.

Phelp's sign: Erosion of carotico-jugular crest in glomus jugulare; can be seen in HRCT.

Rat tailing sign: Seen in achalasia cardia in barium swallow; the lumen is wide in the lower portion of esophagus and tapers suddenly like a rat's tail.

Ring sign: Brain abscess; On CECT, brain hypodense area is seen surrounded by hyperdense area. In the centre of ring is necrosis.

Rising sun sign: Mentioned in two conditions; one during otoscopy in glomus tympanicus where the mass is seen like a sun rising from the floor of tympanum; second during I/L of acute epiglottitis where the edematous epiglottis is seen like a sun rising from hypopharynx.

Raccoon eye sign: Collection of blood in subgaleal plane; cranio facial injuries.

Schwartz's sign: Also called Flamingo red sign. Seen in active phase of otosclerosis where there is reddish hue over the promontory. When this is found immediate surgery is contraindicated.

Steeple's sign: Subglottic edema seen in X-ray of an acute laryngobronchitis patient.

Stankiewick's sign: Protrusion of orbital pad of fat during trauma to orbit in FESS.

Tear drop sign: Protrusion of orbital content into maxillary antral cavity in cases of orbital floor blow out fracture seen in X-ray PNS.

Thumb sign: Swollen epiglottis on X-ray lateral neck film appears like a thumb; seen in acute epiglottits.

Teapot sign: Seen in CSF rhinorrhea from sphenoid sinus; gush of fluid happens when the patient leans forward.

Troisier's sign: GI tract, gynaecological or chest malignancies secondary lymph nodes are palpable in supraclavicular triangle of left side.

Tullio's sign: Transient vertigo and nystagmus on exposure to loud sound or cold air. Seen in cases of Meniere's, labyrinthine fistula, syphilis and operated mastoid cavity.

TRIANGLES IN OTOLARYNGOLOGY

Ear

Macewan's triangle (suprameatal triangle/perforating triangle)
   Surface marking for mastoid antrum.

Boundaries

- *Anterior:* Posterior superior margin of EAC
- *Posterior:* Vertical tangent to posterior margin of EAC
- *Superior:* Suprameatal crest or temporal line

Trautmann's triangle: Bounded by sigmoid sinus, superior petrosal sinus (sinodural angle) and bony labyrinth, through this triangle posterior cranial fossa can be approached in cases of cerebellar abscess.

Neck

Anterior triangle: It is formed posteriorly by the anterior border of sternomastoid, anteriorly is midline and superiorly is mandible.

It is further divided into:

1. *Submental triangle:* Between two bellies of digastric, body of hyoid form the base and apex lie at chin.
   Important contents: Submental lymph node.

2. *Submandibular (digastric) triangle:* Base is formed by mandible. Posteroinferior boundary is posterior belly of digastric and stylohyoid. Anteroinferior boundary is anterior belly of digastric.
   Important contents: Submandibular gland along with lymph nodes, hypoglossal nerve, external carotid artery.

3. *Carotid triangle:* Anterior border of sternomastoid, superior belly of omohyoid and posterior belly of digastric.
   Important contents: CCA, ICA, ECA, IJV, vagus, spinal accessory, ansa hypoglossi, cervical sympathetic chain and lymph nodes.

4. *Muscular triangle:* Superior belly of omohyoid, midline anteriorly and anterior border of sternomastoid.
   Important contents: Infrahyoid muscles.

5. *Posterior triangle:* Formed by posterior border of sternomastoid anteriorly, anterior border of trapezius posteriorly and middle 1/3rd clavicle forms the base.

It is further divided into:

A. *Occipital triangle*: Anterior border of trapezius, inferior belly of omohyoid inferiorly and posterior border of sternomastoid anteriorly.
   Important contents: Accessory nerve, greater auricular nerve, transverse cervical artery, occipital artery and lymph nodes.

B. *Subclavian (supraclavicular) triangle:* Inferior belly of omohyoid, sternomastoid and middle third of clavicle.
   Important contents: Brachial plexuses, third part of subclavian artery, suprascapular artery and lymph nodes.

Beahr's triangle: Two boundaries are CCA and inferior thyroid artery and tracheo-esophageal groove. The significance is to locate recurrent laryngeal nerve in this triangle.

Chaisaignac's triangle: Bounded medially by longus colli, laterally by scalenus anterior and base bounded by subclavian artery. Contents are scalenus nodes and thoracic duct.

SYNDROMES IN ENT

Alport's syndrome: An autosomal dominant progressive glomerulonephritis, nerve deafness and lenticonus. The ear findings are bilateral and symmetrical sensory neural hearing loss. It is synonymous with thin basement membrane nephropathy. Type IV collagen disorder with COL4A5 mutation.

Apert's syndrome: This is due to FGFR2 gene mutation (chromosome 10). Premature fusion of cranial bones (craniosynostosis) leading to disordered neurological development. Limb abnormalities include bony syndactyly. Facial abnormalities include mid-face hypoplasia, shallow orbits, strabismus, down-slanting palpabral fissures, depressed nasal bridge, proptosis, hypertelorism and dental mal-eruption. These features are similar to the ones seen in Crouzon's syndrome.

Alström syndrome: A hereditary syndrome of retinitis pigmentosa with nystagmus and early loss of central vision, deafness, obesity, and diabetes mellitus.

Barany syndrome: A syndrome of unilateral occipital headache with ipsilateral recurrent episodes of deafness, vertigo, tinnitus. Periodic recurrence for days or months. May be corrected by induced nystagmus.

Behçet's syndrome: A syndrome complex consisting of oral ulcers, genital ulcers and iritis. Oral lesions can be severe and heralding lesions of the syndrome.

Branchio-oto-renal (BOR) syndrome: Causes malformation of neck tissues and leads to ear and renal problems. Branchial fistulas/cysts, malformed pinnae with pre-auricular pits or sinuses, sensorineural hearing (cochlear damage)/conductive (ossicular abnormalities) or mixed hearing loss and renal abnormalities that might cause end stage renal disease later in the life.

Charlin syndrome (nasociliary neuralgia): Pain localized to the internal angle of the eye associated with tearing, photophobia, blepharospasm, conjunctival hyperaemia, cheimosis, rhinorrhea and unilateral nasal congestion.

Churg-Strauss syndrome: Bronchial asthma, fever, eosinophilia, allergic rhinitis with chronic sinusitis and nasal polyposis, vasculitis and granuloma. 75% cases of Churg-Strauss syndrome will have ENT presentations.

Cogan's disease: Rare autoimmune disease characterised by sensorineural hearing loss, vestibular symptoms and ocular inflammatory conditions like interstitial keratitis. Caloric test shows canal paresis and PTA shows sensorineural loss at high frequencies.

Crouzon's syndrome (craniofacial dysostosis): Frog eyes (exophthalmos with divergent squint), hypertelorism, parrot-beak nose, prognathism. This is due to premature closure of cranial sutures. They also have mental retardation and conductive hearing loss due to very narrow ear canal. Autosomal dominant inheritance.

Cystic fibrosis: Autosomal recessive trait. Mutation occurs in CFTR gene (trans-membrane conductance regulator). Chronic, multi-system disorder where the patient presents with recurrent chest infections, pancreatitis and sino-nasal and middle ear infections.

Dejean's syndrome (orbital floor syndrome): Exophthalmos, diplopia and anesthesia in the areas innervated by the trigeminal nerve, occurring with a lesion in the floor of the orbit.

Down's syndrome (Trisomy 21): Microcephaly, mental retardation/delayed development, short stature, epicanthal folds (Mongolian slant), macroglossia, stenosis of ear canal, high incidence of serous otitis media and atlanto-axial joint instability.

Eagle syndrome: Syndrome of lateral neck pain due to abnormally long styloid process or its inflammation. This is diagnosed clinically by trans-tonsillar palpation of styloid tip. Radiological investigation of choice is OPG. This can be treated by removal of the long styloid bone.

Frey's syndrome: Also called "auriculotemporal syndrome". Usually the sweat glands are innervated by sympathetic fibres. During parotid surgeries, these fibres are cut during raising the anterior skin flap. Parotid is innervated (secretomotor) by auriculotemporal nerve which loses its target organ after parotidectomy. In this condition it is thought that the auriculotemporal fibres grow into the sympathetic nerve sheaths causing aberrant stimulation of sweat glands. Whenever patient eats spicy food, they start developing profuse sweating.

Garcin's syndrome: Unilateral paralysis all the cranial nerves due to a tumor at the base of the skull or in the nasopharynx.

Gardner's syndrome: Variant of familial adenomatous polyposis syndrome characterised by osteomas of skull and facial bones mainly mandible, multiple epidermoid cysts of skin and polyposis of rectum and colon. It is an autosomal dominant disease.

Goldenhar's syndrome (facio-auriculo-vertebral dysplasia or oculo-auriculo-vertebral [OAV] syndrome): Facial asymmetry, low set ears, atresia of ear canal, cardiac abnormalities, preauricular tags/pits hemivertebrae in cervical region, epibulbar dermoid and coloboma of upper lid; mixed or conductive loss can be present.

Gradenigo's syndrome: Lateral rectus palsy (cranial nerve VI), retro-orbital pain (cranial nerve V) and otorrhoea. This condition is seen in petrous apicitis following CSOM.

Grisel syndrome: Atlanto-axial joint dislocation secondary to infection or surgical procedures like adenoidectomy. They present with severe neck pain and rigidity.

Horner syndrome: It is characterised by ptosis, miosis, anhidrosis due to loss of cervical sympathetic chain tone.

Jervell and Lange-Nielsen syndrome: Repeated syncopes, prolonged QT interval in ECG and SNHL.

Kallmann's syndrome: Anosmia and congenital hypogonadism. GnRH is deficient and they respond to pulsatile Gn therapy.

Kartagener's syndrome: Bronchiectasis, sinusitis, situs inversus and ciliary dyskinesia.

Klippel-Feil syndrome: Short neck, fused cervical vertebrae, spina bifida, atresia of ear canal with SNHL or mixed HL.

Lermoyez's syndrome: Variant of Meniere's syndrome characterised by attacks of tinnitus, sensorineural hearing loss followed by bouts of vertigo. It is seen in younger age group compared to Meniere's and resolves over a period of time without residual hearing loss.

Maffucci syndrome: It is characterised by multiple cavernous hemangioma of head and neck, multiple endochondromas.

Melkersson-Rosenthal syndrome: Triad of facial paralysis, swelling of lips and midline fissured tongue. Seen in childhood or adolescent age group. It is autosomal dominant with variable penetrance.

MEN (multiple endocrine neoplasia)-2A syndrome: Causes familial medullary thyroid carcinoma. There is associated risk for the development of pheochromocytoma, parathyroid neoplasms, mucous neuromas, marfanoid habits and ganglioneuromas of GI tract.

Mendelson's syndrome: Chemical pneumonia or aspiration pneumonia is due to the pulmonary parenchymal inflammatory reaction caused by aspiration of large volume of gastric contents. This usually occurs in comatose patients or when the patient is induced for general anaesthesia without proper nil per oral precautions or insecure airway. If the pH of the aspirated fluid is less than 2.5 and the volume of aspirate is greater than 0.3 ml/kg of body weight (20–25 ml in adults).

Möbius syndrome: Congenital bilateral facial nerve paralysis along with VI nerve and occasional III nerve palsy. Involvement is at the level of nuclei of these nerves.

Mondini dysplasia: Congenital malformation of apical and middle turns of cochlea, vestibular and endolymphatic system. The child will have permanent, profound sensorineural hearing loss.

von Recklinghausen syndrome (neurofibromatosis 2): Familial multiple neuromas; acoustic neuromas are seen more in these patients.

Pendred's syndrome: Discovered by and coined after Vaughan Pendred. Goitre (non-toxic) usually evident before puberty and sensorineural hearing loss. Perchlorate discharge test shows defect in organic binding of iodine SNHL. 60% of the cases are genetic.

Pierre Robin sequence: Triad of micrognathia, glossoptosis and airway obstruction. There can be large U-shaped cleft palate. Often a part of Stickler's syndrome or velocardiofacial syndrome; there can be some external ear malformations.

Ramsay Hunt syndrome (herpes zoster oticus): There is lower motor neuron facial paralysis, painful blisters in the external auditory canal and pinna supplied by sensory roots of facial nerve. There may also be anesthesia of face, giddiness and hearing impairment due to involvement of Vth and VIIIth nerves.

Stickler's syndrome: Small jaw, cleft palate, myopia > retinal detachment, cataract, juvenile onset arthritis along with conductive or SNHL. Usually in combination with Pierre-Robin sequence.

Treacher Collins syndrome (mandibulofacial dysostosis): Anti-mongoloid palpebral fissures, coloboma of lower lid, hypoplasia of mandible and molar bones, malformed pinna and meatal atresia and malformed malleus and incus (stapes normal) causing conductive hearing loss.

Usher's syndrome: Retinitis pigmentosa, night-blindness and congenital SNHL. Pure tone audiogram shows classical U-shaped audiogram.

van der Hoeve's syndrome: Osteogenesis imperfecta with history of repeated multiple fractures, blue sclera, hearing loss (delayed onset) conductive, SNHL or mixed (like otosclerosis).

Vernet's syndrome: This is also called "jugular syndrome". Presents with multiple lower cranial nerves passing through the foramen, namely IX, X and XI. This condition is seen in space occupying lesions of jugular foramen like Glomus jugulare or skull base fracture passing through this foramen.

Waardenburg's syndrome: White forelock, heterochromia iridis, vitiligo, dystopia canthorum and SNHL.

Young's syndrome: Ethmoidal polyps, sino-pulmonary disease and azoospermia. This is due to impaired ciliary motility.

QUICK REMEMBRANCE POINTS IN HEAD AND NECK MALIGNANCIES

Nasal Cavity and Paranasal Sinuses

- Sinus tumors are mostly malignant (75%); squamous cell carcinoma is the commonest followed by adenocarcinoma with maxillary sinus (60–70%) being the commonly involved.
- Risk factors are asbestos exposure, wood dust (mahogany), nickel, leather, etc.
- Inverted papilloma (Ringertz tumor) is a benign tumor which is locally aggressive, with recurrence rate high after surgery. It arises from the Scneiderian membrane in lateral wall of nasal cavity.
- Adenoid cystic carcinoma accounts for 5% of sinonasal malignancies. It shows slow perineural spread to the skull base.
- Olfactory neuroblastoma or Esthesioneuroblastoma is a tumor of neural crest origin arising from olfactory epithelium. Nodal metastasis is a poor prognostic factor.
- Sino nasal lymphomas are the 2nd most common group of extranodal lymphomas in Asian population.
- Fibrosarcoma followed by rhabdomyosarcoma are the common sarcomas of sinonasal cavity.
- Only 10% of sinonasal malignancies are seen with nodal metastasis.
- During maxillary infrastructure malignancy tissue biopsy, Caldwell-Luc approach is avoided due to risk of cancer seeding.
- Surgery is the mainstay of treatment. Approaches are: Lateral rhinotomy, medial maxillectomy, Weber Ferguson, Weber Ferguson with Lynch extension, Weber Ferguson with subciliary extension and Weber Ferguson with sub and supraciliary extension.
- Reconstructive surgery is necessary to fill the surgical defect. Usually done with microvascular free flap—myocutaneous or osseo-myocutaneous.

Skull Base

- Anterior skull base is formed by frontal, ethmoid and sphenoid bones. It is bounded anteriorly by posterior frontal sinus wall, posteriorly by the anterior clinoid processes and roof of sphenoid, laterally by the frontal bone.
- Anterior cranial fossa foramina are foramen caecum for emissary vein, olfactory foramina, anterior and posterior ethmoidal foramina.
- Most of the anterior cranial fossa tumors are extracranial which spread intracranially.
- Middle cranial fossa is bound anteriorly by the lesser wings of sphenoid and anterior clinoid processes, posteriorly by the petrous temporal bone and dorsum sella and laterally by the squamous temporal bone and greater wings of sphenoid.
- Middle cranial fossa foramina are superior orbital fissure, foramen rotundum, foramen ovale, foramen spinosum and foramen lacerum. Note that ICA does not pass through foramen lacerum, whereas vidian nerve and vessels pass through it.
- Middle cranial fossa tumors are mostly neurovascular in origin, e.g. Schwannomas
- Parts of ICA are: Cervical C1, petrous C2, lacerum C3, cavernous C4, clinoid C5, ophthalmic C6 and communicating C7.
- Craniopharyngiomas are epithelial neoplasm in sellar and suprasellar region. They are always benign and have bimodal age distribution: Childhood and elderly.

Lips and Oral Cavity

- Upper lip drains into buccal and parotid lymph nodes.
- Squamous cell carcinoma accounts for more than 90% of oral cancers. Others are minor salivary gland tumors, melanoma, lymphomas, etc.
- In OSMF there is fibrosis of lamina propria with atrophy of the overlying epithelium.
- Lymphatic spread is usually stepwise but skip metastasis to level IV nodes are seen in anterior tongue cancers.
- Mainstay of oral cavity and lip cancers is surgery with or without following chemotherapy or radiation.
- OPG can be used to detect mandibular invasion by the cancer but 30–50% of mineral loss occurs even before the lesion is radiologically evident.
- Single most prognostic factor is neck node involvement: Single node involvement reduces the chances of cure by 50%.
- Sentinel node biopsy can be used to spare the patient from neck dissection in clinically negative node status.
- Adjuvant radiation is indicated in patients with positive margin, lymphovascular or perineural invasion, pathologically positive LN, etc. Dose is 60 Gy or more.

Human Papillomavirus

HPV 16 is found to be associated with oral squamous papilloma, condyloma acuminatum, focal epithelial hyperplasia and esophageal malignancies.

Oropharynx

- Referred otalgia can be the first ever symptom.
- Tonsillar malignancies present very late at stage III or IV.
- LN metastasis is very common.

Nasopharynx

- Nasopharyngeal carcinoma is associated with Epstein-Barr virus, genetic and environmental factors.
- Types are SCC—keratinizing, non-keratinizing and basaloid squamous.
- Definitive RT to nasopharynx and elective RT to neck is the treatment.

Larynx

Tobacco smoking is the main factor in larynx malignancies. Aryl hydrocarbon of smoke is converted by aryl hydrocarbon hydroxylase, an enzyme found in pulmonary macrophage or alveolar cell type 2 into epoxide, the most potent carcinogen in respiratory tract. Epoxide then bring changes in normal cells of larynx or respiratory tract and converts to cancer cells.

It is to be noted that cancer larynx almost always starts from anterior parts of larynx and never originates from posterior parts of larynx, although posterior parts can be involved when cancer spread posteriorly. Reason behind is that pulmonary macrophage also known as policeman of larynx takes round of only posterior parts of larynx and can detect cancer and kills it immediately. But this is not the case for anterior parts of glottis where it does not come in contact with pulmonary macrophage.

- Glottic cancer has least LN metastasis but the supraglottic and subglottic has the chances for even contralateral metastasis.
- Barriers to spread of cancer in larynx are conus elasticus, quadrangular membrane, Broyle's tendon, etc.
- VC fixation is a sign of paraglottic space or arytenoid invasion.
- Voice rehabilitation after laryngectomy: (1) Esophageal speech; (2) TEP and (3) Electrolarynx.

Thyroid and Parathyroid

- Increase in incidence of the disease is due to increased microscopic diagnosis of the disease.
- Differentiated thyroid malignancies are: Papillary, medullary and follicular; undifferentiated—anaplastic.
- Risk assessment strategies for thyroid cancers include grade, age, metastasis, extension, size (GAMES) and recurrence.
- Risk for malignancies are age > 45 years, size > 4.5 cm, anteroposterior diameter of mass more than transverse diameter, microcalcification in USG thyroid and solid mass inside cystic spaces of nodule along with pericapsular indentation.
- For low risk cases lobectomy shows equivalent results to total thyroidectomy.
- For high risk cases, total laryngectomy with central neck dissection is practiced as it facilitates RAI therapy (I-131).
- Medullary cancer is more aggressive and difficult to cure also.
- Parathyroid surgeries should only be done by surgeons with vast experience in thyroid surgeries.
- Minimally invasive parathyroidectomy is done for parathyroid adenoma.

Salivary Glands

- Salivary neoplasms are thought to arise from pluripotent stem cells of the glands' duct.
- Radiation, EBV infection, nickel, rubber industry wastes are a few of the many understood aetiologies.
- 5 Histopathological categories are:
  - *Malignant epithelial* (mucoepidermoid, adenoid cystic and acinic cell carcinoma),
  - *Benign epithelial* (pleomorphic adenoma and papillary cystadenoma lymphomatosum),
  - *Lymphomatous* (Hodgkin's),
  - *Soft tissue sarcomas* and
  - *Metastatic tumors.*
- Incidence of malignancy in parotid, submandibular and minor salivary glands are as follows—25, 50 and 80%.
- Adenoid cystic carcinoma is characterised by high metastasising potential, perineural spread and late local recurrence.
- 5 indications for parotid FNAC, namely to rule out inflammatory lesions, to identify systemic diseases like reticulo, endothelial tumors, to rule out direct invasion or metastasis, to evaluate un-resectable tumors and in poor surgical candidates for surgery.

- Majority of deep lobe of parotid tumors are benign.
- Treatment of choice is surgical resection.

Neurogenic Tumors and Paragangliomas

- Neurogenic tumors constitute to a very small part of head and neck tumors.
- They are usually found in parapharyngeal space.
- Parapharyngeal space is divided into two by the styloid and its attachments: Pre- and post-styloid compartments.
- Schwannomas arise from neuroectodermal nerve sheath of peripheral nerves. Malignant transformation is low but has high local recurrence.
- Neurofibromas can be familial or sporadic. Types are localised, diffuse and plexiform.
- Paragangliomas arise from extra adrenal paraganglionic cells derived from neural crest epithelium.
- Sites of head and neck paragangliomas are: Jugulotympanic region (glomus), vagal body, carotid body, inferior laryngeal paraganglionic tissue, nasal cavity and/or orbit. Most common is carotid body tumor.
- They are benign, slow growing tumors.
- 10% paragangliomas are malignant/multiple/bilateral/familial.
- Benign and malignant paragangliomas are histologically similar and are difficult to differentiate. Only a few features like—local cranial nerve invasions, carotid artery invasion, skull base or other soft tissue destruction or local or regional LN involvement are suggestive of malignancy.

Nutrition

- Daily caloric requirement: 25–35 kcal/kg of body weight.
- Daily protein requirement is 1–1.5 g/kg body weight.
- Daily fluid requirement is 30–40 ml/kg body weight.
- Following head and neck radiation, esophageal stricture might occur leading to dysphagia and malnourishment.
- It can be managed with percutaneous endoscopic gastrostomy. This can be used for a longer duration compared to orogastric or nasogastric tube feeding.
- Prophylactic nasogastric tube should be inserted in patients with more than 5% weight loss in a month, BMI < 18.5, dysphagia, anorexia and dehydration.
- PPN (peripheral parenteral nutrition) and TPN (total) are less effective and expensive than enteral nutrition. Hence, whenever there is possibility for enteral feeding, it should be encouraged.

CHAPTER 51

Pharmacology in ENT

In this chapter we will see a brief introduction to the commonly used drugs in ENT.

Saline nasal mist/spray/drops: This increases the nasal ciliary action. Hence, used in postoperative cases of septoplasty, FESS, angiofibroma, endoscopic DCR. It has a beneficial role in chronic rhinosinusitis. It comes in normal saline formation (0.9%) and also hypertonic formation (3%). Commonly used is 0.66% saline solution.

Nasal steroid sprays or irrigation: Useful in allergic rhinitis and chronic rhinosinusitis. Commonly used drugs are fluticasone furoate, fluticasone propionate, mometasone furoate, beclomethasone dipropionate, budesonide, ciclesonide, triamcinolone, flunisolide, etc.

Out of these fluticasone furoate is better because of its high efficacy as well as less complications due to least systemic absorption. Local complications include nasal dryness and septal perforation.

Irrigation of nasal cavity and sinus can be done with mixture of saline, budenoside and sodium bicarbonate in postoperative period after FESS in fungal rhinosinusitis and polyposis to flushout a toxic byproduct released from eosinophil in blocked sinuses in response to fungal element.

Anti-histaminic drugs: Useful in allergic rhinitis, infective rhinitis.

Oral antihistaminic drugs are:

1. **First generation (highly sedating):** Chlorpheniramine, dexchlorpheniramine, astemizole, terfenadine, hydroxyzine, doxylamine, dexbrompheniramine, triprolidine, pyrilamine, terfenadine, astemizole, loratidine and diphenhydramine cause **QT interval** prolongation.
2. **Second generation (less or non-sedating):** Loratidine, desloratidine, cetirizine, levo-cetrizine, fexofenadine and olopatadine.

   Fexofenadine—second generation; non-sedative; oral formations.

   Azelastine—second generation; available in nasal spray formation.

Anti-asthmatic drugs: ENT practitioners should also possess good knowledge about asthmatic medications as many of our patients have coexisting asthma (ARIA). Commonly used anti-asthmatic drugs are:

a. **Bronchodilators:**
   1. Beta-2 selective agonists like clenbuterol, salmeterol, formetrol, salbutamol, indacaterol, levosalbutamol, etc.
   2. Non-selective beta agonists like epinephrine, isoprenaline, ephedrine, etc.
   3. Parasympatholytics like ipratropium bromide, tiotropium, etc.
   4. Methylxanthines: Theophylline, doxophylline, aminophylline, theocard, etc.
b. **Mast cell stabilizers** are sodium cromoglicate, ketotifen, nedocromil, etc.
c. **Leukotriene antagonists** like montelucast and zafirlucast.
d. **Steroids** in forms of aerosol or powder budesonide, fluticasone, beclomethasone, ciclesonide, triamcinolone and flunisolide. In cases of uncontrolled asthma systemic steroids are also needed, e.g. hydrocortisone and prednisolone.

   Steroid spray is not used in children below 5 years as there is possibility of stunting following their effect on growth centers.
e. **Anti-IgE antibody:** Omalizumab.
f. **Immunotherapy** in allergic rhinitis as well as asthma:
   1. Subcutaneous (SCIT): Multiple allergens can be given at one time.
   2. Sublingual (SLIT): Doses are 30 times more than SCIT. It is the latest technique.

   Along with these medications we might also have to prescribe mucolytic drugs to thin out the sticky bronchial secretions. They can be taken orally or by nebulization, e.g. ambroxol HCL, carbocysteine, N-acetylcysteine, erdosteine, guaifenesin and bromhexine.

   Commonest combination for bronchial asthma is doxophylline orally and formetrol + budenoside in powder form through rotahaler. This is the commonest effective combination. It gives excellent result. Powder form is preferred to inhaled aerosols because it can reduce the inflammation in larger airways also by sticking to their walls. Patients giving non-specific complaints in asthma like irritation and itching in throat get benefitted from powdered form.

Commonly used dressing germicidal solutions are
1. Solutions releasing nascent bactericidal oxygen: Hydrogen peroxide (H_2O_2).
2. Release nascent iodine: Povidone iodine 10% solution for dressing and cleaning. For gargling 1–2% solutions can be used.
3. Release nascent chlorine: EUSOL or chlorine water.

Commonly used epithelializing agents are: Gentian violet solution and acriflavine. They can be used in outer part of mastoid cavity following MRM.

Commonly used bactericidal ointments: Povidone iodine 5%, neomycin, silver nitrate

Commonly used antifungal preparations: Neostatin, tolnaftate, clotrimazole, itraconazole, framycetin sulphate, etc.

Commonly used ear drops: Neomycin, gentamycin, tobramycin, ciprofloxacin, ofloxacin, chloramphenicol, levofloxacin, clotriamazole, itraconazole, etc. Ear drops in combination with steroids can give good results. It should always be kept in mind not to prescribe ear drops containing any ototoxic drugs for long duration.

Commonly used antifungal drugs: Ketaconazole, fluconazole (50–150 mg), itraconazole (100 mg) and voriconazole (intravenous).

Hemostatic dressing materials are classified into:

a. Factor concentrators—absorbs water content in blood and concentrates its protein content thus promoting clot formation. They are organic polymer products, e.g. gelfoam (porcine gelatin), surgical (cellulose).

b. Mucoadhesive agents—they adhere to the tissue surfaces firmly giving no space for bleeding to occur (polyethylene glycol gels).

c. Procoagulant supplements—they provide procoagulant proteins directly to the wound, e.g. dry fibrin, bovine and pooled human thrombin.

Bleeding can occur because of:

1. Defective vasospasm due to:
   a. Nutritional deficiency like scurvy (vasular purpura) due to vitamin C deficiency. Treated with ascorbic acid orally and intravenously.
   b. Genetic disorders like von Willebrand disease major (type 3; rarest) and minor (type 1; 80%). Type 2 (15% of cases; subtypes A, B, M and N) is an intermediate form. Minor and intermediate forms can be treated with recombinant von Willebrand factor, factor VIII concentrate, platelet concentrate, blood transfusion, tranexamic acid and aminocaproic acid. Major form is more dangerous. A simple tooth extraction can cause severe bleeding and can need massive blood transfusion. Treatment options for major form are desmopressin which is a synthetic analogue of vasopressin and purified plasma derivatives of vWF and factor VIII.

2. Thrombocytopenias
   a. Idiopathic thrombocytopenic purpura
   b. Reactionary thrombocytopenia following aspirin, chloroquine and diclofenac in a few patients. These patients need selective COX-2 inhibitors as anti-inflammatory drugs. Cases of reactionary thrombocytopenia are prone to have allergic rhinitis, asthma, renal disease and gastritis. Probably this is due to inhibition of physiological prostaglandins at these sites. Treatment is ethamsylate and tranexamic acid. It could be a mixture of type 1 and type 2 von Willebrand disease.

3. Calcium (IV), factor VIII, IX (plasma thromboplastin component), X, fibrinogen, prothrombin and vitamin K (liver disorder) deficiency; treated by vitamin K injection, management of liver disorders, slow intravenous infusion of calcium, tranexamic acid, ethamsylate, aminocaproic acid and clotting factors concentrate can be used in treatment.

Disseminated intravascular coagulation (DIC) is abnormal initiation of coagulation cascade where all the coagulation factors are used up causing microthrombi in circulation and severe bleeding. Common causes are sepsis (gram negative), viral fever, malarial fever, recent surgeries and anesthetic drugs used during surgery. Diagnosed by measuring blood fibrin degeneration product. Treatment is by replacing coagulation products by fresh frozen plasma (FFP).

Mechanism of action of tranexamic acid: Tranexamic acid is the commonly used drug in ENT bleeding. It is an antifibrinolytic drug. It inhibits formation of plasmin from plasminogen and also displaces plasminogen from the surface of fibrin reticulum. It can also directly inhibit plasmin. It also has minor anti-inflammatory effect and improves platelet function.

Uses of non-selective beta blockers in ENT, e.g. propanolol 2 mg/kg body weight.
- Migrainous headaches
- Cluster headaches
- Vascular malformations and infantile hemangiomas.

Propanalol in combination with steroids give excellent results in hemangiomas and they disappear like a magic.

Intravenous fluids: They can be classified into crystalloids and colloids.

Crystalloids: They are true electrolyte solution which are permeable through cell membranes. They can be hypo, iso or hypertonic based on their osmolarity. However, hypertonic solutions are considered to be volume expanders as they move intracellular and interstitial fluid into intravascular compartment.

A few crystalloids are normal saline (0.9% sodium chloride), Ringer lactate, hypertonic saline (3%, 5%, etc.), dextrose (5%, 10% and 25%), etc.

Colloids: They are high molecular weight solutions which can draw water from extravascular compartment into intravascular by osmotic pressure. They are the best plasma volume expanders.

A few colloids are albumin, hestarch, pentastarch, dextran, etc.

Components of common intravascular fluids are as follows:

Solution	pH	Na^+	K^+	Cl^-	Ca^{2+}	Extra components	Comments
Ringer lactate		130	4	109	3	Lactate–28	Choice fluid in initial resuscitation
Normal saline		154	0	154	0		
5% dextrose and normal saline	4	154	0	154	0	50 g dextrose	Choice immediately postoperative in major surgeries
5% dextrose	4.5	0	0	0	0	50 g dextrose	No role in resuscitation
6% hestarch	3.5-7	154	0	154	0	30 g hydroxy ethyl starch	Coagulation abnormalities
5% plasma protein	7.4	145	<2	0	0	12.5 g protein	Most expensive IV fluid

CHAPTER 52

Reconstructive Surgery in ENT

The necessity for reconstructive procedures arise in cases of tissue loss due to surgeries, trauma, radiation exposure, etc.

Reconstruction can be done based on the nature of tissue lost, like skin grafting, flaps, bone grafts, composite flaps, etc.

Skin grafting: It is a procedure where a portion of skin is transferred from donor site to host site without blood supply. There are two types of skin grafts like

1. Full thickness and
2. Split thickness skin grafts.

Autologous skin of various thickness is used to close an exposed wound. Based on the thickness of the skin taken it is divided into full thickness (Wolfe) skin graft or split skin graft (Thiersch).

Full thickness graft includes epidermis and dermis. This gives excellent cosmetic result as it undergoes least contracture but the take is less. The donor site cannot re-epithelialize and needs primary closure or split skin grafting.

Split skin graft includes epidermis and varied thickness of dermis leaving behind remnants of pilosebaceous system behind in the donor site. Split skin graft contracts significantly but the take is good. The remnant pilosebaceous apparatus in the donor surface leads to complete re-epithelialization. Based on the thickness of the skin taken it is divided into thin (0.005–0.012 inch), intermediate (0.012–0.018 inch) and thick SSG (0.018–0.030 inch).

Nutrition for the graft is provided by the diffusion from the floor. The anchorage of graft is initially by fibrin bridge between the floor and graft. The fibrous anchorage starts by 1 week.

Contraindications for skin grafting are hemolytic bacterial infections like GABHS, bony floor without periosteum, unhealthy granulation tissue, etc.

Hematoma below the skin graft is the main villain in uptake of the graft.

Flaps: It is the unit of autologous tissue transferred from donor site to host site with its own blood supply. The nature of tissue can range from simple skin to composite flaps (skin with fascia, muscle, bone or even viscera). The complexity of the flaps can vary from simple skin advancement to free microvascular flaps. The recipient site can be adjacent to the donor site or can be very remote.

Graft	Flap
Limited to skin transplantation	Can include variety of tissue as discussed
Takes nutrients from host site	Has its own blood supply
Needs pressure bandage to tackle hematoma	No need for pressure damage
Cosmetically inferior	Cosmetically very good
Cannot bridge underlying defects	Can bridge tissue defects

Classification of flaps

1. Based on components—skin, fasciocutaneous, myocutaneous, osseomyocutaneous, other tissues like omentum, etc.
2. Based on method of transfer—advancement, rotation, transposition, interpolation, pedicled and microvascular free flaps,
3. Based on congruity—local, regional, distant, pedicled and island flaps.

Neovascularization of flaps: It occurs by direct ingrowth of new vessels or by anastomosing of capillaries in the flap tissue and the surrounding tissue.

How to decide the nature of flap to be used?

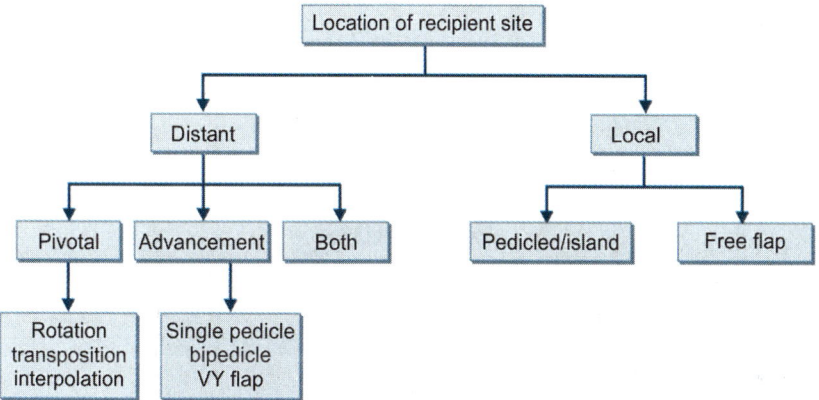

Pectoralis major myocutaneous flap (PMMC flap): Most commonly used myocutaneous pedicled flap in head and neck surgeries. It is based on the pectoral branch of thoracoacromian artery. It is bulky and can cover wide defects. The donor site can be closed primarily. Other myocutaneous flaps in use are trapezius flap based on transverse cervical artery and lattisimus dorsi flap based on thoracodorsal artery and segmental perforating branches of intercostal and lumbar arteries.

Deltopectoral flap: It is a fasciocutaneous pedicled flap including the fascia of pectoral muscles. Medially taken from anterior chest wall without any muscle. Based on 1–4th perforating branches of internal mammary artery.

Forehead flap: It is based on the anterior branch of superficial temporal artery and its accompanying vein. It is mainly used to reconstruct the buccal mucosal or cheek skin defects following a surgery.

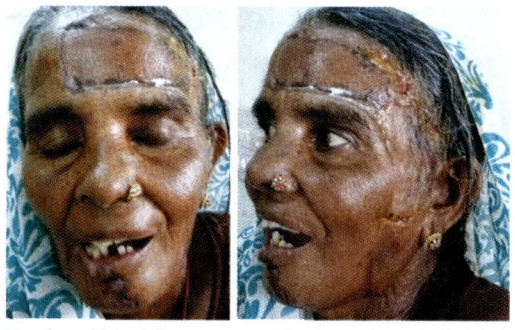

Forehead head flap was used to reconstruct the cheek following carcinoma cheek surgery in this patient.

Distant flaps: They are done in forms of pedicled flaps or free flaps. The pedicled flaps are when the tissue is moved with the blood supply preserved in a pedicle. When the pedicled is buried under the skin it is called "Island flap". Free flap is one where the tissue is detached from its donor site along with feeding artery and draining vein and re-anastomosed at the recipient site. Free microvascular grafts have made the reconstruction of head and neck post-operative wounds with bony defect relatively easy.

Various free flaps are as follows:

1. *Muscle and myocutaneous flaps*: Lattisimus dorsi based on thoracodorsal vessels, rectus abdominis based on deep inferior epigastric vessels, gracilis based on medial femoral circumflex and superficial femoral vessels, serratus anterior based on serratus branch of thoracodorsal vessels.

2. *Fasciocutaneous*: Radial forearm flap (proximal or distal based) based on radial artery and vene commitans, scapular based on subscapular and circumflex scapular vessels, dorsalis pedis flap, groin flap based on inferior epigastric artery, etc.

3. *Osseous*: Fibula based on peroneal artery and vein, iliac crest based on superficial or deep circumflex iliac vessels, outer table of skull, rib based on intercostal vessels, etc.

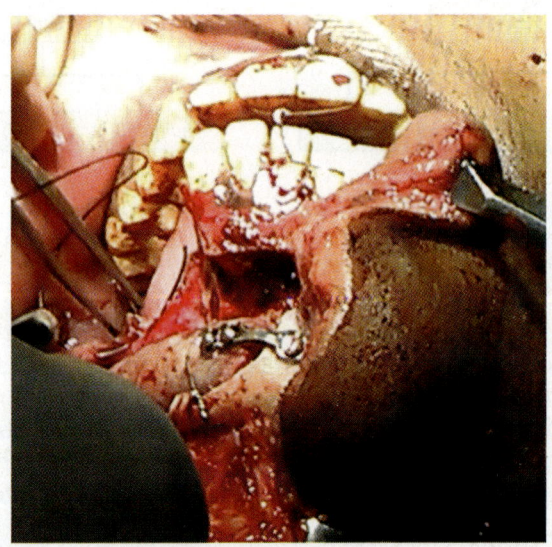

Mandible being reconstructed with rib

4. *Fascia*: Temporoparietal fascia

5. *Viscera*: Greater curvature of stomach with short gastric vessels for tongue, jejunum with jejunal artery and vein arcade for esophageal or oral surface reconstruction, pectoralis minor for facial re-animation, greater omentum with marginal arteries and veins to wrap the bone grafts in head and neck, etc.

Principles of flap surgery—replace like with like, think of reconstruction in terms of units and steps, always have a pattern and backup plan, steal from Peter to pay Paul, never forget to take care of donor area.

Monitoring the flap integrity
1. Color
2. Warmth and skin turgor
3. Blanching over the skin surface and refill time.

Mandibular reconstruction: The harvested bone along with the vessels is remodelled according to the defect and is grafted and vessels are anastomosed to the facial artery and vein. To restore temporomandibular joint, along with tissue transfer we have to use prosthesis also. Final step of mandibular reconstruction is fixing the dentures.

Orbitomaxillary reconstruction: One of the most challenging head and neck reconstructions. The defects encountered in maxillectomy are hard palate, anterior alveolar ridge, anterior maxillary wall and lateral nasal wall; in cases of orbitomaxillectomy, there is absence of orbital floor and orbit also.

Isolated hemimaxillectomy: When the contralateral dentition is normal, palatal defect can be closed by palatal prosthesis to the opposite maxilla. In this condition soft tissue reconstruction with forearm free flap will suffice. In extensive defects, osseocutaneous flap will be needed.

In orbitomaxillectomy, we have to close the defect with rectus abdominis myocutaneous free flap by splitting the skin over the flap into three islands covering skin of eye socket, lateral nasal wall and palate. This will leave only cheek skin and anterior wall of maxilla defects which can be managed by forearm osseomyocutaneous flap easily.

CHAPTER 53

Instruments in ENT

Bull's lamp: 100 W electric light mounted on a stand placed at around 1 feet distance behind and on the left of the sitting patient being examined at the level of his/her ear. The metallic chamber where the light is placed is designed with vents. Light comes out through a port in its front which is directed towards the head mirror of the examiner.

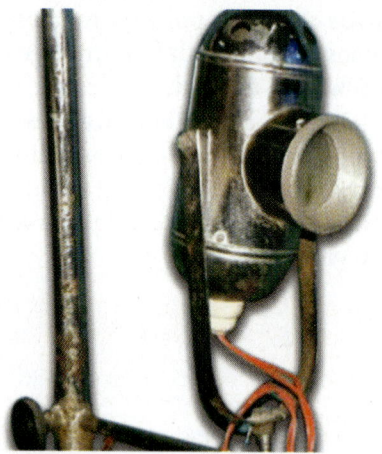

Head mirror: Worn in the head of the examiner sitting in front of the patient. The light from the lamp is directed towards its centre from where it is reflected to the examining zone of the patient. The mirror is tiltable. The diameter of the mirror is 10 cm and of the hole in the centre is 2 cm. Focal length of the mirror is 18–20 cm.

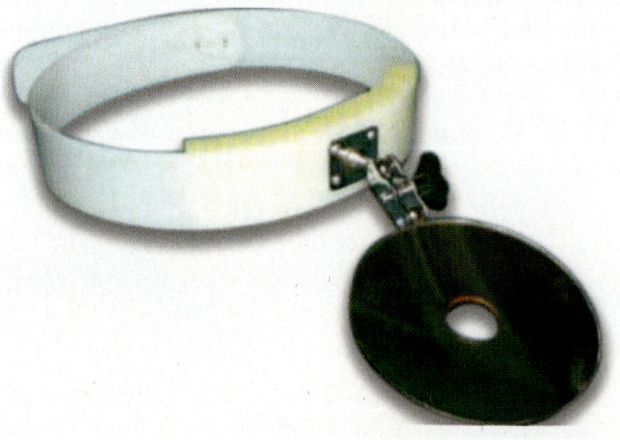

Otoscope: Otoscope has an inbuilt electric light source. Light is projected into the ear through the attached ear speculum. The ear can be examined through the eye-piece which in most models give varying degree of magnification. The intensity of light and the nature of light also varies with different models. There is a port through which a pneumatic bulb can be connected which is useful in siegalization.

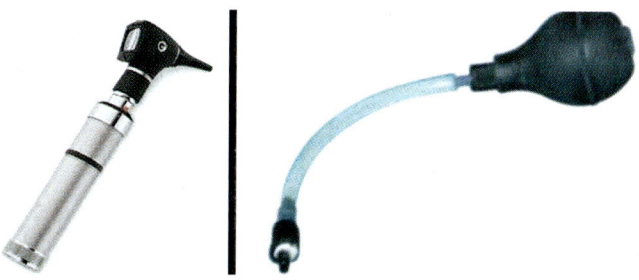

Portable headlight: Battery powered portable headlight of various types which can be used to examine and perform minor procedures in OPD, emergency or minor operation theatre.

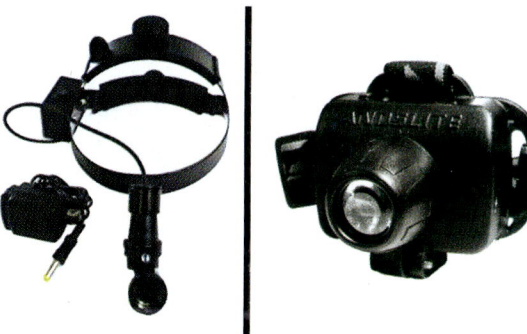

Lac's tongue depressor: Used to examine the oral cavity and oropharynx by depressing the dogs of the tongue with the flattened end. The other end is little curved to balance with the little finger of the left hand of the examiner. This can also be used to elicit Irwin Moore's sign in tonsillitis and while doing posterior rhinoscopy to depress tongue, to perform cold spatula test, etc.

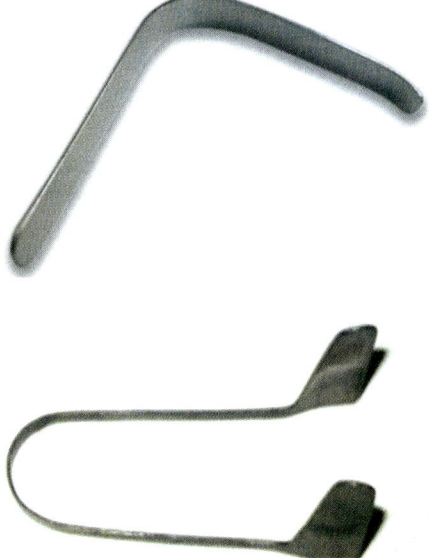

Nasal speculum

A. *Thudicum nasal speculum*: Blade length varies. Held by hooking it around examiner's left index finger. Introduced into the nostril while closed and withdrawn while open. Used to perform anterior rhinoscopy and small procedures like probe tests, nasal packing, etc.

B. *Killian's self-retaining nasal speculum:* Blade size varies. Can be retained in open position with the help of the screw present in the neck. Used in diagnostic as well as therapeutic procedures like septoplasty, polypectomy, nasal packing, etc. Long bladed speculum is also used to fracture the inferior turbinate and push it laterally.

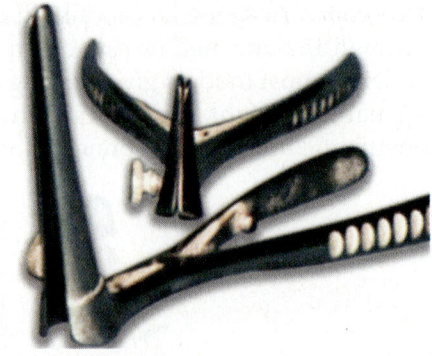

Aural speculums: Used to visualise the tympanic membrane and middle ear for diagnostic purposes. Also used in transcanal tympanoplasty and otosclerosis surgeries. First is Holmgren's self-retaining ear speculum; second is Shea's speculum and third is Tumarkin's speculum.

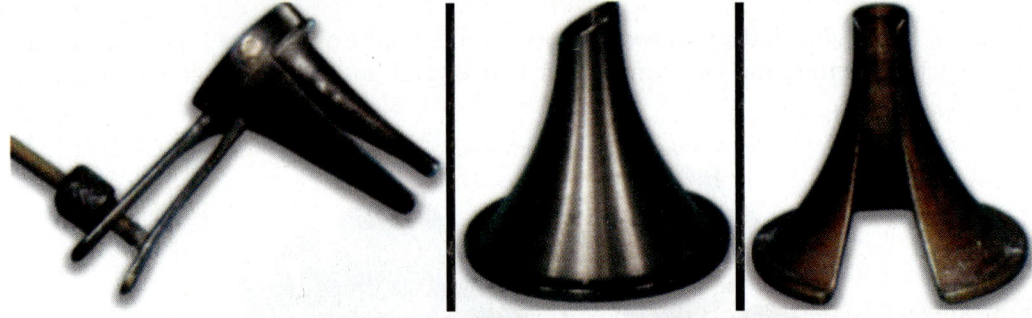

Tuning fork: Used for bedside evaluation of hearing by tuning fork tests. Parts of a tuning fork are prongs, shoulder, stem and base.

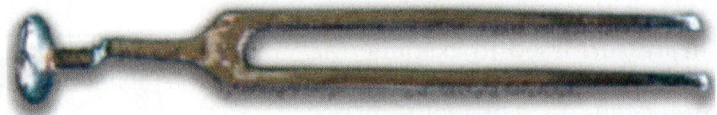

Jobson Horne probe with ring curette: Usually 6 inches long. One end had ring which is used as a curette to remove wax or foreign body from EAC. Other end is a probe which is used to probe any sinuses or to make a cotton swab for aural toileting.

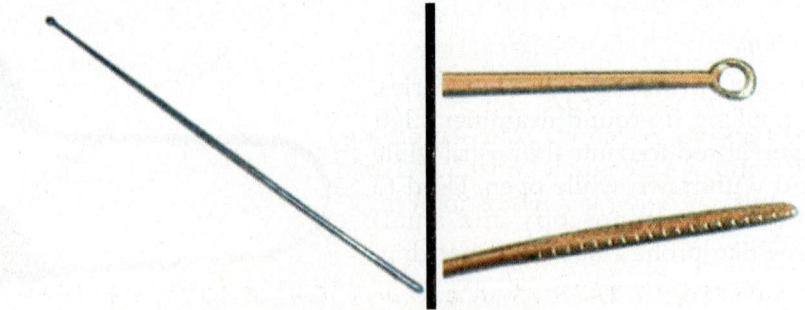

Ear vectis: Used to remove foreign bodies or wax from ear.

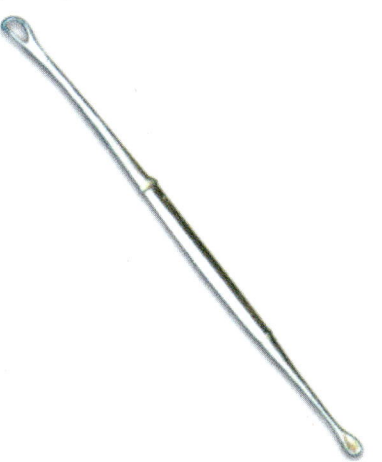

Simpson's aural syringe: Used to remove ear wax from EAC. Jet of lukewarm water should be directed postero-superiorly so that risk of stimulating Arnold's nerve is least. Many a times stringing alone cannot remove the wax. Curetting and mopping should be done along with syringing. Syringing is contra-indicated in TM perforation, dimeric membrane or ASOM.

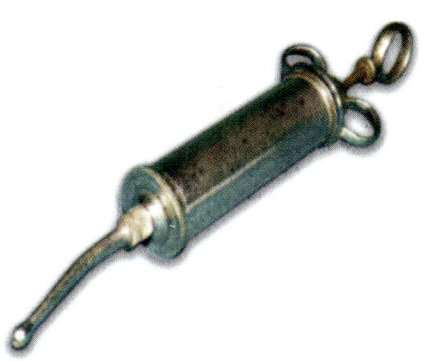

Indirect laryngoscopy mirror: Used to perform indirect laryngoscopy to visualise the larynx, laryngopharynx and hypopharynx. After applying topical anesthetic, tongue of the

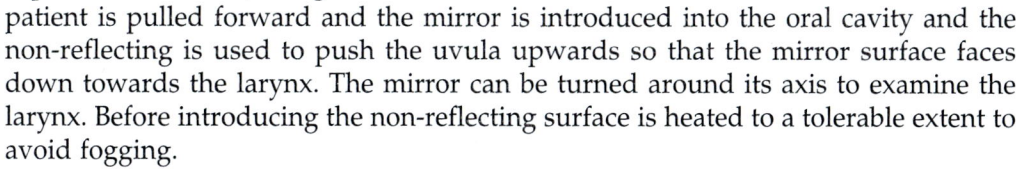

patient is pulled forward and the mirror is introduced into the oral cavity and the non-reflecting is used to push the uvula upwards so that the mirror surface faces down towards the larynx. The mirror can be turned around its axis to examine the larynx. Before introducing the non-reflecting surface is heated to a tolerable extent to avoid fogging.

Posterior rhinoscopy mirror: This is used to perform posterior rhinoscopy. Patient's tongue is depressed and the mirror is introduced into oral cavity with reflecting surface facing the nasopharynx.

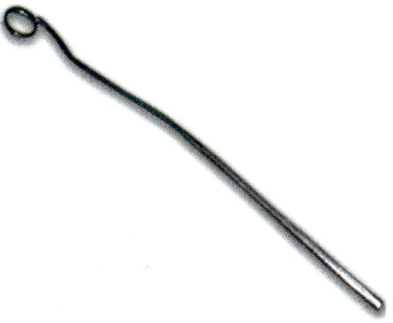

Tilley's nasal packing forceps: Used primarily to do anterior nasal packing but can also be used to remove foreign bodies from nose or ear. Other name for this is Tilley-Hartman forceps. Approximately the length of the blade is equal to the length of nasal floor.

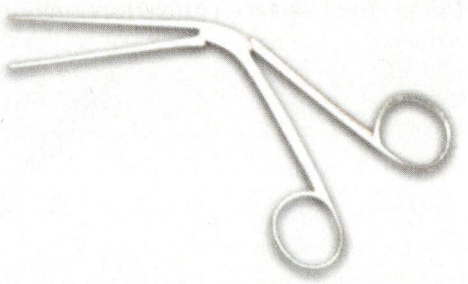

Adson's tooth forceps: Used to hold skin, fascia or soft tissues during dissection or suturing. The teeth are traumatic. For delicate structures non-toothed are used.

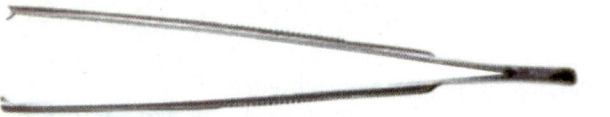

Crilewood needle holder: Used to hold the needle while suturing. It has ratcheted handle. Jaws of the needle holder have criss-cross serrations to avoid slippage of needle. Commonly used is 6 inches long. Needle is to be held at the junction of distal 2/3rd and proximal 1/3rd of the needle.

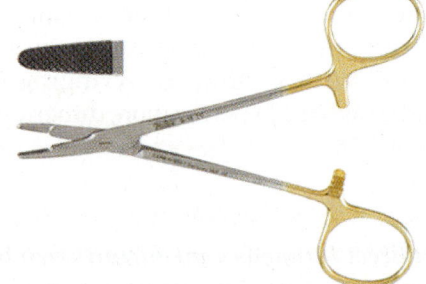

Artery holding forceps—straight and curved: The longer ones are called Birckett and the smaller ones are called Halstead. Smaller arteries are commonly called by the name mosquito forceps. The jaws of the artery forceps are relatively longer than needle holder and the serrations are horizontal. They are used as haemostat forceps.

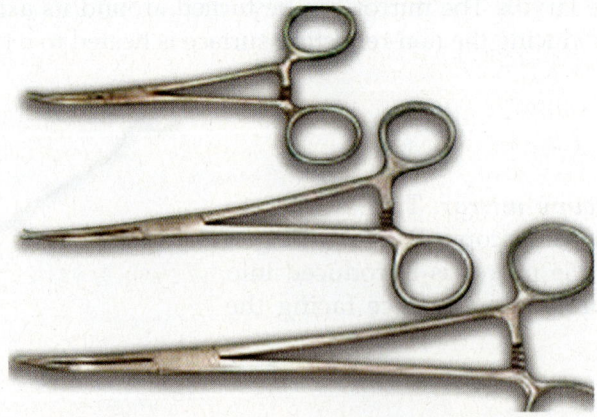

Bard Parker handle (BP handle) and disposable blades: Used to attach disposable blades of various sizes and shapes. Commonly used are size 3 and 4. Scalpel should be held like a pen in the hand. Next picture shows various numbered blades.

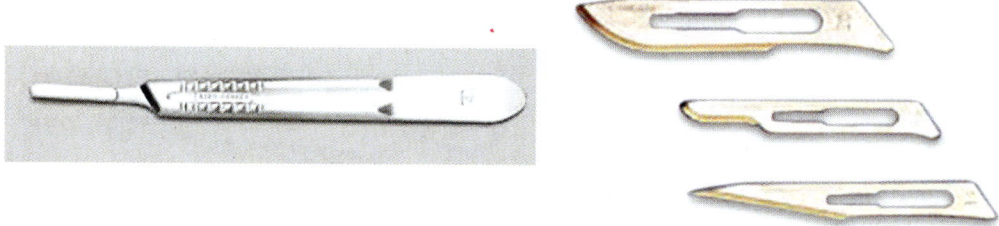

Mayo scissors (curved): Used to cut and dissect soft tissues, sutures, etc. They be curved or straight.

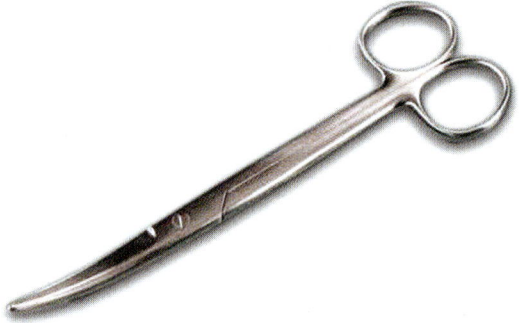

Thin curved scissors are used for dissection of soft tissue, transection of vessels and to cut sutures. Broad straight scissors are used while dressing.

Iris scissors: Used to cut fine tissue like flaps in ear surgery and its main use is in ophthalmology.

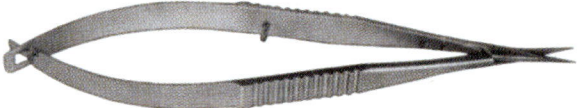

These are fine tipped scissors used in middle ear surgery, originally designed for eye surgeries.

Sponge holding forceps: Used to hold the painting sponge. Tips of blades are fenestrated. Blades are long enough to make sure surgeons arms do not touch the unsterile areas while painting.

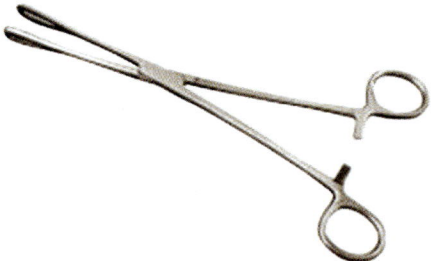

Towel clips: They are used to hold the draping sheets, fix cautery wires and suction tubes in place. Tips of blades are sharp and pointed. Sometimes can be used to pull tongue out in intra-oral surgeries instead of taking sutures.

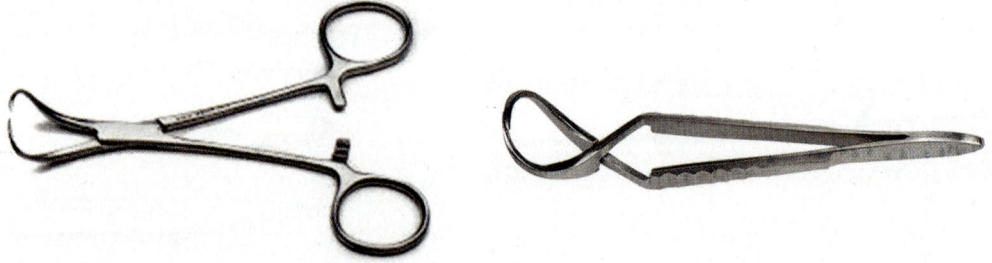

Alley's tissue holding forceps: Used to hold firm tissues like fascial flaps. Traumatic. Ends have no perforations. Ratchet lock present.

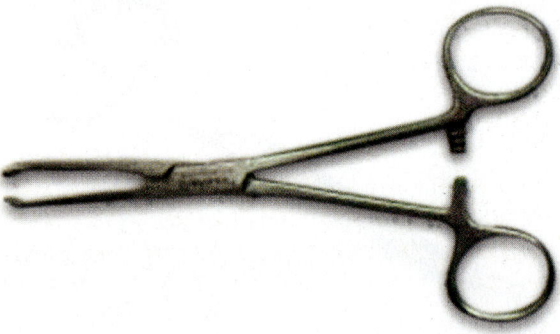

Babcock's tissue holding forceps: Used to catch hold of delicate tissues like thyroid lobe, submandibular or parotid gland during retraction. The end is fenestrated, traverse bars have serrations and non-traumatic.

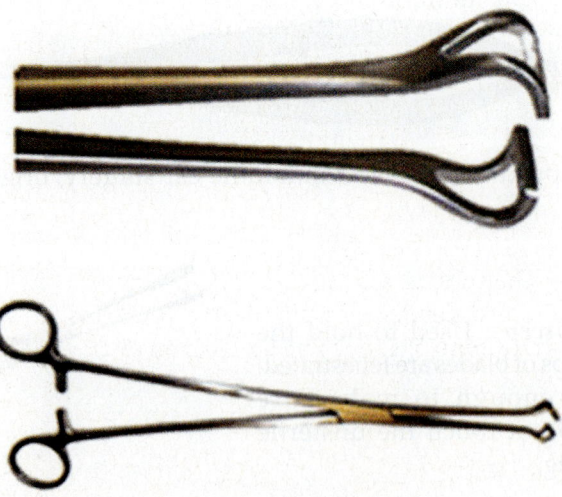

McGill's forceps: Used to pack larynx and hypopharynx in oral/oropharyngeal or nasal surgeries. Used by anesthetists after tracheal intubation to avoid aspiration. Blades are long and uniquely angulated. Ends have perforations and serrations.

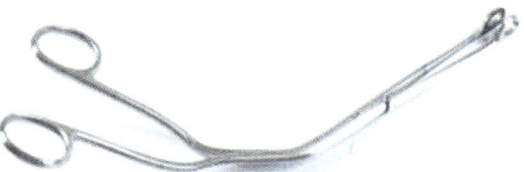

Cheatle's forceps: This is used to handle instruments in and out of the sterile chamber in an operation theatre. They have long and grippy jaws.

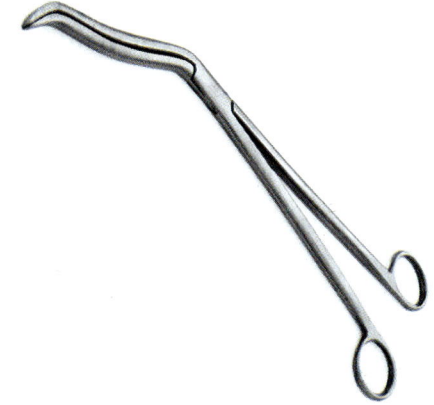

Skin hooks (Gillie's): Used to retract skin while doing subcutaneous dissection in cases like neck dissection, external rhinoplasty or parotid surgeries. When held with so much traction, it can cut through the skin.

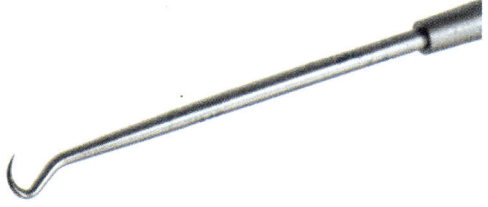

Cat's paw retractor: They are usually double ended; one end is designed like a cat's paw and other is a right-angled slender retractor. All the retractors are to be positioned like a sucker of anopheles mosquito, i.e. they should be at an angle of 45° to the surface.

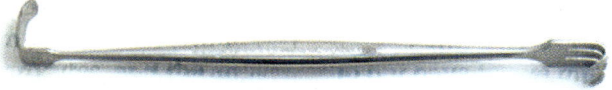

Double hook retractor (Joseph): They are used while taking temporalis fascia graft during tympanoplasty. They can also be used to retract tissues. The tip is blunted but still chances of injury are more than flat retractors.

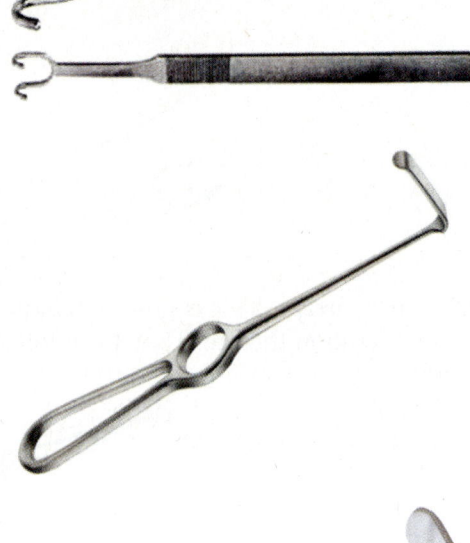

Langenbeck's retractor: They are long bladed flat right-angled retractors. Used to retract strap muscles of neck laterally during thyroidectomy. Used in other neck surgeries also.

Czerny's retractor: Double ended retractor with one right angled flat end and other end has two prongs.

Boyle Davis mouth gag with Doughty tongue blades: Used in oral and oro-pharyngeal surgeries like tonsillectomy, adenoidectomy, styloidectomy, cleft palate repair, etc. The set usually comes with 5 blades, the smallest is called mandible blade which can retract only the mandible and not tongue.

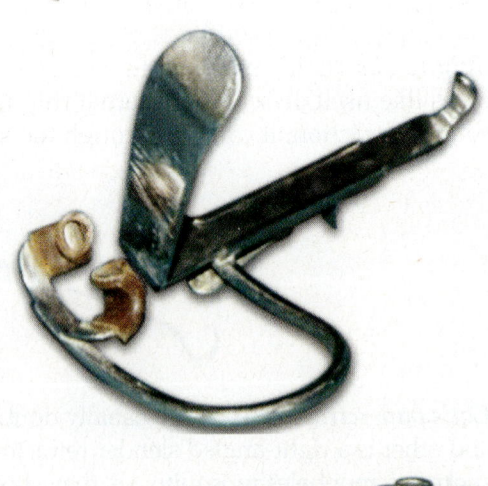

Draffin's bipod: Used to suspend the Boyle Davis mouth gag after positioning it. When placed it forms inverted-V shape.

Magauran's plate: Used to fix the bipod. Kept beneath the patient's neck.

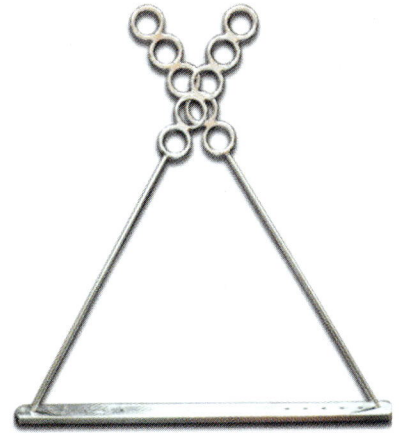

Doyen's mouth gag: The blades are kept between upper and lower jaw dentitions and opened. It is self retaining. Used in oral surgeries.

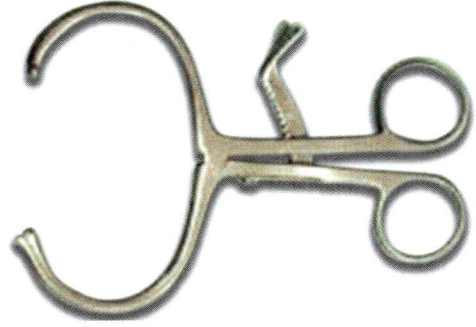

Dennis Browne tonsil holding forceps: This is used to hold the tonsil while dissecting. The jaws are atraumatic and hence does not bite through the tissue. Before starting the dissection, the tonsil is held and medially pulled to locate the extent of upper pole of tonsil. In place of this, some surgeons prefer using tonsillar vulsellum forceps or long Luc's forceps.

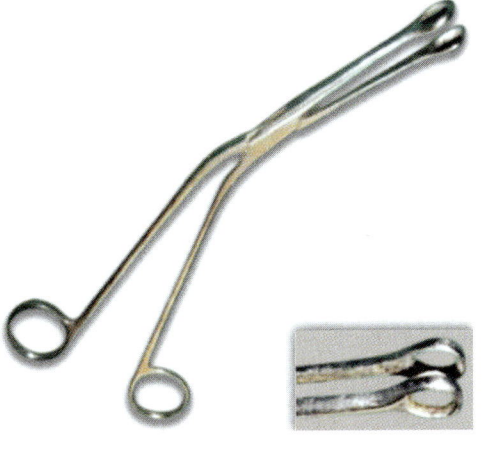

Luc's turbinate forceps: Originally designed for nasal surgeries like SMR, septoplasty, polypectomy, turbinectomy, etc. It is also used in tonsillar surgeries. The jaws of Luc's are equal in length, whereas in Dennis Brown upper one is little short.

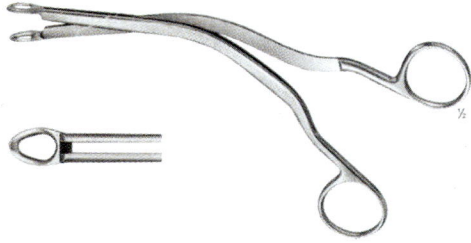

Waugh's tonsil dissecting forceps: They are long slender toothed forceps which is used to make mucosal incision in the upper pole of tonsil as well as dissection from the tonsillar bed. They are also used to hold the soft tissue in oral and oropharyngeal suturing.

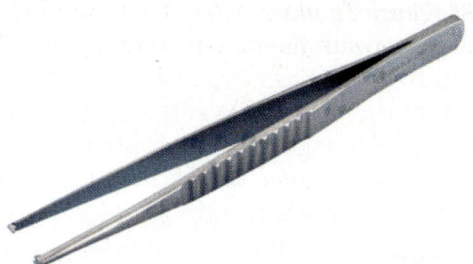

Tonsillar dissector with anterior pillar retractor (Evans): One end is flattened to dissect the tonsil from its bed and the other end is bluntly hooked to retract the anterior tonsillar pillar to identify any bleeders in the bed. The dissector end is used frequently to raise the periosteum over facial bones during surgery to them like mandibulectomy, maxillectomy and plating.

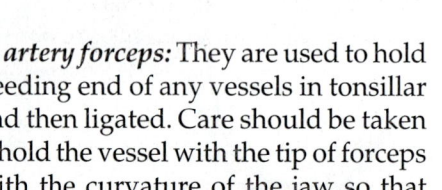

Negus artery forceps: They are used to hold the bleeding end of any vessels in tonsillar bed and then ligated. Care should be taken not to hold the vessel with the tip of forceps but with the curvature of the jaw so that ligature can be placed below that.

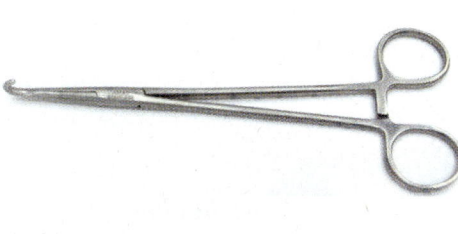

Negus knot pusher: Used to tighten the knot around the Negus artery forceps to ligate any bleeder in tonsillar bed. Can also be used in other oral or oropharyngeal surgeries.

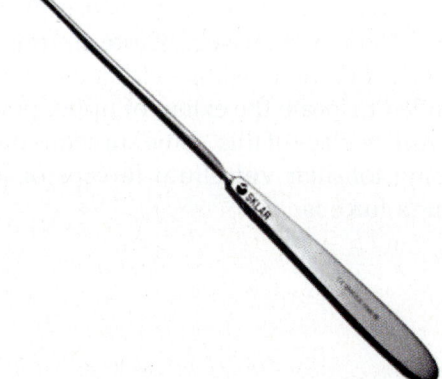

Eve's tonsillar snare: Used to loop around the lower pole of the tonsil to crush and cut it. Because of crushing, the blood vessels go into vasoconstriction and prevents post-operative bleeding. Another method is to catch hold of the pedicle with curved artery forceps and cut with scissors. Then the pedicle is ligated with silk thread. Other methods to remove tonsils are Guillotine method and hot dissection with cautery.

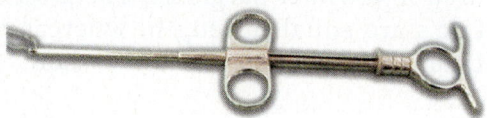

St. Claire Thomson adenoid curette with guard: This is used to perform trans oral adenoidectomy. This is performed in same position as of tonsillectomy, i.e. Rose's position. We can also perform this surgery trans-nasal with endoscopic guidance using a coblator or a microdebrider. The curette is held like a dagger in right hand and adenoid is shaved of. Guard prevents falling off of removed adenoid bits in nasopharynx which can be aspirated. Before performing adenoidectomy, the extent and size of adenoid should be estimated by trans oral palpation.

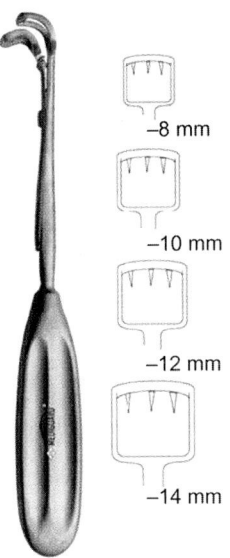

−8 mm

−10 mm

−12 mm

−14 mm

Yankauer suction: Shaped in a way to reach upto nasopharynx. Tip has multiple holes which do not suck directly but sideways so that normally present clots are not sucked away from tonsillar bed.

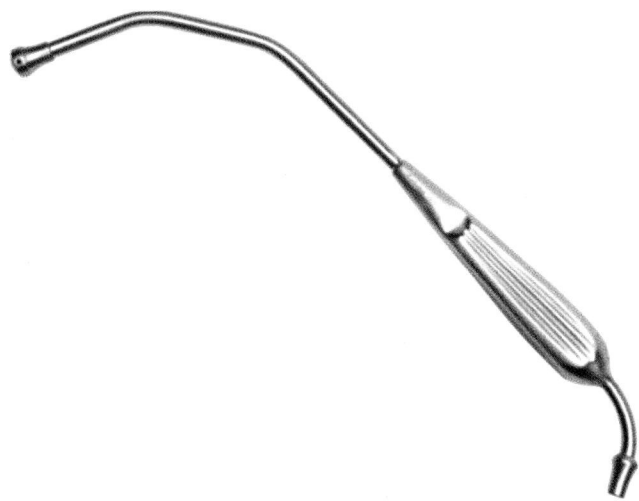

Freer's double-ended elevator: This is used to elevate flap in septoplasty, SMR, endoscopic DCR, etc. One end is straight and one is slightly curved. While elevating the flap, the convex end should face towards the cartilage or bone and not towards flap to avoid rupture of flap. Freer's is also used to make chondrotomies and tunnels. There are modifications to this instrument like suction elevator.

Von Blakesley forceps (straight, 45°, 90°): Commonly called nasal crocodile forceps. They are used in septoplasty, FESS, etc. Sometimes they are used in places of biopsy forceps to take punch biopsy.

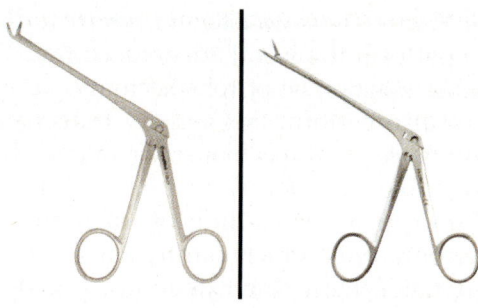

Heyman turbinectomy scissors: Used to do inferior or middle turninectomy, concha bullosa uncapping, etc.

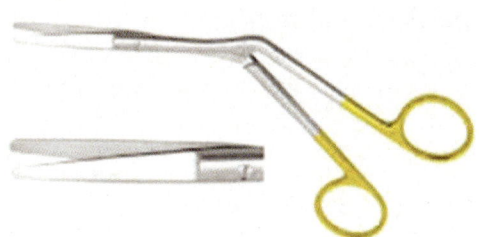

Chisel, Mallet and osteotome: Chisel is used in septoplasty. Osteotomes are used in mandibulo(ec)tomy, maxillectomy, etc. Mallet is used with doubte tap method for controlled fracturing. Centre picture is chisel; note the bevelling is found in only one surface. Last picture is of osteotome; note both surfaces are tapered and bevelled.

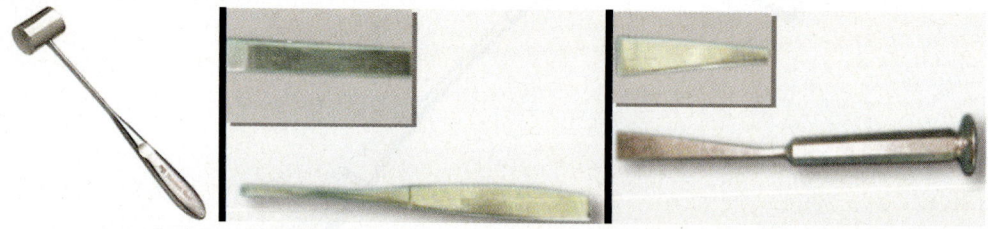

Bone gouge: Used in mastoidectomy. Powered micro drill has replaced their role quite a lot. But still many surgeons prefer gauze to remove mastoid tip cells and to decrease the height of mastoid cavity.

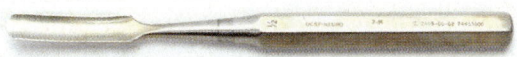

Ballenger swivel knife: Used to cut septal cartilage after creating swinging door. This removes the cartilage in single piece.

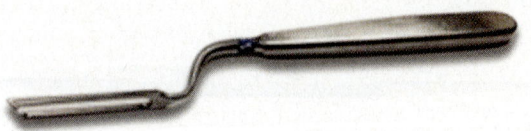

Tilley-Litcwitz antral puncture trocar and cannula: Used to perform maxillary sinus puncture and lavage. Puncture is made in the medial wall of maxillary sinus through the inferior meatus. This is the thinnest point in maxillary sinus wall. After

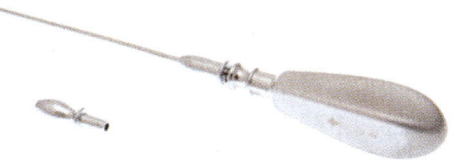

puncturing, the trocar is removed and wash is given through the cannula till water coming out becomes clear.

Nasal suctions (straight and curved): They are connected to suction apparatus. There are malleable suctions also available. Curved suctions are used to perform suction in maxillary and frontals.

They are connected to a central suction or small suction machine and can be used to perform suctioning during surgeries or in minor OT.

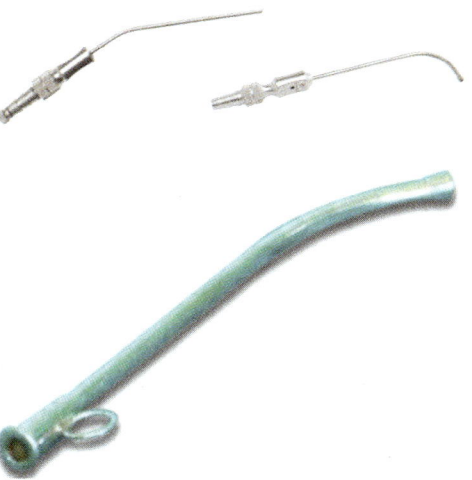

Rose eustachian catheter: Used to dilate eustachian tube pharyngeal orifice. Nowadays rarely used due to risks of iatrogenic stricture. The direction of end of the catheter is identified by the presence of a ring at the outer end of the catheter.

Backbiting forceps: Used to perform uncinectomy, widening of maxillary sinus ostiumetc. Usually the tip is rotatable 360°.

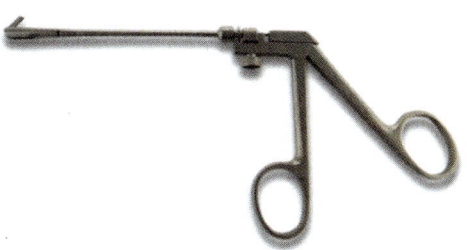

Nasal sickle knife: Used to do uncinectomy. Care should be taken not to damage lamina papyracea. Hence before making an incision in the uncinate, with the help of nasal probe, the attachment of uncinate should be defined.

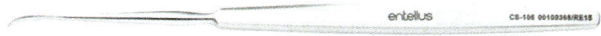

Nasal probe: Used to probe for the sinus ostia, to feel the tissue before proceeding for further steps, etc. Usually curved at both ends. End has ball like point to be atraumatic.

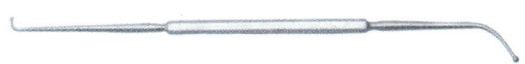

Yoon or Moriyama through cutting forceps:
They are used to make straight punches.
Usually used to connect natural osmium of
maxillary sinus to fontanelles. As it
punches through the tissue the chances of
mucosal injury by avulsion is lesser than
Blakesley forceps.

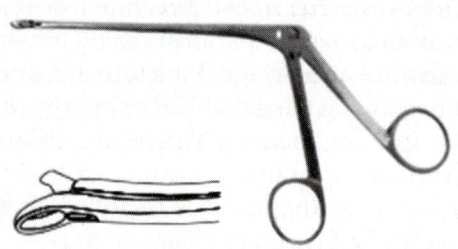

Antral grasping forceps: The tip is uniquely curved so that it can reach the anterolateral wall of maxillary sinus under angled endoscopic guidance. Used to remove
polyps or cysts from maxillary antrum.

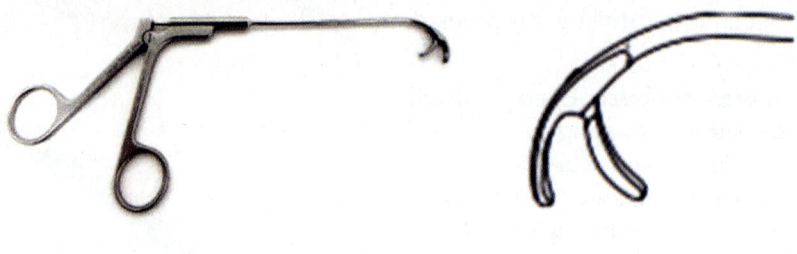

Giraffe forceps for frontal sinus: Designed
in such a way that it reaches the frontal
recess and sinus. Usually the angulation is
about 55°.

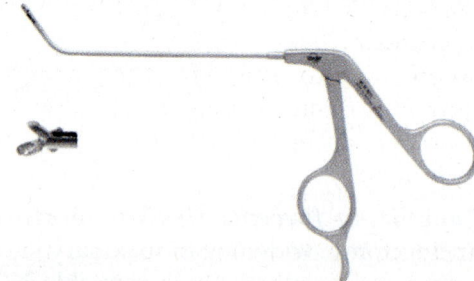

Mushroom forceps: Used to widen frontal
and sphenoidal sinus ostia. In cases of
frontal sinus angled forceps is used as
shown in picture. Sphenoid sinus ostium
needs straight forceps.

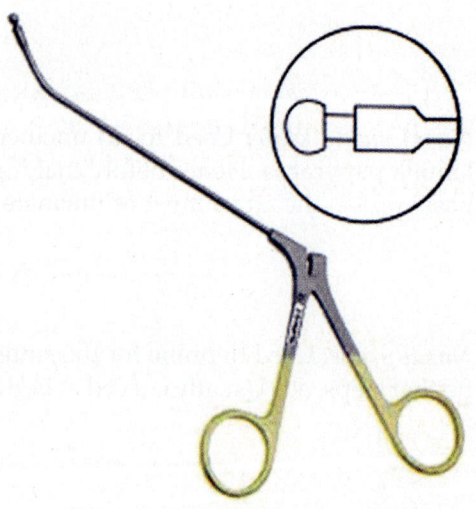

Kuhn's curette: Also called as J-curettes as there is angulation to make it look like a J. Used to curette out the contents of sinuses like polyp or fungal debris. Note the tip is designed like a scoop. Originally designed to uncap agger nasi.

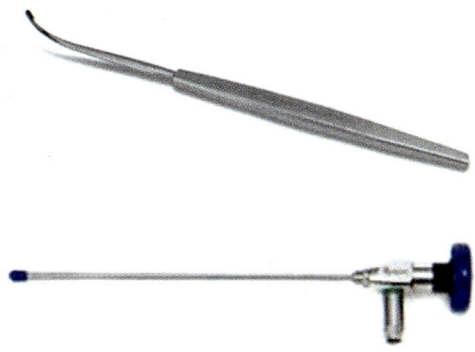

Rigid endoscopes: Rigid endoscopes of varying angled rod lens of Hopkin's type. The diameter of the endoscope varies from 2.7 mm to 4 mm. The subjective end can be connected to a camera system which can be connected to surgical quality monitors for better visualisation. Endoscopes play a vital role in endonasal, micro-ear, micro-laryngeal surgeries and laryngeal diagnostic purposes. Short and thin 0 degree endoscope can be used for oto-endoscopy.

Asch's septum forceps: Used in reducing the nasal septal fracture. The curvature should be directed towards the floor of the nasal cavities and septum should be held between the blades and fracture reduced and septum brought to midline.

Wulsham's forceps: Used to reduce fractures of nasal bone. Care should be taken not to damage the lacrimal apparatus. Many a times a rubber sheath is used to cover the outer jaw to prevent such injuries.

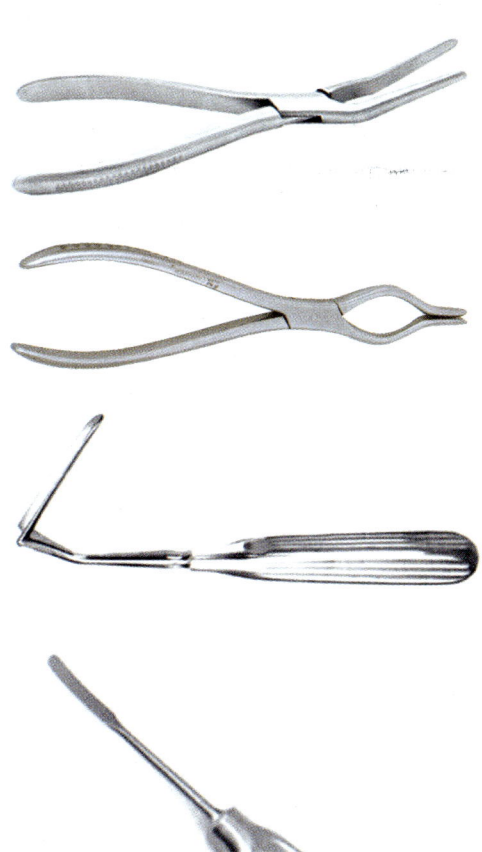

Aufricht nasal retractor: Used to retract nasal skin external rhinoplasty. When placed correctly, the surgeon can visualise whole of the dorsum of nose.

Cottle periosteal elevator: Used to elevate the periosteum over the nasal bone. Following this rasping or osteotomy can be done.

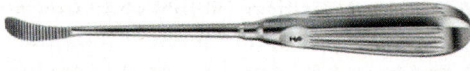

Aufricht nasal bone rasp: Used to remove bony nasal hump.

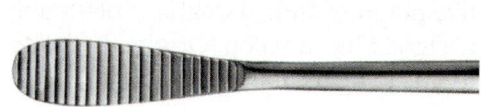

Microdebrider: Microdebrider console along with foot-controller and hand piece. Hand-piece has two ports—one for irrigation and one for suction. The blade can be straight or angled. Most recent models have high speed drill system also. Useful in FESS, adenoidectomy, anterior skull base surgeries.

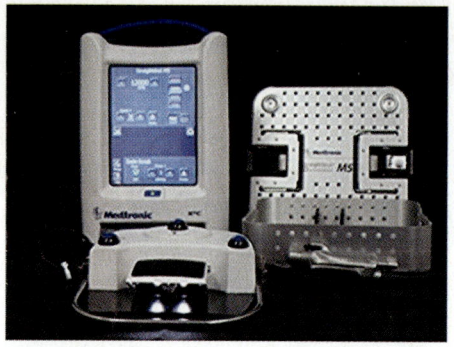

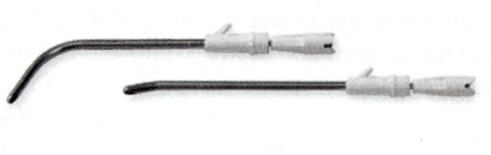

Coblator: Coblator console along with wand. Useful in daycare tonsillectomy, adenoidectomy, angiofibroma surgery, laryngeal papillomatosis, etc. Temperature produced is very less compared to electro-cauterisation thus causing less charring and less postoperative pain.

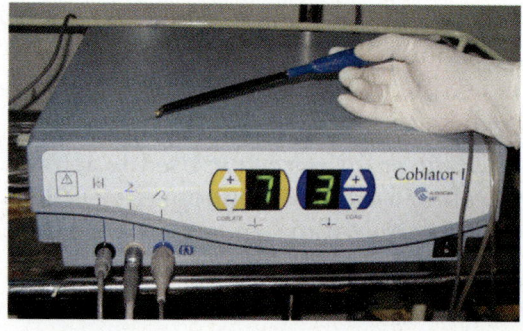

Mollison self-retaining haemostatic mastoid retractor: Used to expose the mastoid region in postaural mastoid and middle-ear surgery. The claws help to cause hemostasis. Lock keeps in retained

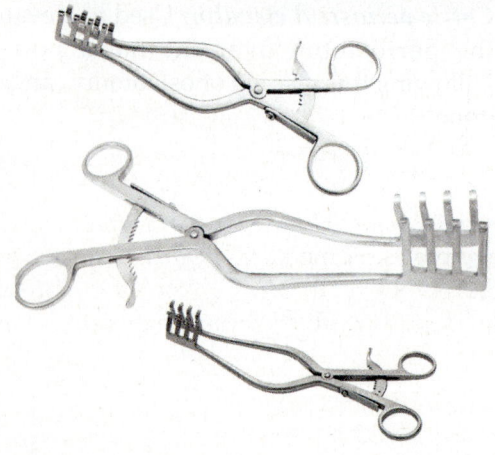

in retracted position. Picture shows various sizes of the retractor.

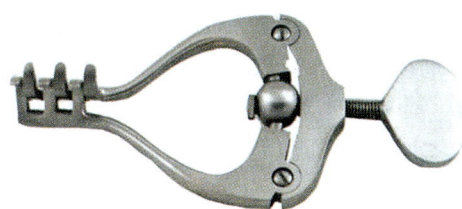

Jansen's mastoid retractor: Used for same purpose like Mollison retractor.

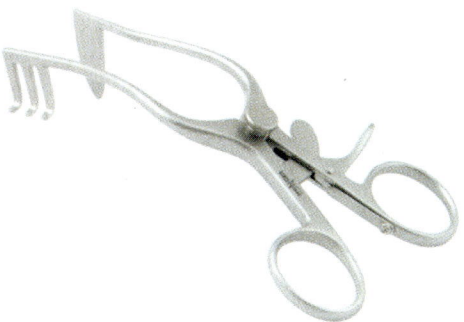

Plester Jansen mastoid retractor: Can be used to expose mastoid as well as to retract the incised posterior canal wall skin anteriorly to expose tympanic membrane and medial EAC.

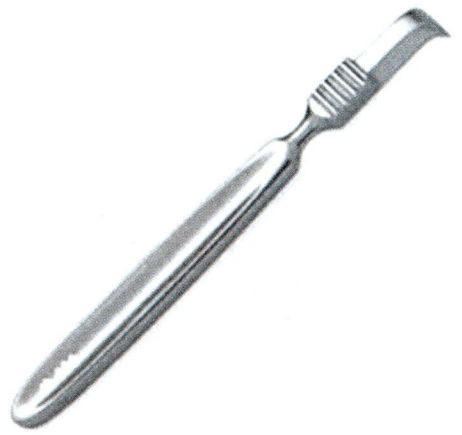

Farabeuf's periosteal elevator: Used to elevate the periosteum over the mastoid bone before starting mastoidectomy procedure. Before elevating the periosteum, sharp incision should be made over it. Other places where periosteal elevator is used are mandible plating, maxillary plating, etc.

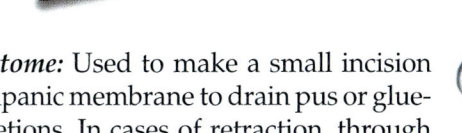

Myringotome: Used to make a small incision over tympanic membrane to drain pus or glue-like secretions. In cases of retraction, through the incision a grommet can be placed.

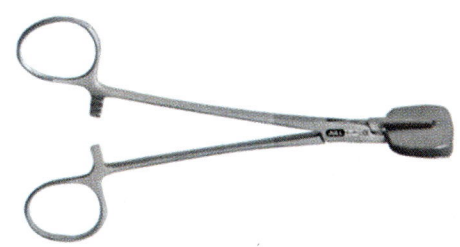

House's graft punch: Used to flatten the graft harvested for tympanoplasty. Graft is spreaded between the flat surfaced jaws and closed tightly with the help of ratchet.

Rosen's circular knife: This is used to elevate the tympano-meatal flap till the annulus. The surface of the knife may be perforated to allow suctioning from behind it.

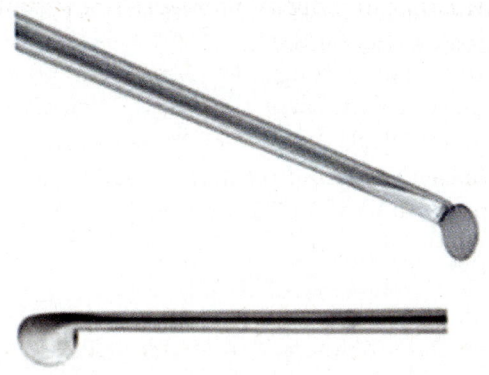

Plester's side/flag knife: Used to make incisions in the EAC skin at usually 12 and 6 O'clock. The sites of incision are variable with different types of perforations and techniques.

Sickle knife: Used to freshen the margin of perforation to render them raw. Other uses are to free the adhesions in middle ear, skeletonizing the handle of malleus, to incise facial nerve sheath, etc. In cases of rounded margin squamous cell from medial surface of the TM should also be scrapped off. This can be done with a sickle knife or a side knife.

Ball probe: Used to spread and tuck the graft, negotiate the tympanomeatal flap, place gel-foam, probe aditus, check ossicular mobility, etc. The ball like end is atraumatic and does not cause any injury to the promontory.

Annulus elevator and repositor: Both straight and curved are available. Used to elevate and separate the annulus from posterior part of tympanic sulcus during intermediate (lateral) tympanotomy. Can be used to deposition the elevated flap over the graft in underlay method.

Posterior tympantomy is facial recess approach. Anterior tympanotomy is through the anterior annular tunnel done to perform anterior tucking of graft.

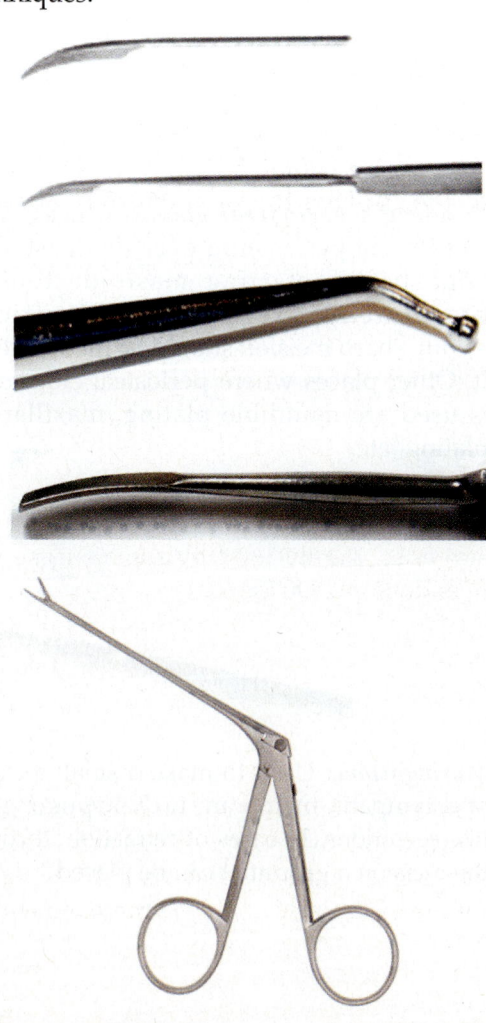

Microaural crocodile forceps: The jaws are like that of crocodile. Used to introduce graft into the bed, remove granulations, polypoidal mucosa, to crimp the loop of piston around incus long process, etc. This is also useful in catching hold of the graft and pulling it inside the anterior tucking flap.

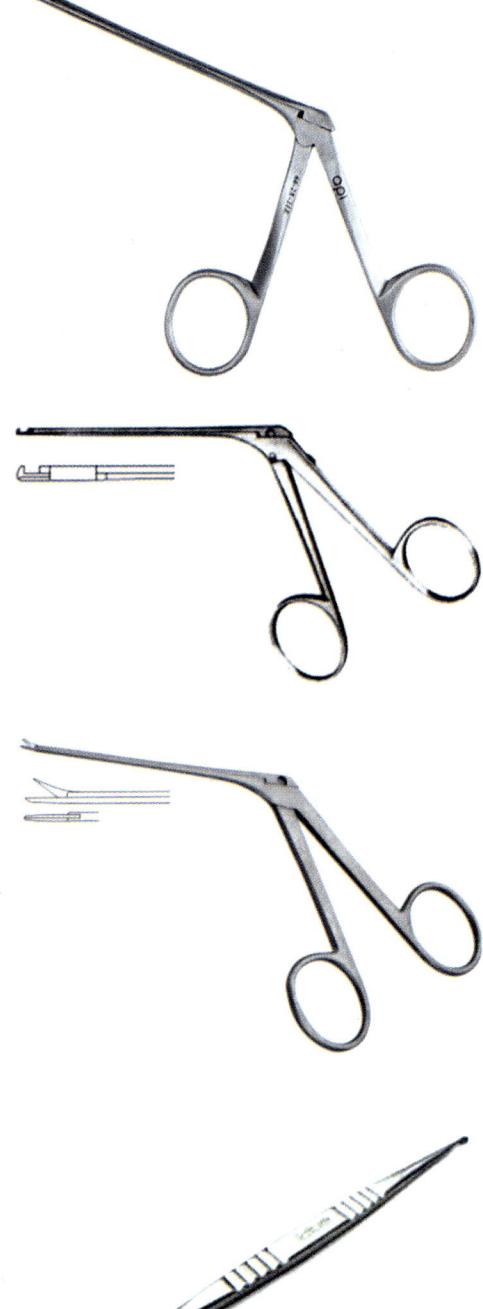

Microaural cup forceps: Used to remove the tags of margin of perforation after incising them with sickle knife. They can be used in alternate with crocodile forceps in many a place.

Malleus head nippler: Used to cut the head of the malleus to approach the disease medial to it. If the head is not eroded, it can be used in ossicular reconstructions.

Microaural scissors: Used in middle ear surgeries. Rarely used by some surgeons in endoscopic DCR also.

House curette: Used to remove posterior bony canal overhangs, thin bone over-hanging the incudal fossa from the side of mastoid antrum, etc. Bone is removed with a controlled scooping action directed laterally. Also used to remove granulations and debulking cholesteatoma.

Microdrill system and drill burrs: This is used to drill the bone in ear as well as nose surgeries. The speed (rpm) of drill and direction of rotation can be adjusted. Drill burrs used are cutting and diamond. Cutting burrs are used for rapid bone removal. They are traumatic. Diamond are used for smooth and slow bone drilling. Used in meticulous places like facial nerve canals, labyrinth and venous sinuses. They come in various sizes and lengths. Drilling causes local increase in temperature and thus needs continuous irrigation to avoid nearby neuronal injuries.

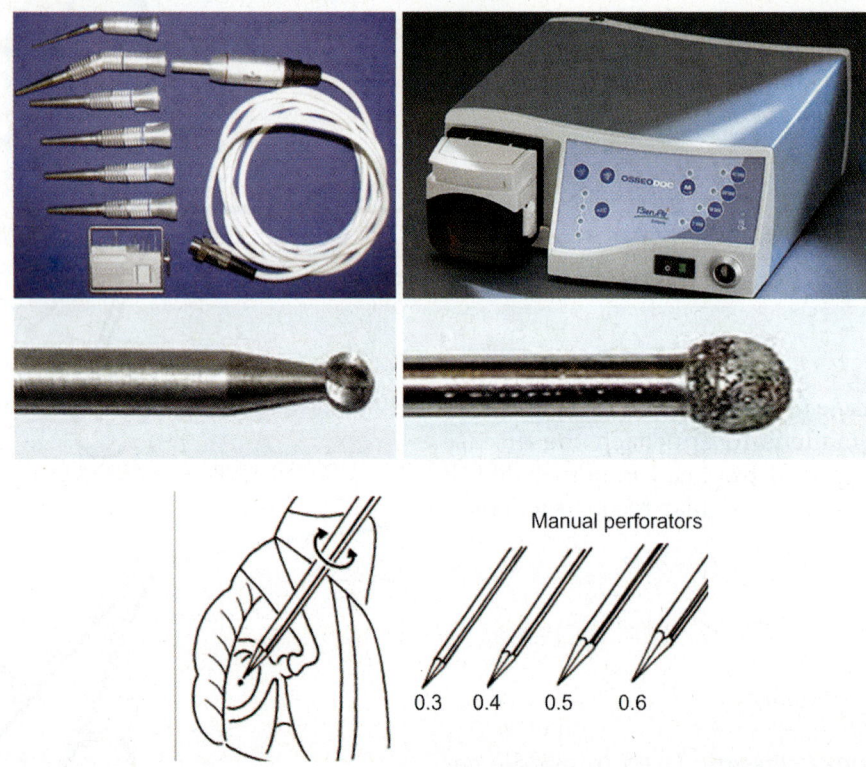

In an order the picture shows various hand-pieces and micro-motor, motor console, cutting and diamond burrs.

Perforator: Used to perforate the fixed stapes footplate to introduce the piston. Obliterative type stapes needs drilling also.

Tracheostomy tubes: They come in various types like metallic and silicone; cuffed and uncuffed; single lumen and double lumen; fenestrated and non-fenestrated.

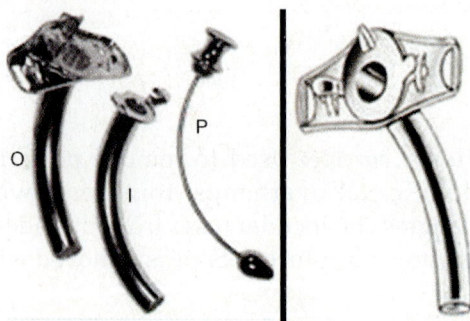

A. *Jackson tracheostomy tube is a metallic tube, non-fenestrated.* Has outer (O), inner tubes (I) and obturator (P); inner tube can be removed, cleaned and replaced easily. While introducing tube initially, obturator is placed so that the insertion remains atraumatic.

B. *Fuller's tube is a metallic, fenestrated tube.* It has hole on the outer curvature of the tube. This can help the patient to vocalise to an extent by closing the tube.

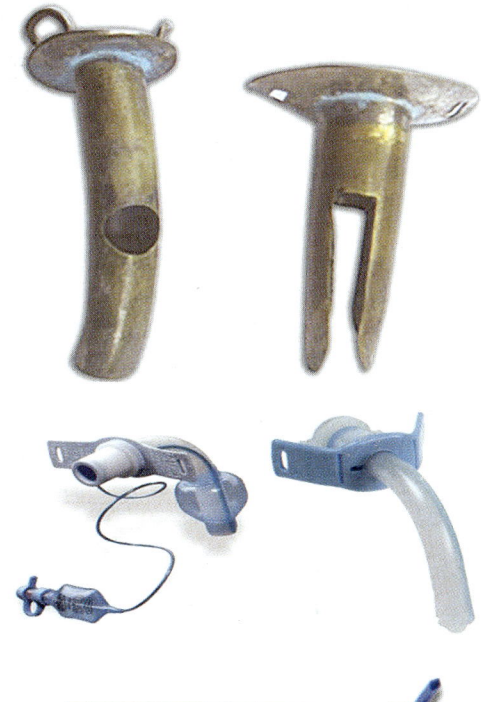

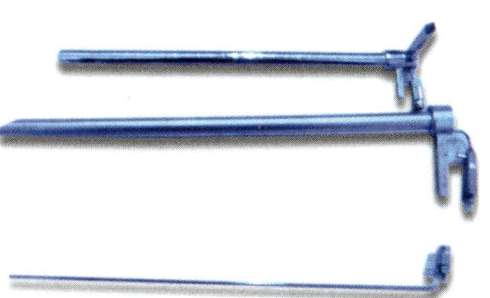

C. *Portex cuffed tube is made of silicone, MRI-friendly, connectable to ventilator. Cuff prevents aspiration in comatose patients. Cannot be used in age < 12 years.*

D. *Portex uncuffed tube is used in children and conscious patients who do not need ventilatory support.*

Rigid esophagoscope: It is an instrument to visualise the interior (lumen) of esophagus.

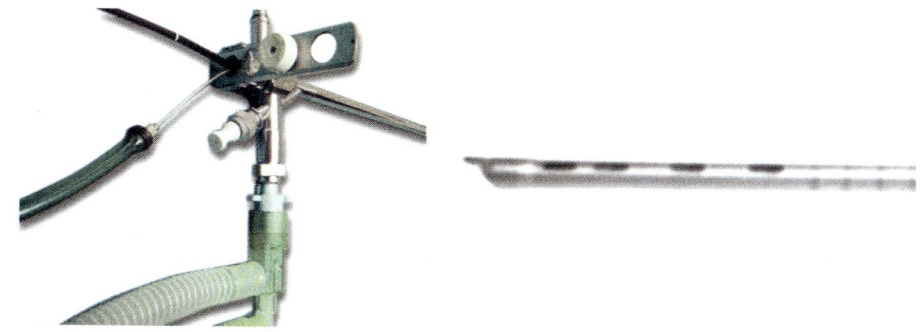

It is used for diagnostic (visualization and biopsy) as well as therapeutic purposes (foreign body removal and dilatation). It is similar to bronchoscope, made of stainless steel but it can be differentiated from bronchoscope as it has markings along the outer surface of the lumen, has no vents at the lower end of tube and it is horizontally oval in cross section.

Rigid bronchoscope with jet ventilator port: It consists of a hollow steel tube for the purpose of aeration and visualisation of the trachea and bronchi. The tube has side vents at the lower end. The size and length of the bronchoscope can be selected according to the age and stature of the patient. It has both diagnostic (bronchoscopy and bronchial biopsy or lavage) and therapeutic roles (removal of FB, suction and clearing mucous plugs). The observer end has a jet ventilation port attached to it which helps to ventilate the patient during the procedure itself allowing for longer procedures without risk of hypoxia.

There are two types of illumination for rigid scopes, viz Jackson and Negus. The differences are:

Features	Jackson type	Negus type
Location	Distal	Proximal
Brightness	Less	More
No. of illuminants	One	Two
Visibility of forceps tip	Good	Poor
Chances of secretions covering illuminant	Frequent	Occasional
Vision	Relatively poor	Better
Introduction	Easy	Relatively difficult

CHAPTER 54

Local Anesthesia in ENT

Local anesthetics act by reversible nerve blockade by binding to Na^+ gated channel. Usually the local anesthetics commonly used are chemically either amides or esters. Amines contain 2 "i" in their names, e.g. lignocaine and esters contain 1 "i" in their name, e.g. cocaine.

Factors affecting the efficacy are
1. Lipid solubility,
2. Degree of ionisation and
3. Protein binding.

Excreted by kidneys and minimal percentage by biliary system.

Cocaine is the preferred topical local anesthetic and lignocaine is the most common injectable local anesthetic drug.

When used in mixture with adrenaline (1:200,000), the duration of infiltrated local anesthesia increases, local absorption decreases and local bleeding decreases.

Fastest LA is lignocaine (30 seconds); longest LA is ropivacaine (8–13 hours), bupivacaine (5–6 hours).

Earliest sign of local anesthetic drug toxicity is tachycardia and palpitations. Treated with barbiturates, benzodiazepines and beta blockers.

Type 1 hypersensitivity to LA is mainly due to reactions against the additives present in the solution.

1. *Local anesthesia in laryngology:*
    a. Topical administration to pyriform sinus, vocal folds, epiglottis by keeping topical anesthetic drug soaked pledgets ties to thread or by using sprays.
    b. Percutaneous infiltration and blocking superior laryngeal nerve by injecting 3 ml of LA 1 cm caudal to the greater cornu of hyoid by 1 cm deep.
    c. Transtracheal injection of 4 ml of LA through cricothyroid membrane in midline after checking the position by aspirating tracheal air.
2. *Temporomandibular joint:* Needed for procedures like reduction of TMJ dislocation. Achieved by injecting in the glenoid fossa by anteriorly locking the TMJ by keeping mouth open. Direction should be towards condyle. 2 ml of drug will suffice.

3. *Trigeminal nerve block:* Maxillary division of trigeminal nerve.
   Can be accessed at the pterygopalatine fossa near foramen rotundum.
   Mandibular division of trigeminal nerve.
   Accessed at the foramen ovale; difficult to block when compared to maxillary division.
   Superficial cervical plexus branches.
   By injecting along the posterior border of sternocleidomastoid.
   Trigeminal block is useful in reduction of facial skeleton fractures.

4. *Otology*
   Myringotomy: Inject at bony cartilaginous junction of EAC at 12, 2, 4, 6, 8, 10 O'clock positions.
   Stapedotomy: Similar like myringotomy + infiltration of tympanomeatal flap.
   Tympanomastoid: Preferred to be done under GA. If the patient status does not permit GA, then tympanomastoid can be considered to be done under LA. In addition to EAC and flap injection, postauricular and conchal infiltration should be done. If tragal cartilage is to be harvested that region should also be infiltrated.

5. *Rhinology*
   Polypectomy: By keeping 4% lignocaine with vasoconstrictor drug-soaked cotton pledgets along nasal mucosal surface, as well as around sphenopalatine ganglion.
   Septorhinoplasty: Cotton pledgets as above and infiltration around floor (incisive canal), lateral wall, vestibule (mucocutaneous junction), inferior orbital nerve, sphenopalatine nerve (through greater palatine foramen transorally with a curved needle) and septum.

   Sinus surgery
   Caldwell Luc surgery: Block infraorbital, sphenopalatine and posterior superior dental nerve along the buccal sulcus. Further topical nasal pledgets to be used.
   Middle turbinate and uncinate: Injected at the neck of middle turbinate near axilla. This will spread along the plane to infundibulum and uncinate as well.

Index